AND
NURSING

HUMAN DYNAMICS AND NURSING

PSYCHOLOGICAL CARE IN NURSING PRACTICE

Stewart Hase RN RPN DNE BA

Lecturer in Nursing, Tasmanian State
Institute of Technology

Andrew J. Douglas RPN

Psychiatric Nurse Consultant, Royal
Hobart Hospital

Churchill Livingstone

MELBOURNE EDINBURGH LONDON AND NEW YORK 1986

CHURCHILL LIVINGSTONE
Medical Division of Longman Group UK Limited

Distributed in Australia by Longman Cheshire Pty
Limited, Longman House, Kings Gardens, 95 Coventry
Street, South Melbourne 3205, and by associated
companies, branches and representatives throughout
the world.

First published 1986
 Reprinted 1988

ISBN 0-443-03224-6

British Library Cataloguing in Publication Data
Hase, Stewart
   Human dynamics and nursing.
   1. Psychiatry   2. Psychiatric nursing
   I. Title   II. Douglas, Andrew J.
   616.89'0024613   RC454

Library of Congress Cataloging in Publication Data
Hase, Stewart.
   Human dynamics and nursing.
   Includes bibliographies and index.
   1. Psychiatric nursing.   2. Nurse and patient.
I. Douglas, Andrew J.   II. Title.   [DNLM: 1. Nursing
Process.   2. Psychiatric Nursing. WY 160 H346h]
RC440.H345   1986   610.73'68   86-9764

Produced by Longman Singapore Publishers (Pte) Ltd.
Printed in Singapore.

Preface

At the time of writing this introduction it is worth noting that it is only 76 years since the death of Florence Nightingale and only a few more years since the modern rebirth of nursing on the battlefields of the Crimea. Within this relatively short time nursing has grown as a science and an art seeking to establish itself as a profession with the rights and obligations of independent practice. The essential goal is a meaningful contribution to health care and improved health for the community.

Traditionally based on an illness model, following the tenets of medicine, nursing has tended to concern itself primarily with the diseases that confront those people called 'patients'. In the face of an ever increasing body of scientific knowledge, nursing has, like medicine, become highly specialized so that it is no longer feasible to simply use the term 'nurse'. Instead we more accurately distinguish between the geriatric nurse, oncology nurse, orthopaedic nurse, renal nurse, intensive care nurse, infection control nurse and stomal therapy nurse, etc.

Mental health nursing has traditionally been a specialty with a programme of study outside that of the general nursing stream, and in an area of practice historically separate from general nursing. Mental health nurses are seen to possess special knowledge of behavioural sciences, helping skills, psychopathology, and psychological distress. By contrast these subjects have, in the past, received only scant attention in the general curriculum, where the emphasis has been on physical problems. With nurse education moving into tertiary institutions, this state of affairs is, however, changing.

In recent years more and more evidence has been gathered to suggest that there is a very close relationship between physical illness and psychological influences. Similarly, physical illness affects the psychological state of the individual. Ill health in general and hospitalization in particular are important stressors, very special nursing intervention strategies being required to restore or maintain physical and mental health. The incidence of psychological problems among hospitalized persons is very high, with the result that in any one day the nurse may be confronted with someone who is disoriented, confused, intoxicated, anxious, depressed or hallucinating.

This book is intended for the general nurse in either the community or hospital setting and attempts to provide guidelines for the management of people with a variety of common psychological problems.

We have not utilized a specific nursing model as a framework for this text and believe that the essential guidelines for nursing assessment, planning, and implementation can be incorporated into any theoretical model. Moreover, our approach is largely eclectic, relying heavily on cognitive, behavioural, and humanistic techniques wherever a particular theoretical or practical strength applies. One might suspect that in the future this approach may be supplanted when conclusive evidence for one particular psychological explanation of behaviour appears. It is noteworthy, however, that we have chosen to move away from using a disease model of mental ill-health, and avoid utilizing diagnostic psychiatric labels, in an attempt to individualize nursing care. We have, however, included chapters on diagnostic criteria and labels, since nurses can expect to be confronted with the illness model, and it cannot be ignored as a means to treating what are called 'mental illnesses'.

We have refrained from using the word 'patient' throughout the text. The role of patient, we believe, has come to be associated with an illness role rather than a health seeking role, and implies dependency and passivity. To call someone a 'patient' presupposes that the person is simply the receiver of care or illness interventions, and is somehow not responsible for his or her own health or ill-health. By contrast, our view suggests that the health of the individual is primarily his or her own responsibility, and is principally affected by his or her own actions.

The text is presented in two distinct sections. In Part One we deal with essential background information and some theoretical issues. Part Two presents a number of commonly encountered psychological problems, an explanation of each, and guidelines for nursing action based on a problem-solving approach — the nursing process.

We would like to thank all the friends and colleagues who inspired and assisted us in the development of this text. In particular Judy Waters is to be congratulated on her faith, patience, and the intelligent use of her pen. Special thanks go to Sandra Tolra for typing the manuscript with admirable enthusiasm and ability.

Hobart 1986   S. H.
                                               A. J. D.

Publisher's note
No gender-specific incidence of ill-health is implied in the use of pronouns throughout this text. For clarity and convenience, however, the 'patient' is usually referred to as male.

Contents

PART | # ONE

Approaching the Problem

If sanity and insanity exist, how shall we know them?

Rosenhan, 1973

1

Mental health and mental ill-health

NURSING PRACTICE AND PSYCHOLOGICAL CARE

One of the effects of technological development and the enormous increase in knowledge in the 20th century has been compartmentalization and specialization. In medicine, areas of specific care are directed towards particular body systems or organs so that, for example, we have cardiac surgery, vascular surgery, cardiology, neurology, and respiratory medicine. Nursing has followed this trend, giving rise to a wide range of education programmes and areas of practice. An important partitioning has been that of physical and psychological care, so that an emphasis is placed on one or the other depending on the diagnosis and the expertise of the care-giver.

Fortunately, in recent years the notion of holistic care has emerged, with the accent on recognition of the functioning of the total person rather than on just the diseased organ or system. Workers such as Wilson-Barnett (1983) and Dossey (1982) have increasingly stressed the relationship between the psychological state of the individual, the disease, and the outcome of treatment. Moving away from what can be described as the 'germ theory' of health care, more emphasis now is being placed on the psychosocial aspects of illness and illness behaviour. In particular these include: the role of mental health in the causation of physical disease; the psychological effects of illness; the psychological effects of treatment; and the maintenance of mental health in the prevention of physical illness. Additionally there is an increasing tendency to consider the ill person in terms of significant others, the home setting, cultural background, work, and lifestyle. From a more strictly psychological point of view we must take into consideration such factors as individual reactions to stress, stressors, locus of control, needs, drives, self-awareness, growth, and cognitive ability.

APPLYING PSYCHOLOGICAL CARE

There are a number of contexts in which psychological care may provide health benefit for the individual. Firstly, it can be applied as a means of preventing illness by maintaining or building psychological strength. This may be achieved by education or by early intervention. Achievement of potential through growth, decision-making, alteration to lifestyle, assertiveness training, and other ways of dealing with stressors are possible strategies. Secondly, illness or change in health status produces any number of psychological problems that in turn may interfere with future attainment of full health. Thirdly although an individual may present with physical illness, a psychological problem may be acting as a significant cause or may manifest *conjointly* with the particular disorder. In this case intervention will be directed as much towards the psychological problem as the physical disease. Lastly, illness may become manifest in some individuals as overt mental ill-health rather than as physical illness. In this instance the focus of care is directed almost entirely towards psychological management.

On a day-to-day basis then, nurses are likely to encounter individuals who are anxious, depressed, confused, disoriented, hallucinating, angry, withdrawn, grieving, self-destructive or abusing substances. Caring for people with such problems requires special knowledge, understanding and skills, and in this book, we aim to help the reader attain these. This chapter introduces a number of

concepts regarding mental health and mental ill-health to provide a basis for an approach to nursing practice that emphasises the importance and power of the nurse-patient relationship, and its role in maintaining health or recovery from illness.

MENTAL HEALTH AND MENTAL ILL-HEALTH

HISTORICAL PERSPECTIVES

This history of society's attitudes towards, and treatment of, deviant behaviour is largely one of fear and persecution. This is not difficult to understand when we consider the complexity of human behaviour, and the difficulty of explaining in simple terms phenomena such as hallucinations, delusions, thought disorder, or mania. Such mysteries have been accounted for in terms of evil spirits, magic and witchcraft (Szasz 1974). This account also provides a means of dealing with the problem.

The mystery of 'madness' has its basis in antiquity, with stone-age man carrying out trephining — making a hole in the skull, presumably to let out spirits. Early Hebrew, Chinese, Egyptian and Greek thinking involved the notion of possession by demons, which was treated by exorcism. It is interesting that Hippocrates rejected this idea and gave a more rational flavour to the understanding of abnormal behaviour. His treatment for melancholia was a prescription of tranquillity, sobriety, a good diet, continence, and exercise (Davison & Neale 1978, Coleman 1972). It is worth noting that some of the elements of this prescription are features of modern health measures. However, this somatogenic treatment was not to last and the Middle Ages saw a resurgence of demonology. Exorcism was effected by insulting the possessing devils, and later, by torturing the body to make it an unpleasant host. By the late 15th century the belief in witchcraft became established to the extent that a manual, the *Malleus Maleficurm*, was published describing how to detect, examine, and deal with witches. Confessions of witchcraft were extracted by torture and followed by a sentence of death and burning of the body.

From the 16th to 19th centuries the mentally ill were incarcerated in institutions (asylums), while social attitudes changed very slowly towards the notion of disease and away from that of demonic possession. However, treatment was still harsh, involving inmates being chained and straight-jacketed, with bleeding and purgatives commonly used to cleanse the body of 'madness'. A favourite pastime for socialites in London during this period was to wander through the asylum 'Bedlam' and watch the antics of the 'mad' (Foucault 1965).

As recently as the late 1950s and early 1960s the most common method of managing the mentally ill was to place them in large institutions behind high walls, the emphasis being on keeping the 'mad' contained and out of society. Modern psychiatric drugs and treatment have only a short history coinciding with a softening of public attitudes, and a less punitive and custodial approach to care and discharge arrangements.

Another important element in our thinking about abnormal human behaviour has been the 'disease' or 'illness' model. Following the precepts of the 'germ theory' this model assumes that, given a certain set of signs and symptoms, it is possible to determine the manifestation of a particular illness. Once defined, a certain treatment pattern, usually medication, can be set in motion to 'cure' the so-called 'illness'. This concept is of course the one used for rationalizing treatment and causation in physical illness.

Although obviously useful, this model tends to emphasize the categorization of behaviour as a means of distinguishing abnormality from normality. Do we assume, for example, that a person is mentally healthy simply because there is an absence of certain symptomatology? It may also be argued that a disease model is inappropriate to describe emotional and behavioural problems that are not necessarily linked to a disorder of the nervous system (Szasz 1960). This notion is discussed further on page 6. The very positive effect of the medical model was to humanize the

treatment and understanding of people with psychological problems.

The increased sophistication of psychology has contributed, in recent years, to a number of alternative perspectives regarding psychopathology. In turn this has led to the availability of a variety of treatment methods, other than physical treatments and the traditional psychotherapies. A view that has increased gradually in popularity since the mid-1970s is that of the mind-body relationship, which holds that the two are interrelated and not separate entities. Implicit in this assumption is that the consciousness of the individual is a vital factor in determining physical health and that disease is not simply the result of misbehaviour between molecules, but something more (Dossey 1982). Stress, for example, has become a major area for research, particularly in regard to its role in the causation of disease and recovery. Emanating from this theme have come strategies to reduce stress, such as relaxation, problem-solving, massage, reducing dependency, assertiveness training, and diet changes.

These changing attitudes and notions about mental health and mental ill-health also affect nursing activities and roles. No longer are nurses forced to adopt a principally custodial role or one of distance from the psychological problems that confront those in their care. The therapeutic function of the nurse becomes more than restoring and maintaining biological health, more than treating disease. Many tools are now available for nurses to utilise in their relationship with others. This theme is central to this book and will be expanded within the context of specific mental health problems.

THE CONCEPT OF MENTAL HEALTH

The value of a definition lies in its precision, so that certain properties can be measured accurately and decisions made about what can or cannot be subsumed under it. One of the major problems in defining mental health is the risk of being precise but narrow to the point of inaccuracy, or of being so broad that measurement is virtually impossible.

A very narrow view is one which attempts to describe mental health as the absence of mental illness or psychiatric symptomatology. This is a convenient method of measurement and the criteria are straightforward for those who have skills and knowledge. Otherwise described as the 'medical model' using the criteria of disease, this approach has been criticised on a number of grounds: as a myth (Szasz 1974); as a providing medical answer to an essentially social problem (Szasz 1970); and as having poor validity (Rosenhan 1973). Studies have shown that the number of people who have potentially diagnosable mental illness far outweigh those who have treatment. That fact that these untreated people manage to survive without help raises questions as to the reliability and validity this model of mental illness (Ullman & Krasner 1969). Despite these criticisms, the model remains the most common method of differentiating the mentally ill from the mentally healthy. The principal focus is on the restoration of health, which presumably means achieving the absence of symptomatology. Chapter 2 discusses in detail the major medical classifications of mental illness.

Another way of looking at mental health is in terms of optimal functioning, towards which the individual can be seen as striving. As Haber et al (1978) point out, the use of such terms as 'self-actualization', 'fulfilment', and 'creativity' make the boundaries around mental health fluid and diffuse. Peplau (1980), for example, has described health as being:

'. . . conditions that facilitate forward movement of personality and other ongoing human processes in the direction of creative, constructive, productive, personal and community living.'

Humanistic theories tend to consider health as a dynamic process involving growth and self-awareness in which any person may engage. Instead of mental illness it is possible to think in terms of degrees of optimal functioning.

Stress or adaptation models view mental health as the psychosocial ability to cope with stress so that human needs can be met and the person can function within a culture (Pasquali et al 1981). A reasonable extension to this definition would be the inclusion of physical responses to stress; this takes into account the mind-body relationship; a holistic view.

Whatever the definition, the problem remains one of who makes the judgement about whether or not health has been attained. A person might feel good, believing he or she is functioning appropriately, but in fact may be operating outside acceptable social boundaries, or may be having difficulties in carrying out the normal activities of daily living, to his or her own detriment. It is clear from the historical perspective that social mores are an important determinant of what is acceptable or normal behaviour.

Another aspect of mental health which is frequently not considered by definition is that of time. Mental health, like physical health, is a dynamic state that may change from moment to moment and may vary according to situational circumstances. It is difficult to imagine a person functioning at an optimal level all of the time and in all situations. In the same way it may be a mistake to view a particular behaviour as indicating an enduring abnormality or as a prominent feature of personality.

Despite these problems in defining mental health in any succinct or accurate way, most people would have a fairly good idea of their own and others' normality using criteria gained from experience and socialization (Haber et al 1978). Mosak (1976) suggests that individuals evaluate their own normality on a number of criteria:

1. *Frequency criterion*. A behaviour or feeling is normal if the majority act or feel in the same way.
2. *The other as referent*. Normality is evaluated by the way in which a person *thinks* other people behave.
3. *Therapist as referent*. The therapist, or helper, is seen as being a standard for normality.
4. *Self as referent*. One sees oneself as

normal and others as abnormal if they think otherwise.

5. *Pre-morbid criterion*. This involves comparing how one used to be with how one feels now.
6. *Conformity*. Normality is behaving according to the generally accepted standard of what is good or correct bahaviour.
7. *Mediocrity*. Some see normality as being average.
8. *Boredom*. In antithesis to mediocrity some view average as being boring and resist it to be what they consider to be normal.
9. *Perfection*. Normality for some involves being able to operate to perfection and anything less is abnormal.
10. *Symptomatology*. Like psychiatrists these people believe normality is based on being symptom-free and undiagnosed.

Psychological functioning

Given the complexities of arriving at a universally acceptable definition of mental health, it is perhaps more worthwhile to attempt, by description, to evaluate the ways in which an individual's psychological functioning is reflected. Five broad groups of functioning can be identified:

— feelings and emotional behaviour
— interpersonal behaviour
— activities of daily living
— intellectual activity
— physical well-being.

Feelings and emotional behaviour. Being mentally healthy means feeling good about and within oneself. It is not merely the absence of depression or anxiety or other bad feelings, it is a sense of emotional well-being. Attaining such a state rests on our ability to be aware, to be in control and to be accepting of ourselves. Awareness (sometimes referred to as 'insight') involves self-knowledge, the ability to know our needs and how to attain them in order to feel good. It also involves being honest with self. Awareness enables us to acknowledge our feelings and to face up to them rather than engaging in avoidance.

Some people, for example, find it difficult to respond in emotionally appropriate ways (with love, joy, anger or with grief), which may affect behaviour, overall functioning or physical health.

Control stems from awareness and involves being able to act when feelings are negative and not beneficial. A person might find that he responds with anger every time he has to relate to a work colleague. When this feeling results in negative behaviour and makes the individual feel bad, control enables him or her to find a reason for the anger and resolve the problem.

Developing a sense of personal acceptance or simply being comfortable with ourselves is not as easy or as universal as we might at first think. Many of us are programmed through our childhood experiences with feelings about ourselves which tend to lead to negative behaviour. A sense of guilt is an excellent example; another involves expectations. We learn to feel bad (or guilty) for being imperfect and it is quite possible to spend a great deal of time either feeling bad or striving to be perfect; meeting the expectations that others have set. Accepting oneself is being aware of limitations and also acknowledging our very own personal wishes and desires. It also involves being aware of strengths and maximising them, which ultimately results in positive self feelings. Nurses are very good examples of victims of the 'guilt trap', tending to perpetuate guilt programming by rationalizing it through the notion of dedication. Hence nurses will work overtime for nothing, accept poor working conditions and worry if everything hasn't been done, despite poor staffing and even lack of expertise.

Another perhaps less obscure example might involve a marriage in which the wife plays out her role as a child-carer and home-help. At first comfortable with the expectations of such a role, she gradually becomes disillusioned, feeling bored and cheated. Depression and anxiety may ensue, and are dealt with in the usual way with tranquillizers, antidepressants and alcohol. No longer living out the fairy-tale existence popularized by folk-lore, media and novels, she carries on because her programming is quite clear in interpreting the importance of being 'responsible' and not questioning the status quo. Marriage after all is made and sanctified in heaven! Unless this woman engages in some self-evaluation, she is never likely to experience a positive self-image, and will fail to achieve her emotional potential.

In short, the emotionally healthy person achieves a personally satisfying level of potential and behaves in emotionally appropriate ways.

Interpersonal behaviour. A great deal of what we do involves interacting with other people either in small or large groups. These transactions can range from very simple relationships with minimal verbal, physical and emotional interaction, to very complex relationships, such as those in the family. The ability to relate appropriately to other people enables us to meet our needs, to make our wishes known, to achieve, and to generally obtain satisfaction. There is both a cause and effect relationship between interpersonal behaviour and mental health. On the one hand mental health may be reflected by behaviour, and on the other, failure to relate well to others may result in poor adjustment and self-evaluation.

Argyle (1978) has identified eight needs which people attempt to fulfil by relating to other people.

1. Biological needs — hunger and thirst, eating and drinking, co-operation and competition, and emergence of other drives.
2. Dependency — acceptance, help, protection and guidance, especially from people in positions of power and authority.
3. Affiliation — physical proximity, eye contact, warm and friendly responses, and acceptance by peers and groups of peers.
4. Dominance — acceptance by others, and groups of others, as the task leader, being allowed to talk most of the time and make the decisions, and being referred to by the group.

5. Sex — physical proximity, bodily contact, eye contact, warm, friendly and intimate social interaction, usually with attractive peers of the opposite sex.
6. Aggression — harming other people physically, verbally or in other ways.
7. Self-esteem and ego identity — the need to have other people make approving responses and to accept the self-image as valid.
8. Other motivations which affect social behaviour — needs for achievement, money interests and values.

Human society is complex and there are many rules and sanctions that guide us in how to go about fulfilling these needs in our relationships with others. We learn these skills as we grow up, and later modify them through experience to achieve a sense of well-being within ourselves and with the world about us. For most people successful interpersonal interaction leads to good feelings. The opposite is also true, so that when things go wrong bad feelings may result.

Some people have learned poor relating skills and have difficulty in meeting the needs described above. On the one hand this may result from poor communication skills, or on the other there may be an overdeveloped trait which tends to affect interactions. For example, an individual may be extremely aggressive and dominant. This is perceived as an asset in the business or political scene and would probably lead to success; however, using the same skills in a caring relationship could be disastrous. Successful interpersonal behaviour requires a balance.

Activities of daily living. There are a great number of behaviours in which humans habitually engage on a day-to-day basis. These activities of daily living primarily involve biological and social functions which enable people to maintain themselves satisfactorily as individuals and as members of the group. Mental health is reflected by achieving a balanced commitment to these activities:

— hygiene

— nutrition
— exercise
— recreation and relaxation
— sleep
— goal-directed behaviour
— sexual fulfilment.

Goal-directed behaviour includes such activities as work, which is the way in which modern man is able to maintain himself or survive in the world. This would be akin, in animals and stone-age man, to activities such as foraging, finding shelter and keeping warm. These basic survival needs, however, are now achieved by engaging in myriad and complex processes, such as employment, obtaining goods and chattels, and using money. Added to this of course is the notion of achievement, so that some people attempt to obtain bigger and better caves to live in as a means to personal satisfaction and positive self-regard. The measure of satisfaction varies from person to person, with some attempting to achieve at a high level and others being less motivated. Mental health may well be the ability to be satisfied with one's level of attainment.

In recent years an increasing amount of attention has been devoted by those involved in health care to the importance of nutrition, sleep, relaxation and exercise in day-to-day living. This has largely been due to a growing interest in preventive medicine. A particularly prominent theme has been that of stress management and stress prevention, stress having been identified as a major pathophysiological agent resulting from everyday living.

Intellectual activity. Psychological health may also be reflected through intellectual or cognitive functioning — the ability to make decisions and to think rationally. This notion does not necessarily imply that mental health is a function of intelligence. Instead we should think in terms of the level of performance required for a person to operate in order to meet his or her needs and to function within society.

It is, however, difficult to consider cognitive functioning without being confronted by the notion of intelligence. In particular, the value of testing and the meaning of intelligence quotients is a debatable issue within psychology and beyond the scope of this book. Despite difficulties with the concept of intelligence, there are some intellectual abilities that may be useful in evaluating human performance. These are: abstract thinking, problem-solving, the ability to plan, attention, adaptability, educatability, insight, and grasping of relations. A more general definition that is useful has been proposed by Wechsler (1958):

'. . . the aggregate or global capacity of the individual to act purposefully, to think rationally and to deal effectively with his enviroment.'

Subsumed under the abilities described above are factors such as memory, orientation, concentration, perception, and thought content, all of which reflect mental health and are required intact for successful living. These are common parameters used in the diagnosis of mental illness by psychiatrists (see Ch. 2).

Physical functioning. Here we are highlighting a very important consideration in the description of mental health: the mind-body relationship. The division may be seen as artificial although perhaps academically useful. It would seem that there is a strong relationship between psychological processes and physical health (described in detail in Ch. 4). The suggestion here is that mental health may be reflected by physical health, or at the very least by a sense of physical well-being.

It is also true that certain physiological changes such as trauma to the brain or excesses of toxic substances in the blood may impair psychological activities.

MENTAL ILL-HEALTH

So far we have described a number of ways in which it is possible to describe a mentally healthy individual. Mental ill-health and mental health may best be thought of as a continuum, a linear scale on which an individual moves throughout life, from moment to moment, and varying according to situational circumstances. Judgement about the degree of health may be either subjective (the individual's own assessment), or it may be objective (determined by others).

At one end of this scale the person may be seen as operating at an optimal level with satisfying interpersonal relationships, a sense of well-being, engagement in self-fulfilling activities, management of stress, and with properly developed intellectual capacity. At the other end of the scale there is a gross failure to function in one or more of these measures. Between these two extremes there are varying degrees of mental well-being (Fig. 1.1). It is important to note that this is a conceptual framework since at this stage it is not possible to accurately measure or predict particular levels of well-being.

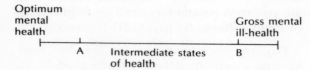

Fig. 1.1 Continuum between mental health and mental ill-health.

Despite this constraint, let us hypothesize that an individual is at point A on the continuum illustrated in Figure 1.1. This person may feel generally dissatisfied with his or her level of achievement and as a result is excessively stressed, is not sleeping well, and is having difficulties with relationships at home. Despite this, functioning within the social context and management of the activities of daily living are completely satisfactory. (In fact we may well be describing a picture that exists fairly commonly in our society.) This person may resolve the problem and grow, with or without external help, or may become more mentally unhealthy.

Let us suppose that this stress leads to a chronic use of excessive amounts of alcohol to the extent that: relationships completely break down; work performance deteriorates; the person's self-image becomes extremely negative; nutrition deteriorates; physical health becomes endangered; and memory

and orientation become mildly impaired. The person is now at point B on Figure 1.1. Again the possibility of moving up or down the scale exists but clearly the degree of mental ill-health, compared with that in healthy behaviour, is much greater, and fairly basic activities are impaired.

This simple description of mental ill-health has a number of important features and corollaries:

1. Normality is not easily defined, nor is it a black-white notion, and is probably not a useful concept.
2. Mental ill-health can be thought of as something more than the presence of certain symptomatology or deviation from what is considered as average.
3. It is possible for society to consider a person mentally unhealthy yet, subjectively, he or she feels very well and is largely unaware of any problems. This dilemma is highlighted by writers such as Goffman (1961) and Szasz (1960). R. D. Laing '. . . regards the psychotic's experience of an alien reality as something akin to a mystical apprehension . . . the faithful reflection of another actuality which is concealed from us by the blinkers of our mundane civilization' (Sedgwick 1971). Laing's view is a controversial yet interesting notion to consider in this age of human rights.
4. The concept of health, rather than disease, is stressed, implying that intervention may occur at any point where optimal functioning is not being achieved.
5. Transient states of mental ill-health do occur, and may be considered to be expected reactions to life events, during which the individual may require help in some way to regain optimal functioning.

This conceptualization of mental ill-health is utilized in two ways in the course of this book. In the first place it attempts to demonstrate an alternative to the idea of mental ill-health as madness and that once mad, always mad. Secondly, although nurses need to understand the disease model, because it is so commonly used as a basis for diagnosis and treatment, intervention does not always require a person to be diagnosed as sick. Our view is that nurses need not be locked in by a disease model, and can be more concerned with helping people overcome difficulties or distress than with treating disease.

UNDERSTANDING ABNORMAL BEHAVIOUR

The current status of psychological theory and research is one in which there are a number of explanations for human behaviour rather than one universally accepted paradigm. At this stage it seems reasonable to consider an eclectic approach to understanding human behaviour — one of multiple or interactive causation. In some cases two or more paradigms can be seen to be useful in explaining behaviour, while some may explain some behaviours but not others. What follows is a brief review of some paradigms of abnormal behaviour and their treatment corollaries, chosen because of their prominence in the literature and in research.

The medical model

The medical model assumes that abnormal behaviour can be explained in terms of disease or illness. This notion is, of course, linked to the physical disease model in which particular signs or symptoms are reasons for believing certain pathophysiological processes are operating. A further step is to then categorize signs and symptoms into patterns, followed by labelling a specific disease. Thus, the label 'schizophrenia' is given to a certain set of signs and symptoms, and treatment is applied according to the diagnosis.

Linked to the medical model are physiological explanations of mental ill-health which stress genetic, hormonal and nervous system malfunctions. There is evidence to suggest, for example, that: schizophrenia has some genetic component; depression is the result of abnormal neurotransmitter function; and anxiety exists in individuals who tend to have

easily arousable automatic nervous systems (Davison & Neale 1978). Electrolyte imbalances and brain damage certainly affect behaviour in quite significant ways, a fact that most nurses working in the general hospital setting would recognize. A whole classification, organic brain syndromes, is given to these sorts of problems.

The psychoanalytic model

In very simple terms psychoanalytic theory makes a distinction, in describing the function of the human mind, between conscious and unconscious processes. Freud described a theory of three major systems or organizational components of the mind: the Id, the superego and the ego.

The Id consists of unconscious drives or instincts and supplies the energy required for the functioning of the psyche. The two basic instincts are Eros and Thanatos, being the life and death forces respectively. The energy for the life-continuing force is called 'libido' and in Freud's theory is largely sexual. The Id constantly seeks gratification, and when this is not provided tension results. When the Id is satisfied, a conscious sensation of pleasure occurs that reinforces further pleasure-seeking behaviour. Thanatos accounts for phenomena such as suicide, aggression, sadism and masochism.

The ego consists of the thinking, knowing, problem-solving branch of the personality. Operating on the reality principle, the ego attempts to gratify unconscious drives by using reality, which may at times mean delaying the instant need for gratification which characterises the Id. The ego for instance is aware that instant gratification is not always practical nor desirable and that there are better ways of going about things.

Lastly, the superego is the conscience, which derives from parental teaching about right and wrong. The Id seeks gratification, the ego decides how to go about it in a rational way, and the superego sets limits on behaviour within the boundaries of what it believes are the social norms and values. The superego is the origin of guilt, or moral anxiety, and of all the 'shoulds' ('I should do this or that') that we internalize from others, and which direct much of our behaviour.

A central issue in psychoanalytic theory is that of anxiety (Freud 1936) which comes about due to the awareness that unconscious energy may manifest itself beyond ego control. Three types of anxiety may be described: phobias — anxiety focused on a particular object; free floating anxiety which has no obvious external cause; and moral anxiety which arises due to the superego. Mental defence mechanisms (described in detail in Ch. 7) operate to protect the organism or ego from anxiety. Whether the Freudian notion of defence mechanisms is entirely accurate may be a matter for debate, but they can be seen to operate in people threatened with a potentially overwhelming situation.

Freud also postulated that the child goes through, and has to successfully negotiate, a number of psychosexual stages during which sexual gratification is directed at particular parts of the body. These are the oral, anal, phallic, latent, and finally the genital stages. It is thought that the child may become fixed at one particular stage (due to problems), this fixation resulting in particular behaviours later in adult life (Table 1.1).

A psychoanalytic theory which has achieved a degree of popularity in recent years is that of transactional analysis. Transactional analysis involves the conceptualization of the ego as having three components: Parent, Adult and Child. It is primarily involved in analysing the transactions (interpersonal behaviour) that occurs between people. The interested reader is referred to Berne (1968) and Harris (1973). These books are easy to understand and offer a very practical interpretation of psychoanalytic theory.

Psychoanalysis is directed towards assisting the person to develop insight into repressed conflicts. The principal goal is to make conscious the unconscious, so that it may be examined in terms of its effect on behaviour. There are many variations on the psycho-

Table 1.1 Freudian stages of psychosexual development

Stage	Age	Child behaviour	Fixation adult behaviour
Oral	0–2	Sucking; ingestion	Dependency. Oral suggestion such as sarcasm, cynicism.
Anal	2–6	Holding back and giving up	Messy, dirty, extravagant or neat, clean, stingy, compulsive
Phallic	3–6	Masturbation; sexual desire directed at opposite parent (Oedipus complex and penis envy)	Guilt, poor sexual identity, anxiety
Latency	6–12	Asexual development	
Genital	12–	Adult heterosexuality	

analytic theme, but the principle of developing insight and resolution of conflict is central.

An important concept arising from psychoanalytic theory is that of transference. This involves an individual or client transferring feelings, held towards an important person in his life, to the therapist. These feelings may be either positive or negative, and are sometimes extremely intense. The therapist uses the transference in insight development, since when it occurs it signifies repression and conflict.

Learning theories

In contrast to psychoanalysis, the behaviour therapies, rather than dealing with unconscious material, tend to deal with problems that consciously confront the individual. This is achieved by relearning behaviour or responses to situations to achieve a more positive pay-off.

According to behaviourists there are two principle methods of learning: classical conditioning, and operant conditioning. In both these processes the individual makes connections, from experience, between events which occur in the environment. These connections are known as 'stimulus-response bonds', and, when learned, lead to particular stimuli in the environment evoking particular responses.

Classical conditioning involves the association of two stimuli with a particular response, and is demonstrated by an experiment conducted by its originators, Ivan Petrovich Pavlov. If a dog is given food it will salivate as the digestive tract prepares itself, quite automatically and without learning. The food is called the 'unconditioned stimulus' and the salivation is the 'unconditioned response'. Consider now what happens when a bell is rung prior to the presentation of the food. Eventually the dog associates the bell with the food and starts to salivate at the sound of the bell. The bell is termed the 'conditioned stimulus'.

Three important learning principles arise from experiments in classical conditioning. Firstly, the conditioned stimulus needs strengthening by 'reinforcement' or repeated trials in which the conditioned stimulus is followed by the unconditioned stimulus. Secondly, learning can be extinguished when the unconditioned stimulus is repeatedly withheld following the conditioned stimulus. However, at a later date spontaneous recovery will occur unless many trials without the unconditioned stimulus have taken place. Thirdly, it has been shown (Kimble 1961) that similar stimuli to the conditioned stimulus can cause the response to be elicited. For example, one might expect the dog to salivate at the ringing of a doorbell or bicycle bell.

The relevance of this type of learning to understanding human behaviour becomes clearer when we consider the behaviour therapies. Phobias are conditioned responses to objects or situations (conditioned stimuli) which are associated with anxiety (unconditioned stimulus). Of similar importance is the notion of vicarious learning or 'modelling' described by Bandura & Rosenthal (1966). Here the individual develops a conditioned emotional response by watching the negative reactions of others to various stimuli (snakes, spiders, sharks, minority groups, etc.).

Operant conditioning involves the principle that if a response produces a reward it is likely to be repeated. Similarly, negative consequences are likely to prevent repetition of a particular act. In humans rewards may be money, material possessions, attention, praise, food, sex, or achievement. Operant conditioning has been applied to modifying behaviour in mental hospital patients (Ayllon & Azrun 1968) by providing rewards for socially acceptable behaviour. It has also been used with some success (Ayllon & Kelly 1972) in the training of retarded children.

In recent years behaviour therapists have incorporated the role of thinking and reasoning into their framework for understanding disturbed behaviour. These theories are labelled as 'cognitive', and in treatment attempt to alter the person's patterns of thinking about self and the world. Cognitive therapies tend to concentrate on overt symptoms and are highly structured (Beck 1970). Ellis' 'rational emotive therapy' (1962) is an example of a modern cognitive theory operating on the assumption that psychological ill-health stems from irrational patterns of thinking. According to Ellis, what the person says to himself has a major effect on the way he feels and acts. The treatment involves assisting the individual to change these self-verbalizations as a means to changing behaviour. Put simply by Ellis (1975):

'People afflicted with neurotic behaviour have potential capabilities but do not realise how self-defeatingly they act. Or they understand how they harm themselves but, for some irrational reasons, persist in self-sabotaging behaviour. Since we assume that such people have potential capabilities, rather than have inborn stupidity, we also assume that their emotional problems arise because either they do not know how to, or know how but do not try to think more clearly and behave less self-defeatingly.'

Social skills

'Social skill' refers to the ability to perform successfully at an interpersonal level which enables the person to obtain rewards from interacting with others and to ultimately feel good about himself or herself. 'Social inadequacy' refers to the failure to affect the behaviour and feelings of others in the way intended and which society accepts (Trower et al 1975). For example, people who are boring, annoying, uninteresting, cold, destructive, bad-tempered, inept, and destructive are likely to be quite unrewarding to other people. The result is rejection and isolation which leads eventually to psychological problems. Being socially skilled requires a firm grasp of the verbal and non-verbal communication skills which enable us to interact well with other people.

These skills are (or are not) learned in childhood from those around us, such as parents, peers, and teachers. Argyle (1978) likens social skill learning to that of learning motor skills. Treatment then is largely educational and is a process of teaching a person how to communicate more effectively by direct skill training which may also include dealing with situational anxiety. The basic principles of teaching apply, e.g. modelling, behaviour-shaping, prompting, reinforcement and practice.

Humanistic theories

Under this heading we will consider the views of Carl Rogers and Fritz Perls who are responsible for client-centred and Gestalt therapy respectively. These therapies are basically insight-oriented in much the same way as is psychoanalytic theory, but with an emphasis on the notion of free will or freedom of choice (Davison & Neale 1978).

Rogers suggests that people can be understood only in terms of their own personal thoughts and feelings. The person is the expert on himself and, when given the opportunity, can solve his own problems. Therapy is designed to help the person become healthy by becoming aware of his behaviour and its effects. The role of the therapist is to provide an environment which facilitates this development of awareness. In fact, 'facilitator' describes the role of the therapist in assisting the client to solve problems by being accepting and completely non-judgemental. Some other skills involved in

Rogerian methods include: clarification of feeling, listening skills, positive regard for the client, empathy, and reflecting, all of which take place within a warm therapeutic relationship.

From the point of view of understanding people, Rogers postulates that behaviour is directed towards the tendency to self-actualize. This may be described as self-development, the learning of new things, growth, and the realization of full potentials.

Three important themes in Gestalt therapy are wholeness, awareness, and getting in touch with the present. To Perls, health '. . . is an appropriate balance of the coordination of what we are' (Perls 1969). Ill-health occurs then when the person alienates parts of himself or blocks out parts of his experience and resists becoming aware of self. The sorts of attitudes that Gestalt therapists see as being important in living now are as follows:

1. The past is gone and the future is yet to come so be concerned with the present.
2. Concentrate on what is actually here rather than what is absent.
3. Experience things rather than imagine them.
4. Feel rather than think.
5. Express feelings freely without justification.
6. Be aware of pain as well as pleasure.
7. Avoid the word 'should'.
8. Accept responsibility for actions, thoughts and feelings.
9. Accept and be yourself.

OVERVIEW

In this chapter we have attempted to illustrate the complexities involved in describing and explaining mental ill-health. Although only an overview, it is intended as a starting point in the rationalization of the nursing care discussed in Part Two. Many related ideas about the cause of psychological problems are discussed in following chapters. In particular we consider stress to be a central issue (see Ch. 4). We would also like to draw attention to the nursing models presented in Chapter 6, which are an attempt to draw together many of the concepts discussed here.

It should also be apparent that there is a tremendous richness available from which to draw understanding about people and their behaviour. Our view on effective approaches to people with behavioural disturbances is somewhat eclectic, tending to draw the best substantiated techniques from the various therapies, and those backed by research or a sound theoretical framework. The chapter on interpersonal skills (Ch. 4) draws heavily on Rogerian techniques, and that on depression (Ch. 8) uses a number of cognitive ideas. If anything, our stance tends towards the cognitive-behaviourist techniques, although with some humanist approaches.

REFERENCES

Argyle M 1978 The psychology of interpersonal behaviour. Penguin, Harmondsworth

Ayllon T, Azrun N M 1968 The token economy: a motivational system for therapy and rehabilitation. Appleton Century Crofts, New York

Ayllon T, Kelly K 1972 Effects of reinforcement on standardized test performance. Journal of Applied Behavioural Analysis 4

Bandura A, Rosenthal T L 1966 Vicarious classical conditioning as a function of arousal level. Journal of Personality and Social Psychology 3

Beck A T 1970 The care problem in depression: the cognitive triad. In: Masserman J (ed) Depression: theories and therapies. Grune & Stratton, New York

Berne E 1968 Games people play. Penguin, Harmondsworth

Coleman J C 1972 Abnormal psychology and modern life. Scott Foresman, Glenview

Davison G C, Neale J M 1978 Abnormal psychology. Wiley, New York

Dossey L 1982 Consciousness and caring: retrospective 2000. Topics in Clinical Nursing, Jan3

Ellis A 1962 Reason and emotion in psychotherapy. Lyle Stewart, New York

Ellis A, Harper R A 1975 A new guide to rational living. Wilshire, Hollywood

Foucault M 1965 Madness and civilization. Vintage Books, New York

Freud S 1936 The problem of anxiety. Norton, New York

Goffman E 1961 Asylums. Penguin, Harmondsworth

Haber J, Leach A M, Schudy A M, Sideleau B F 1978 Comprehensive psychiatric nursing. McGraw Hill, New York

Harris T A 1973 I'm OK — you're OK. Pan, London

Kimble G 1961 Hilgard and Marguis' conditioning and learning. Appleton Century Crofts, New York

Mosak H M 1976 Subjective criteria of normality. In: Allman L P, Jaffe D T (eds) Readings in abnormal psychology: contemporary perspectives. Harper & Row, New York

Pasquali E A, Alesi E F, Arnold M M, DeBasio N 1981 Mental health nursing: a bio psycho-cultural approach. Mosby, St Louis

Peplau H 1982 In Foreword to: Fitzpatrick J, Whall A, Johnston R, Floyd J Nursing models and their psychiatric mental health application. R J Brady, Maryland

Perls F 1969 Gestalt therapy verbatim. Real People Press, Utah

Riel J P, Roy C 1980 Conceptual models for nursing practice. Appleton Century Crofts, New York

Rosenhan D C 1973 On being sane in insane places. Science 179

Sedgwick J 1971 Anti-psychiatry. Penguin, Harmondsworth

Szasz T S 1960 The myth of mental illness. American Psychologist 15:2

Szasz T S 1970 The manufacture of madness. Palladin, London

Szasz T S 1974 The myth of mental illness. Harper & Row, New York

Trower P, Bryant B, Argyle M 1975 Social skills and mental health. Methuan, London

Ullman L P, Krasner L 1969 A psychological approach to abnormal behaviour. Prentice Hall, Englewood Cliffs

Wechsler D 1958 The measurement and appraisal of adult intelligence, 4th edn. Williams & Wilkins, Baltimore

Wilson-Barnett (ed) 1983 Patient teaching. Churchill Livingstone, Edinburgh

2

Classification of mental disorders

This chapter is disease-oriented, describing mental illnesses in terms of cause, clinical features, and treatment. Although this method of describing mental illness is incongruous with our general theme and approach, its inclusion in the text is justified: it depicts a model of mental illness which can be contrasted with the nursing model described in Chapter 6, and it provides necessary factual information for the nurse.

Many aspects of a nurse's day-to-day practice are performed independently of members of other associated health-care disciplines. However, to promote genuine holistic care, and to assist the ill person with the management of his health most effectively, all personnel need to combine their particular expertise in a team approach. It is as a member of this team, and often as co-ordinator of care, that the nurse needs to perform certain dependent functions. To perform this role effectively it is necessary to have a knowledge and understanding of the theories and practice on which psychiatrists, and others within the medical profession, base their diagnosis and management of the person's problem. Fundamental to this practice is a diagnostic classification of mental disorders. Such a classification enables signs and symptoms of illness to be grouped under diagnostic categories, and people to be described as suffering from a particular mental illness or an amalgamation of mental disorders. The authors of an internationally accepted classification, the '*Diagnostic and Statistical Manual of Mental Disorders*', state the purpose of their classification as being to '. . . provide clear descriptions of diagnostic categories in order to enable clinicians to diagnose, communicate about, study, and treat various mental disorders' (American Psychiatric Association 1980).

This chapter is a concise synthesis and categorisation of the basic disorders of mental health. It provides the nurse with an introductory, factual knowledge base necessary to understand the psychopathology of people's disturbances, and to communicate competently and effectively within the health team. The nurse is the member of that team who has most continuous contact with the ill person and, as such, will soon discover that a textbook description will not always apply to a person's individual problem or problems. Categorisation of mental illnesses tends to de-emphasize the individuality of the person and the importance, to him, of his particular problem. It is this nursing concern for the individual, rather than the illness, that calls into question the necessity for nurses to have a knowledge of psychopathology, and the consequent inclusion of a chapter on mental disorder in a book concerned about nursing interventions with the ill person, rather than management of mental illness. Apart from the previously mentioned purpose of facilitating interdisciplinary communication, a further justification is summarized by Kreigh & Perko (1979)

'. . . knowledge of the pathological process is important only in so far as it contributes to furthering the nurse's assessment or appraisal of the individual patient's need system.'

The classification of the clinical conditions examined in this chapter is based on the categories described in the Third Edition of the *Diagnostic And Statistical Manual of Mental Disorders* (DSM III). Terminology and descriptive phrases are those used in DSM III and quotations have been used to define and describe various conditions. Description is in the traditional form, detailing definitions,

aetiology, clinical features and medical treatment.

Nursing management is not considered here, as this aspect is examined by an individual symptomatic approach in Part Two. The categories of mental disorders described are only a selection of the total range of possible classified disturbances to which individuals are subject. We describe those disorders which occur most often in the general population, are most serious in terms of effect on the individual's functioning, and are most likely to be encountered by the nurse in a general hospital or community setting. They include:

1. Organic mental disorders.
2. Affective disorders.
3. Schizophrenic disorders.
4. Other psychotic disorders.
5. Anxiety disorders.
6. Personality disorders.
7. Substance-use disorders.
8. Somatoform disorders.

ORGANIC MENTAL DISORDERS

Definition

'The essential feature of all these . . . [organic mental disorders] . . . is a psychological or behavioural abnormality associated with transient or permanent dysfunction of the brain.'

(DSM III)

This dysfunction produces syndromes in which a number of abnormalities may exist, including impairment of

- orientation
- memory
- comprehension
- calculation
- learning capacity
- judgement.

Associated with these abnormalities may be a disturbance in the person's mood, and an exaggeration of personality traits. Variations in the locality of the dysfunctional neurones of the brain, the onset of the dysfunction, the progression and duration of the disturbance, and the nature of the underlying pathophysiology produce different syndromes. The most common organic brain syndromes are grouped here under the two general categories of acute disturbance (delirium), and chronic dementia.

DELIRIUM

States of delirium are probably the most frequently occurring psychotic mental disturbance seen by nurses in general hospitals. 'Psychotic', as defined in DSM III, is:

'a term indicating gross impairment in reality testing. It may be used to describe the behaviour of an individual at a given time, or a mental disorder in which at some time during is course all individuals with the disorder have grossly impaired reality testing. When there is gross impairment in reality testing, the individual incorrectly evaluates the accuracy of his or her perceptions and thoughts and makes incorrect inferences about external reality, even in the fact of contrary evidence . . .'.

The term 'delirium' is now adopted to classify all disturbances previously described as acute brain syndromes or toxic confusional states.

Definition

Delirium may be defined as an altered state of consciousness, usually of short duration, involving reversible changes in the metabolic processes of the brain, and characterized by

- a clouding of awareness of the environment
- confusion
- disorientation to time, place and person
- perceptual disturbances
- increased or decreased psychomotor activity
- disturbance of the sleep-wakefulness cycle.

Aetiology

Delirium can occur at any age but is more common in infants, young children, and the elderly. The most common cause is infection, particularly pneumonia in the elderly. Holding

& Kay (1984) report the occurrence of delirium, during the course of an illness, in 15–20% of hospitalized elderly people.

Apart from infection, the causes most frequently seen in the hospital setting include

- postoperative states
- metabolic disorders such as hypoxia, hypercarbia
- hypoglycaemia
- electrolyte imbalance
- hepatic or renal failure
- thiamine deficiency
- concussion and recovery from unconsciousness following head injury
- excessive intoxication of substances
- withdrawal from toxic states, as in alcohol withdrawal syndrome (delirium tremens), or other drug withdrawal (e.g. from barbiturates or benzodiazepines)
- idiosyncratic reaction to almost any prescribed medication
- exposure
- fatigue and sensory deprivation
- severe constipation.

Clinical features

The altered state of consciousness and associated clouding of sensorium produce difficulty in concentrating on external environmental stimuli. The person is easily distracted, his attention wanders, and he experiences problems in maintaining reasonable thinking, manifested by alteration in the rate and coherence of speech. Difficulty is experienced in following arguments or ordinary events going on in the immediate surroundings, leading to bewilderment and confusion. In more severe cases total disorientation occurs, the person being unable to state accurately the day, date or time, or even to remember very recent events. The confusion becomes worse at night in almost every form of delirium except that caused by encephalitis. The degree of confusion is liable to vary from hour to hour.

Often the prevailing mood is one of anxiety or fear; however, the mood is likely to change rapidly, with anxiety being replaced by irritability and anger. In some cases, people experience heightened, happy moods or become erotically inclined. A typical feature of delirium is a rapid change, not only in emotional state but also in intensity of feelings.

Perceptual disturbances common in more serious delirium are misinterpretation of external stimuli (illusions), and sensory perceptions for which there are no external stimuli (halluncinations). The hallucinations are typically threatening, giving rise to an increase in fear and perhaps the development of delusional ideas. (A delusion is a fixed, false, personal belief firmly held despite evidence to the contrary, not amenable to logical argument, and not in keeping with the person's culture, intelligence, religious beliefs or education.)

Motor (physical) activity is often increased, the person becoming restless and overactive. He may become violent as an act of self-preservation against the threat arising from the content of his hallucinations and delusional thinking. The person may, alternatively, demonstrate a decreased level of psychomotor activity, with drowsiness and lethargy progressing to a stuporose state. As with mood, psychomotor activity often fluctuates from one extreme to the other.

Duration

Delirium, by definition, is a disturbance of short duration. Onset is generally rapid, with the delirious state lasting from a few hours to one week. The total duration of the disturbance often is dependent upon the cause, the speed at which the cause can be identified and treated, and the sufferer's rate of response to treatment.

Treatment

Management of delirium involves

1. Determining the cause and initiating appropriate treatment — this may, for instance, necessitate rehydration of the person, correction of electrolyte imbalance, or commencement of antibiotic drugs.
2. Alleviating excitement and promoting rest — achieved by administration of central nervous system depressing drugs supported by the provision of a quiet environment.
3. The maintenance of the person's strength by a high fluid intake (except in cardiac failure) — small, frequent, highly nutritional meals, and supplementary doses of B group vitamins, if necessary.
4. The prevention of complications and injury to the person.

DEMENTIA

Definition

DSM III states:

'the essential feature is a loss of intellectual abilities of sufficient severity to interfere with social or occupational functioning. The deficit is multifactorial and involves memory, judement, abstract thought, and a variety of other higher cortical functions, Changes in personality and behaviour also occur.'

This syndrome occurs due to structural damage to brain tissue resulting from pathology or trauma.

Aetiology

Dementias may arise from a number of causes and, although occurring predominantly in the elderly, some precipitating factors may produce the disorder at any age. These factors include

- subdural haematoma
- normal pressure hydrocephalus
- viral encephalitis
- meningitis
- intracranial neoplasm
- hypothyroidism
- Parkinson's disease
- Huntington's chorea
- brain injury
- vitamin deficiency (B_{12} or folate)
- chronic alcohol and other toxic substance abuse.

Incidence

Although dementia should not be considered synonymous with ageing, it is present in 20% of the population over the age of 79; and of all cases, those occurring in old age, principally senile dementia Alzheimer type and multi-infarct dementia, represent 80% of the total (Holding & Kay 1984).

Course

The onset and course of a dementing process are dependent upon the nature of the aetiological factors involved, being rapid or insidious, and progressive, static or reversible. Primary degenerative dementia (senile dementia Alzheimer type), for instance, may be presenile in onset, occurring before age 65, or senile, occurring after age 65 but mainly in the over 75s, the onset of clinical features being insidious and gradually progressive until death occurs after an average of 5 years.

An example of a less insidious onset is seen in dementia arising from normal pressure hydrocephalus, where the process can be reversed following treatment. The degree of resolution is dependent upon the amount of permanent damage that has occurred.

Head trauma or neurological disease will produce a sudden onset of features with little or no further progression, the degree of dementia remaining static.

Regardless of the age of the individual at the time of brain damage, the subsequent dysfunction is still classified as a dementia.

Clinical features

The presence of clinical features of dementia is not always related to the degree of pathological change in brain tissue. Many individuals will demonstrate severe impairment with only slight changes in brain structure, while others with prominent changes noted postmortem will show few or no signs during their lives. This phenomenon would suggest an involvement of social, environmental, personality and intellectual factors in the development of dementia arising in the absence of neurological disease or brain trauma. Such factors might be loneliness and lack of interpersonal contact leading to voluntary withdrawal into a twilight of confusion.

These factors influence the individual's ability to cope with the deficiency in cerebral functioning and this is in turn governs the extent and severity of the presenting features of dementia.

Memory

The prominent feature of any dementia is an impairment of memory. This may vary from an initial forgetfulness, progressing through an inability to remember proper names and daily events, to a total absence of memory of relatives, important life events, and even the individual's own name.

This memory impairment leads to problems in daily living and produces potentially dangerous situations for the person in an unsupervised environment: forgetting to switch off electrical appliances, leaving taps running, and misusing prescribed medications are only a few of the many hazards to which a sufferer of dementia is susceptible. The hospitalised individual may demonstrate this impaired memory by continuous repetition of requests or repeated telling of a story, being totally unaware of having previously recounted it. Preceding events during the day are forgotten, as is often the memory of the most recent meal. Short-term memory, the recall of new information, is most severely impaired, but many people will be able to recall events in their early lives and will describe them as if they had recently taken place, often filling gaps in their memory with fictitious details.

Disorientation

Accompanying the memory impairment is a state of disorientation. In severe cases of dementia there is a total disorientation to time, place and person. The individual is unable to state the approximate time of day, the day of the week or the date; does not know who he is; and is unable to correctly identify the people in his environment.

Judgement

Impaired judgement is a characteristic feature, evidenced by unrealistic expectations for the future, inability to make decisions and becoming generally socially disinhibited. This often results in a decline in personal appearance, self-degenerating and socially unacceptable behaviour, inappropriate comments, and the use of coarse language — all of which may be completely uncharacteristic traits of the individual's previous personality. A change in the general character may take place, a previously outgoing individual becoming withdrawn and apathetic, or a quiet, retiring person becoming uncharacteristically loud. The former occurs more commonly and is noticed early by relatives and friends, especially as the range of social involvement narrows progressively. Alternatively, there may be an exaggeration of previous personality traits.

Abstract thinking

A major deficit in intellectual functioning is apparent in the capacity for abstract thought. Cognitively unimpaired individuals of average intelligence are able to generalise from concrete facts. One way in which this is demonstrated is in the interpretation of proverbs. If, for example, a person is asked to explain the meaning of the proverb 'Too many cooks spoil the broth', he will be able to give a concrete reply such as 'Too many cooks over the same pot or in the same kitchen will spoil the soup.' He will also, however, be able to abstract from the statement ideas or thoughts that can be applied to other situations as well. For example, 'If there are too many people engaged in some project they will get in each other's way and achieve little of value'; or 'If too many people tackle the same project they may have such divergent and conflicting ideas about the project that no definite plan can be put into operation.' It is the inability to perform abstract thinking that is characteristic

in dementia and renders the ill person unable to process new information, be decisive, and undertake tasks that require a logical problem-solving approach.

Mood

Associated with the essential features of dementia is a change in general mood state. Depending on the degree of dementia, mood may vary from anxiety and depression to extreme suspicion, paranoia, and jealousy. In the early stages of a primary degenerative dementia, the individual may be aware of deteriorating intellectual functioning, causing substantial feelings of lowered self-esteem, justifiable worry, agitation and anguish. A significant number of people with dementia do have concurrent symptoms of depression which will respond to treatment. These alterations in mood may also be present in static dementias resulting from head trauma or a neurological disease. With a deterioration in intellectual functioning, memory, and abstract thinking, develops a suspicion of the actions and motives of those around, which can progress to fleeting delusions of paranoid intensity resulting in verbal and physical attacks on others. These outbursts arise from falsely held beliefs and accusations, or exaggerated feelings of jealousy towards other people.

Interpersonal relationships

A loss of feeling and sympathy for others, accompanied by irritability and petulance, are features of a demented person's character commonly encountered by those caring for the person. These factors, in conjunction with previously mentioned changes in mood and behaviour, often give rise to unpredictable response from the person, and general problems in interpersonal and intergroup relationships.

Speech

The problems are compounded if the features of dementia indicate involvement of higher cortical functioning. Such involvement is dependent on the degree of pathology and, when present, can affect ability to communicate and express thoughts verbally. Speech may alter in both form and content, becoming rambling, repetitive, and degenerating eventually to incoherence.

These clinical features apply particularly to disorders occurring in old-age. However, although ageing and physical deterioration are usually synonymous, intellectual performance need not inevitably decline with age. Moreoever, the presence of clinical signs does not necessarily indicate the degree of brain damage or atrophy, but only represents a measure of the person's capacity to function in the presence of cerebral damage.

Treatment

The presenting signs of dementia necessitate thorough investigation to establish the causal factors. The underlying cause may be amenable to treatment resulting in the halting or reversal of otherwise progressive deterioration. An example is the presence of normal pressure hydrocephalus which, when corrected, can produce almost total amelioration of symptoms. The progression may also be halted or slowed in cases arising from cerebrovascular disease, where steps can be taken to lessen the chance of further cerebrovascular accidents occurring.

Generally speaking, there are no specific pharmacological treatments which can prevent or reduce the pathological changes present in primary degenerative dementia; however, recent orthomolecular psychiatric research has found levels of zinc in diet to be an important factor (Burnett 1981). Management through medical intervention concentrates on any concurrent physical illness and on the pharmacological control of psychiatric symptoms such as agitation, depression, insomnia, confusion, and paranoia. As these are only palliative measures, emphasis should be placed on the defective social performance occurring in dementia, and interventions undertaken to permit and encourage the

person to function at his maximum potential. Such interventions should be supported by providing a stimulating environment that will not compound the propensity for confusion, disorientation, wandering, agitation and depression. Without symptom-relief and social stimulation, the rate of deterioration is more rapid.

Hospitalization of the person with advanced dementia typically necessitates provision, by nursing staff, for all aspects of physical and mental health including hygiene, nutrition, protection, sleep, management of acute confusional episodes and wandering, and continual interaction. Fundamental to this physical care is the need to maintain the demented person's dignity, pride, and individuality.

AFFECTIVE DISORDERS

Definition

Before proceeding with description of some of the disorders considered under this category, a distinction between the meaning of the terms 'affect' and 'mood' needs to be made.

Affect and mood

Affect is an expressed and observable feeling state. Mood is a prolonged emotion, a purely subjective, sustained feeling state.

Affect must be distinguished from mood and not used as a synonym. However, generally the mood and the affect, i.e. the way a person feels and the way he appears to others to feel, are the same. For example, a person may have a depressed mood; when this feeling state becomes observable, he is described as also having a depressed affect. Occasionally the outward expression of mood, the affect, differs from the actual emotion being experienced by the individual: for example, a person may feel sad and in despair, but may appear angry and be outwardly aggressive.

Disorders in which the principle feature is

a disturbance in the feeling state of an individual are described as 'affective disorders' rather than 'mood disorders', as the disturbance is apparent to others and not solely a subjective disturbance of which only the sufferer is aware.

Normal feelings versus pathological state

The range of human emotions allows mood states of varying type and degree to occur at various times, in response to appropriately provoking stimuli. These fluctuations in feeling can be experienced by anybody, regardless of societal, cultural, economic or intellectual differences. Apart from the fluctuations in mood states, each healthy person has an individual, prevailing mood. In one person this might be an objective social withdrawal, a passive desire to spend life quietly and uncomplicatedly, but this would not necessarily indicate an unhappy feeling state. This is in objective contrast to the person with seemingly insatiable gaiety and energy who is an automatic leader and centre of attraction when in a group, again not necessarily indicative of continuous, worry-free happiness. The prevailing mood in these cases is synonymous with, or at least a component of, the individual's personality.

The two extremes, or poles, of mood variation are profound depression and mania; but what constitutes acceptable human emotion within these variations, and when does it reach the stage of a pathological state? There are four main criteria to be taken into consideration when examining a mood state: the intensity of the mood, the duration, the precipitating event and the quality of the individual presenting features (Klerman 1971). Consideration of these criteria individually and collectively determine whether the mood state is exceeding the boundaries of acceptable emotional variance and has become a pathological condition. Regardless of these criteria, the occurrence of certain features immediately indicates the presence of a pathological state; such features may be hallucinations, delusions, thought disorder, a serious alteration in body weight, persistent suicidal ideation, bizarre behaviour.

Aetiology

There are several theories as to why people develop affective disorders, discussion of which is outside the scope of this book. However, mention will be made of some of the causal factors which have been the subject of research, to provide some understanding of the puzzling question of why people develop these disorders.

One overall explanation incorporates the current philosophy of a biopsychosocial causation in which the occurrence of a disorder has components of a biological, psychological and sociological nature, and cannot always be attributed to a single identifiable cause.

The following are some of the factors considered to be involved in these biological, psychological and sociological components of both depressive and manic disorders.

Loss or separation

Although considered by a large number of the general population to be the obvious precipitant of depression, loss or separation, in fact, account for no more than 25% of depressive illnesses.

Stress

Apart from loss or separation, which are extremely stressful events, other life events, the accumulative responses to which exceed the individual's threshold of coping, can precipitate the development of an affective disorder. Excess stress alone is most likely to precipitate a relapse or recurrence of symptoms in an individual with a history of previous episodes of depression or mania.

Biogenic amines

'Biogenic amines' is the term generally used to describe three substances — dopamine, noradrenaline and serotonin — which function as neurotransmitters in the brain. Alterations in the levels of these essential neurotransmitters have been found to be present in affective disorders. However, studies to date have indicated that deficiencies of these substances alone will not necessarily produce a disturbance in mood. Excess stress, genetic make-up and significant life events will produce changes in biogenic amines which, in combination with other factors, can lead to the development of an affective disorder.

Neuro-endocrine activity

The hypothalamic-pituitary-adrenal axis has received much study in regard to the responses evoked by physical and psychological stress. Since this axis comes under the control of the central nervous system, and in particular the hypothalamus (which is also considered to be influential in dictating and controlling emotions), disturbance in emotional state can be assumed to be associated with the activity of the components of this axis.

Electrolyte disturbance

The concentration of intracellular sodium increases in depressive and manic illnesses, with a corresponding accumulation of extracellular potassium.

Genetics

There is a definite familial tendency in the occurrence of affective disorders in the general population (Price 1968). This tendency is considered to be due to an inherited factor, although the mode of genetic transmission is not known.

Psychological development

Experiences and events occurring during an individual's formative years have considerable bearing on psychological and emotional development. These factors strongly influence the susceptibility of an individual to the occurrence of an affective disorder in later life.

DEPRESSION

Classification of depressive disorders

Over the years, there have been many attempts to organise the varying presentations of depression into some uniform classification. These endeavours still exist, there now having been in excess of fifty different classifications attempting to describe the phenomenon. This text will attempt to avoid classifying depressions but concentrate on describing the range of presenting signs and symptoms that may be seen in, or experienced by, individuals suffering from a depressive disorder. One very broad distinction between depressions should be mentioned here, as it is particularly significant when considering the presentation of depression in a general hospital setting. This differentation is between primary and secondary depressions. In general terms, a primary depression is an illness occurring in an individual who otherwise was previously well, or if unwell, the illness was a previous affective disorder. The depressive state, therefore, is not distinctly related to any other physical or psychological disturbance; the majority of depressions (60–70%) are primary depressive illnesses.

A secondary depression is generally a symptom of either another mental disturbance or physical disease. Other mental illnesses may be schizophrenic disorder, alcohol or other drug abuse, or dementia; precipitating physical illnesses include endocrine disorders, central nervous system disorders, nutritional deficiencies, anaemias, viral infections, cardiovascular disease, and some cancers. Depression can also be induced chemically by pharmacological agents prescribed for the treatment of a physical disorder. Antihypertensive drugs and steriods, for example, often cause secondary depression.

Clinical features

People suffering from a major depressive illness present with multiple symptoms which are abnormal, for them, and persistent. The essential feature is a dysphoric mood or loss of interest in almost all usual activities. This is associated with several of a large range of symptoms, the multiplicity of which can dominate the presentation and detract from the underlying depressed mood. This range includes

- feelings of worthlessness, guilt, helplessness and hopelessness
- anxiety
- tearfulness
- suicidal thoughts or self-harming acts
- loss of interest, loss of affectional feelings
- social withdrawal and an impaired capacity to perform everyday social functions
- psychomotor retardation or agitation
- increased incidence of, and attention to, bodily complaints including anorexia, weight loss, constipation, headache, dry mouth, loss of libido, and insomnia.

Where the depression is of psychotic depth, there may also be delusional ideas of a depressive nature, for example, individuals believing they are responsible for some tragedy that has occurred, that they have committed a terrible sin for which they will be punished, or that part of their body, particularly their bowels, is dysfunctional or missing altogether ('nihilistic delusion').

The diagnostic criteria set down in DSM III for the diagnosis of a major depressive episode include the presence of a prominent, persistent dysphoric mood or loss of interest in all usual activities, and at least four of the other multiple symptoms previously mentioned, present nearly every day for at least two weeks.

The aforementioned obviously describes a severe depressive illness in which there would be extremes of symptomatology. However, a great number of people suffer from an episode of depression or chronically recurring episodes where the degree of severity and the extent of symptoms are not as debilitating. Although hospitalization for such a condition is not as often required as for a more severe disorder, many people admitted to hospital for investigation and management of a physical disorder may be suffering from a

depressive illness of this kind. Such a disturbance, referred to as a 'dysthymic mood disorder' and previously as a 'depressive neurosis' or 'neurotic depression,' is described in DSM III as being constituted by the following criteria.

A. During the past two years (or one year for children and adolescents) the individual has been bothered most or all of the time by symptoms characteristic of the depressive syndrome but that are not of sufficient severity and duration to meet the criteria for a major depressive episode.

B. The manifestations of the depressive syndrome may be relatively persistent or separated by periods of normal mood lasting a few days to a few weeks, but no more than a few months at a time.

C. During the depressive periods there is either prominent depressed mood (e.g. sad, blue, down in dumps, low) or marked loss of interest or pleasure in all or almost all, usual activities and pastimes.

D. During the depressive periods at least three of the following symptoms are present.
1. Insomnia or hypersomnia.
2. Low energy level or chronic tiredness.
3. Feelings of inadequacy, loss of self-esteem, or self-deprecation.
4. Decreased effectiveness or productivity at school, work or home.
5. Decreased attention, concentration, or ability to think clearly.
6. Social withdrawal.
7. Loss of interest in or enjoyment of pleasurable activities.
8. Irritability or excessive anger (in children, expressed toward parents or caretakers).
9. Inability to respond with apparent pleasure to praise or rewards.
10. Less active or talkative than usual, or feels slowed down or restless.
11. Pessimistic attitude toward the future, brooding about past events, or feeling sorry for self.
12. Tearfulness or crying.
13. Recurrent thoughts of death or suicide.

E. Absence of psychotic features, such as delusions, hallucinations, or incoherence, or loosening of associations . . .'

MANIA

Definition

The term 'mania' is associated with varying conditions other than affective disorder. Two meanings with which the term is commonly associated by people outside the health professions are

1. Any mental disorder, 'madness', especially when characterized by violent, unrestrained behaviour.

2. When used as a suffix, a morbid preference for or an irrepressible impulse to behave in a certain way, e.g. kleptomania (Campbell 1981).

The disturbance with which we are concerned here is related to the third meaning of the term, which deals with mania as a pole or extreme of emotional variance opposite to depression. This form of affective disorder is characterized by a predominantly elevated or euphoric, although unstable mood and associated increase in mental and physical activity giving rise to alterations in the individual's speech behaviour and general social functioning, and work performance.

Clinical features

Some of the DSM III criteria for a manic episode include

A. One or more distinct periods with a predominantly elevated expansive, or irritable mood. The elevated or irritable mood must be a prominent part of the illness and relatively persistent, although it may alternate or intermingle with depressive mood.

B. Duration of at least one week (or any duration if hospitalization is necessary), during which, for most of the time, at least three of the following symptoms have persisted (four if the mood is only irritable) and have been present to a significant degree:

1. Increase in activity (either socially, at work, or sexually) or physical restlessness.
2. More talkative than usual or pressure to keep talking.
3. Flight of ideas or subjective experience that thoughts are racing.
4. Inflated self-esteem (grandiosity, which may be delusional).
5. Decreased need for sleep.
6. Distractibility, i.e. attention is too easily drawn to unimportant or irrelevant external stimuli.
7. Excessive involvement in activities that have a high potential for painful consequences which is not recognised, e.g. buying sprees, sexual indiscretions, foolish business investments, reckless driving . . .'

Most people who are manic, or showing signs of becoming so, have little insight into the fact that they are unwell. Frequently they are referred for treatment as a result of concern, by others, over their inability to work effectively, insomnia, overactivity, disinhibited behaviour, unusual alcohol abuse or wild spending sprees.

'Hypomania' is the term used to describe a less intense form of mania in which the person may be full of energy, have many bright ideas and eagerness to talk, but lacks the extremes of overactivity, overtalkativeness, flight of ideas, and disruptive behaviour characteristic of a manic episode.

Bipolar and unipolar affective disorders

Severe and prolonged disturbances of mood are classified, for diagnostic purposes, as being either bipolar or unipolar affective disorders.

The two poles, or extremes, of mood are mania and depression. A bipolar affective disorder is characterized by recurring severe episodes of mood disturbance involving both depressive and manic phases. Between episodes the individual functions well and there is no deterioration in personality. A unipolar affective disorder is one in which the disturbance of mood is only of depression; the depressive illness can either be a single episode or recurrent.

Treatment

Initial treatment of affective disorders primarily concentrates on amelioration of the major presenting symptoms. Associated causative factors, other than any concurrent physical illness, are usually attended to when the acute situation has been brought under control; such causative factors may be of a familial, sociological, or environmental nature.

Depression

The primary treatment for depressive illnesses, especially those of psychotic depth, is the use of antidepressant drugs, details of which are described in Chapter 3. Electroconvulsive therapy is another available treatment, and indications for, and details of, this treatment are provided in Chapter 3 also. Hospitalization is not necessarily the rule in the treatment of depressive illnesses. If possible, the person is treated as an out-patient, the need for hospitalization being dependent upon a number of factors such as the severity of the illness, the ability to comply with medication regimes, available and capable family support, and community support resources. Later, additional treatment may include educational and supportive interviews with close relatives aimed at identifying and addressing factors which may have been significant in the development of the illness. Individual psychotherapy with the person who has suffered the depressive illness can provide the individual with the means to avoid or prevent future depressive illnesses from occurring.

Mania

Hospitalization is usually necessary in cases of mania to protect the individual from causing himself, and others, excessive harm in his work situation, interpersonal relationships, and financial situation. Neuroleptic drugs (see Ch. 3), particularly haloperidol, are indicated to rapidly diminish the symptoms of mania and prevent the person further compromising his physical health and psychosocial functioning.

Maintenance prophylactic medication is frequently indicated when a depressive or manic illness is considered to be an episode of either a bipolar or recurring unipolar affective disorder.

SCHIZOPHRENIC DISORDERS

Definition

The term 'schizophrenia' has been the source of a great deal of misunderstanding both in the health care professions and the population generally, over a long period of time. Many false or misdirected perceptions have been rife regarding origins, presentation, prognosis and treatment, leading to fear, embarrassment and stigmatization in the sufferers, and relatives of individuals with a diagnosis of schizophrenia. The traditional concept of schizophrenia being a single illness phenomenon has been replaced by the idea of a disease entity or group of disorders, the different features of which constitute a syndrome. This has led to the often used, more technically accurate terms, 'schizophrenic disorders', or 'the schizophrenias', although common usage still refers to 'schizophrenia'.

DSM III describes schizophrenia as a group of disorders, the essential features of which are

'. . . the presence of certain psychotic features during the active phase of the illness, characteristic symptoms involving multiple psychological processes, deterioration from a previous level of functioning, onset before age 45, and a duration of at least six months. The disturbance is not due to an Affective Disorder or Organic Mental Disorder. At some phase of the illness Schizophrenia always involves delusions, hallucinations or certain disturbances in the form of thought.'

Schizophrenia is in no way associated with the multiple personalities or split personalities described in novels and depicted in films. There is a change in the sufferer's personality but it takes the form of a fragmentation due to the disturbance and disorganisation in the processes of thinking, perceiving feeling and behaving. In other words, the personality is 'fragmented' or randomly broken up, rather than 'split' into recognisably differing entities.

Epidemiology

The incidence of schizophrenia in the general population is approximately 1%, ranking the illness as occurring as frequently as other more familiar illnesses such as epilepsy and diabetes. Thus, schizophrenia is not a rare condition affecting a very few people. However, like diabetes and epilepsy, schizophrenia varies in intensity and presentation and covers a wide spectrum of behavioural patterns ranging from what may appear as moderate eccentricity to chronic disturbances necessitating hospitalization and involving severe personality deterioration. The disorder occurs in all countries of the world, with little variation in the incidence in differing cultures or socioeconomic groups. The incidence is higher in unskilled and low status workers, the unmarried and those living alone. However, studies suggest that schizophrenics, incapacitated by early symptoms, drift into these sociocultural areas, and are thus seen to be over-represented in these settings (Goldberg & Morrison 1963, Hare 1967).

Aetiology

The comparatively high incidence of schizophrenia, and the traditional resemblance of the illnesses to prototypical images of insanity, have resulted in a great deal of research and speculation regarding causation. To date, the causes are not known, but several factors have been demonstrated to be involved in the development of an illness. It is the interaction of these causative factors which appears to determine the development of an illness in a particular individual. Of the many aetological theories proposed, research has heredity, environment and biochemistry as significant causative or precipitating factors, as described below.

Heredity

Although the exact mode of genetic transmission is still not clear, a definite hereditary component does exist, giving an individual an inherent vulnerability to the development of a schizophrenic disorder. The actual occurrence of an illness in an individual is dependent on many other factors, one of the most important of which appears to be environmental. Many studies, notably those of Kety et al (1973) and Gottesman & Shields (1976), have successfully demonstrated the relationship between hereditary and environmental factors. The results of studies in this area are summarized by Leff (1978).

'The work discussed . . . has suggested that the contribution of genes to the eventual development of 'schizophrenia' is approximately 50%. Whatever the size of the proportion, it is clear that environmental factors play a substantial part in aetiology. Some of them . . . are likely to be somatic in nature. Others are psychological or social.'

The empirical risk of schizophrenia occurring in the relatives of schizophrenics, as a result of genetic transmission, is as follows (Gottesman & Shields 1976):

— In children with one schizophrenic parent — 12%.
— In children with both parents schizophrenic — 25%
— In siblings of a person with schizophrenia — 8–14%.

Environment

Environmental factors associated with the development of schizophrenic disorders involve three areas: family influences, significant life events, and sociocultural factors. Of the many theories on the influences of family members, few have been confirmed by research. Only a small number of general observations can be stated as being useful, following studies based on these theories.

These observations are considered by Hirsch & Leff (1975) to be

1. Sufferers of a schizophrenic disorder are more likely to have psychiatrically disturbed parents.
2. Parents of schizophrenics show more conflict in their thinking and communication than parents of other people.
3. Mothers of schizophrenics may show more over-concern than parents of other children.

One aspect of the influence of family members that has been found to be significant in the relapse rate of schizophrenics is the incidence of 'high expressed emotion' in the sufferer's home. Studies (Brown et al 1972, Vaughan & Leff 1976) have shown that in homes where the sufferer was subjected to hostile criticism by his relatives or where relatives were over-involved in his welfare, both the rate of recurrence of schizophrenic symptoms and the readmission rate to hospital were significantly increased.

Significant stressful events occurring in the lives of schizophrenics influence the time of first onset of a disorder and the occurrence of relapses at later dates (Brown & Birley

1968). The events are not objectively excessively devastating nor necessarily unpleasant, but are perceived as stressful, and do seem to require a sudden change in the individual's daily living pattern. This additional stress exceeds the level of stress with which the individual can cope and subsequently can precipitate symptoms of a schizophrenic disorder in someone predisposed to the development of such an illness.

Biochemistry

As with other disturbances of mental health, a single biochemical cause of schizophrenic disorders has not been found. However, of the many theories postulated, three appear to be most plausible. The first, the 'dopamine hypothesis', suggests that a disturbance of dopamine metabolism in a specific area of the brain may produce the psychotic symptoms of a schizophrenic disorder (Bird et al 1977). The second, the 'toxic metabolite' theory, involves the presence of a substance produced in the brain, the toxic effects of which give rise to psychotic symptoms. The third theory of biochemical causation, which is still the subject of continuing research, relates to the involvement of brain endorphins, prostaglandins and prolactin in the production of psychotic symptoms.

Clinical features

The features of schizophrenic disorders present as disturbances in

- personality
- thinking
- perception
- behaviour.

Personality

The fundamental change in personality is a noticeable degeneration in social functioning, associated with a deterioration in academic or work performance and interpersonal relationships. These disturbances are characterised by an overall withdrawal from everyday activities, a loss of volition and drive, ambivalence, and negativism.

Thinking

Disturbances in thinking are manifested by the way in which the sufferer speaks or writes. Speech may be rambling and circumstantial, using many words and providing much irrelevant information to state an idea. Conversation is often hard to follow as there appears to the listener to be little logical connection between expressed ideas, or the actual flow of speech is suddenly interrupted, then continued on a completely different topic. Other disturbances in the content of thinking include ideas that the person's thoughts are being controlled by some external force, that thoughts are being placed in his mind, or that his thoughts are leaving his mind and travelling to other people's.

Perception

Perceptual disturbances involve delusions and hallucinations. The types of delusions characteristic of schizophrenic disorders are: grandiose, in which sufferers believe they are someone important, or a well-known figure, or have special powers or significance; religious; or persecutory. The belief that information received from radio or television, or from newspapers, magazines or books, specifically relates to them is a delusional idea often held by sufferers of a schizophrenic disorder.

The most commonly reported hallucinations are auditory, in which the sufferer hears, for instance, the voice of a third person continually commenting on his thoughts and actions; or the voice may issue commands which he obeys. Other hallucinations can involve unpleasant smells (olfactory) or the sensation of strange taste (gustatory). Disturbances of perception through the skin give rise to the claim that the person feels he is being bombarded by 'rays' or electricity.

Behaviour

A person with a schizophrenic disorder may demonstrate disturbances in behaviour which are often associated with the nature and intensity of existing thinking and perceptual disturbances. Such behavioural disturbances include repeating peculiar gestures, adopting unnatural postures, grimacing, and exhibiting generally bizarre, unpredictable behaviour.

Prodromal phase

The preceding clinical features are found individually or in various combinations during an acute or active phase of a schizophrenic disorder. Apart from this period of acute symptoms, there may be a prodromal or residual phase (DSM III, p. 189), the symptoms of which are described as

1. Social isolation or withdrawal.
2. Marked impairment in role functioning as wage-earner, student, or home-maker.
3. Markedly peculiar behaviour.
4. Marked impairment in personal hygiene and grooming.
5. Blunted, flat or inappropriate affect.
6. Digressive, vague, overelaborate, circumstantial, or metaphorical speech.
7. Odd or bizarre ideation, or magical thinking.
8. Unusual perceptual experiences.'

The DSM III diagnostic criteria for a schizophrenic disorder require evidence of illness over at least a six-month period in which there has been an obvious deterioration in social functioning, and an active phase in which one or more acute symptoms have been present, with or without a prodromal or residual phase.

Treatment

Treatment of the schizophrenic disorders is, by necessity, multifaceted, concentrating on the various factors which have been established as precipitating or contributing to the development of an illness. Management thus includes the areas of psychopharmacology, social rehabilitation, psychotherapy and family support.

Psychopharmacology

The introduction of the phenothiazine group of drugs was a major advance in the treatment of acute symptoms. Chlopromazine and trifluoperazine, for example, are widely used and particularly effective, in diminishing the intensity and duration of the psychotic symptoms of schizophrenic disorders. More recent development of slow-release, long-acting, intramuscular phenothiazine preparations (fluphenazine decanoate) has almost precluded the need for maintenance on daily multiple doses of oral medications. This slow-release preparation ensures compliance and enables symptoms to be controlled while the person remains in the community, thus avoiding the need for lengthy periods of hospitalization and the inherent problems associated with institutionalism.

Social rehabilitation

The drugs used in the treatment of schizophrenic disorders are undoubtedly effective in diminishing and stabilising the more distressing behavioural and thought disorders. However, they have little direct effect on the progressively disabling deterioration in social functioning. Adequate long-term management and social rehabilitation is, therefore, equally important as pharmacotherapy. Individual rehabilitation programmes aim at retarding the rate of social withdrawal and degeneration in functioning. To achieve this, social support systems are utilized to enhance the ability of the person to cope adequately with everyday living and make the best use of his diminished abilities. The importance of securing a suitable, non-stressful job or other esteem-raising occupation is emphasised, as is resocialisation into group activities and creative leisure pursuits. Suitable accommodation needs to be arranged for the person, often, initially, away from the family. Following an active phase of an illness or discharge from hospital, some form of supervised or sheltered accommodation is often advisable. This may be in the form of a hostel, 'half-way house', day-centre or a shared household with others, supervised by an appropriately skilled person.

Psychotherapy

A further essential component of management is regular contact between the person and a therapist. These sessions provide on-going support for the person at which help and advice are given to assist in coping with problems that confront the individual in every day living. They also serve the purpose of reinforcing the need for compliance with treatment regimes, management programmes and observation of the degree and extent of any symptoms that may be present or emerging. Participation in group therapy sessions is also beneficial in the process of resocialization.

Family support

Relatives of people with a schizophrenic disorder also require help and support from members of the professions involved in the person's management. This assistance is provided by making the relatives aware of the characteristics of the person's illness so that they may more easily understand and cope with the disturbances in behaviour which they may well find distressing and embarrassing. They need to be able to express the feelings evoked by this behaviour and to discuss their own reactions to it. Advice is given on how best to manage situations, help the individual function at his maximum potential, and avoid further deterioration or exacerbation of acute symptoms.

Community-based care

The trend towards avoiding lengthy hospitalization, and encouraging the management of people with schizophrenia in the community has seen the establishment of community psychiatric services, and outreach services, resources, and contacts such as the Richmond Fellowship. The aim of such agencies is to minimize the disruption of the family unit which otherwise occurs when a family member is hospitalized for long periods; they also offer support to both the person with schizophrenia, and his relatives.

Community-based care thus enables large numbers of people with schizophrenia to be managed at relatively low cost in the community. However, for this method of management to be completely successful, extensive community facilities are necessary; unfortunately the extent of such facilities is at present inadequate. The results of community-based care and the practice of community psychiatry has been viewed with scepticism. Hirsch (1976) states that such practices have become

'euphemisms for the undesirable process by which a group of persons are converted from their former status as chronic institutionalised patients to a new equally undesirable status as lonely, single persons, homeless or inadequately housed often residing in flop homes, prisons or the park bench with a high prevalence of unemployment and self-neglect.'

Caring for a schizophrenic person in the community can also have detrimental effects on the health of relatives and cause disturbances in the way of life of the family (Brown et al 1966).

Orthomolecular theories

'Orthomolecular therapy' is a term coined by Pauling (1968) to describe the practice of preserving good health and treating disease by varying the concentration of substances normally present in the body and required for health. A number of psychiatrists, mainly in North America, are utilizing this idea to formulate schizophrenia treatment programmes centred around the use of megadoses of B group vitamins. Two of the leading proponents of orthomolecular psychiatry, Abram Hoffer and Humphrey Osmond, believe schizophrenia is basically a physical illness caused by disturbances in the biochemical balance of the body, and that these are determined by genetic disposition. In their book on the subject (Hoffer & Osmond 1974), an orthomolecular treatment programme is described as incorporating

'. . . all the treatments (for schizophrenia) in use today . . . but as secondary or adjunctive to a proper consideration of nutrient therapy. This means that optimum diets are used combined with supplementation with vitamin B₃ (nicotinic acid and/or nicotinamide), with ascorbic acid, with thiamine, pyridoxine, and other vitamins which may be indicated.

For each patient, once he is well, the non-nutrient chemicals (tranquillizers, etc.) are gradually withdrawn until the patient can remain well on nutrient and dieto-therapy alone.'

The use and efficacy of this mode of practice is still viewed sceptically, and it is not used by the majority of psychiatrists.

Prognosis

Traditionally, schizophrenic disorders have been considered to have a poor prognosis. However, the worst prognosis, in which the person maintains acute symptoms, follows an unremitting social degeneration, and requires frequent, lengthy periods of hospitalization, exists in only approximately 11% of cases. The remaining cases have better outcomes: 35% suffer some residual symptoms but are able to maintain a reasonable level of functioning in the community; the remaining 54%, having recovered from an active phase, apparently experience little or no disturbance to their premorbid personality and return to everyday living without further exacerbation of their original symptoms (Brown et al 1966). Bleuler (1974) considers that over the last century the symptoms of schizophrenia have become less severe, and that a better prognosis is becoming more frequent.

OTHER PSYCHOTIC DISORDERS

Definition

Disorders classified under this heading are the psychotic disturbances which do not meet the criteria of organic, schizophrenic, or affective disorders. DSM III specifies three categories: schizophreniform disorder, brief reactive psychosis, and schizoaffective disorder.

SCHIZOPHRENIFORM DISORDER

Clinical features

The features are identical to those of a schizophrenic disorder, differing only in the duration of the illness. The onset and resolution are generally acute, with a total duration of 'more than two weeks but less than six months' (DSM III). A return to premorbid levels of functioning is more likely than in a schizophrenic disorder.

BRIEF REACTIVE PSYCHOSIS

Clinical features

As stated, in DSM III, 'The essential feature is the sudden onset of a psychotic disorder of at least of few hours but no more than two weeks duration, with eventual return to premorbid level of functioning. The psychotic symptoms appear immediately following a recognizable psychosocial stressor that would evoke significant symptoms of distress in almost anyone. The clinical picture involves significant emotional turmoil and at least one of the following psychotic symptoms:

- incoherence or loosening of associations
- delusions
- hallucinations
- behaviour that is grossly disorganized or catatonic . . .

SCHIZOAFFECTIVE DISORDER

Clinical features

This disorder consists of features of both schizophreniform and affective disorders and is diagnosed when there is difficulty in making a differential diagnosis between these two disorders.

ANXIETY STATES

Definition

Anxiety states are non-psychotic disturbances in which there are combinations of physiological and psychological manifestations of anxiety, not attributable to real danger. The states can be acute in onset, and severe in intensity, or chronic, and fluctuating in severity. The anxiety is usually diffuse, not being attached to any object or situation.

Description

Anxiety is a feeling state experienced by any individual who perceives that he is somehow threatened. The threat can be to the individual's physical integrity or to his ego or emotional state. These threats produce a proportionate degree of disease which exists until the particular threat diminishes or is removed. In pathological states of anxiety there is not usually any obvious threat to the individual; rather there exists a generalized, non-specific feeling state which results in significant disturbances in the individual's daily living. The physiological responses to threat arising from increased autonomic nervous system activity are still present in anxiety states despite the fact that the individual is not in any actual jeopardy.

Aetiology

The factors responsible for the development of anxiety are detailed in Chapter 7.

Clinical features

Anxiety states may be either infrequent, episodic attacks, or a chronic recurring, almost continuous state. In either case, the prevailing feeling is one of inner tension, intense foreboding and fear of impending doom which can reach the stage of panic or overwhelming terror.

The person worries continuously, ruminates over actual or potential problems and has an unremitting fear of something bad happening to him or to a relative. He may, for instance, fear he is going to have some form of heart attack, faint, or otherwise suddenly become seriously ill, and become preoccupied with these thoughts to the exclusion of usual concerns of daily living. Associated with these thoughts are somatic symptoms originating from autonomic nervous system activity and exaggerated and perpetuated by the state of anxiety. Characteristic somatic symptoms include palpitations due to increased heart rate, a tightness across the chest, and pericardial pains, hyperventilation, epigastric discomfort, diarrhoea, sweating, dry mouth, frequency of micturition, muscle tension, pallor, tremor and headache. The headaches are frequently described as 'tight bands' around the head, or 'queer sensations' in the head and lead to the person expressing fears of going insane. A continual state of arousal and muscle tension produces fatigue, an inability to relax, and decreased ability to concentrate on any task. Irritability, depressive feelings, anorexia and insomnia are also characteristic features of anxiety states. Where hyperventilation is a predominant feature of the anxiety, respiratory alkalosis occurs resulting in tingling and parasthesia in the extremities, dizziness and muscle spasms involving the face, limbs, and respiratory and abdominal muscles.

Classification

Apart from the generalized anxiety disorder described above, there are also more specific disturbances classified as anxiety states; these include panic disorders, phobic disorders, obsessive compulsive disorders, and post-traumatic stress disorders (DSM III).

Panic disorder

This is a disorder characterized by recurrent, sudden, severe anxiety attacks in which the physiological and psychological feelings of anxiety are intense. Particularly prominent symptoms are palpitations, chest pain, choking, dizziness, trembling, feelings of unreality, and a fear of dying or losing control.

Phobic disorder

In a generalized anxiety disorder, the anxiety is usually diffuse, not arising from any particular situation. When symptoms of anxiety or a panic attack occur in association with a particular object or situation, the disturbance is referred to as a 'phobia' or 'phobic disorder'. The persistent and irrational fear of a specific object or situation produces a panic attack. The person therefore adopts a pattern of behaviour which prevents this situation from occurring.

Phobic symptoms are a common source of psychic distress, occurring in approximately 20% of all people with disturbances of mental health (Marks 1969), and present as symptoms of a primary illness, such as depression. When the phobia is the predominent feature and the major cause of distress, the resultant illness is a phobic disorder. Phobic disorders comprise approximately 3% of all disorders occurring in psychiatric out-patients (Marks 1973).

The three more commonly occurring phobic disorders are agoraphobia, social phobia, and simple phobia.

Agoraphobia. Originating from the Greek 'agora' meaning the market place or place of assembly, agoraphobia in its narrowest sense means a fear of open spaces. This fear is experienced in everyday life in such situations as shopping, using public transport and crowds. DSM III defines agoraphobia as a disorder in which

A. The individual has marked fear of and thus avoids being alone or in public places from which escape might be difficult or help not available in case of sudden incapacitation.
B. There is increasing constriction of normal activities until the fears or avoidance behaviour dominate the individual's life.'

Agoraphobia is the most common and most handicapping phobic disorder, the majority of people being intensely frightened of leaving their own home, using public transport or going shopping. The consequent social isolation from being house-bound can be severe and handicapping, and may lead to the development of further illnesses such as depression, alcohol and other substance abuse, and generalized anxiety.

A major life event, such as marriage, serious family illness, bereavement, often leads to the development of agoraphobia, as can a significant organic brain trauma, e.g. encephalitis, neurosurgery, or tumour (Marks 1969).

Social phobia. DSM III defines social phobia as

'a persistent, irrational fear of, and compelling desire to avoid, situations in which the individual may be exposed to scrutiny by others. There is also fear that the individual may behave in a manner that will be humiliating or embarrassing.'

The behaviours and situations typically include eating, drinking, speaking and writing in the presence of other people; the consequent avoidance behaviour leads to diminished or completely absent social contact and a reclusive life-style.

Simple phobia. This is said to be present when the phobic situation is other than agoraphobia or social phobia; the fear is attached most commonly to animals or situations such as heights, darkness, closed spaces, air travel, or underground trains, although a great range of other situations may generate individual phobias.

Obsessive compulsive disorders

Obsessions are recurrent, persistent, distressing thoughts, images or impulses which produce anxiety in the individual.

Compulsions are behaviour patterns arising from action in response to obsessions. The behaviours may be performed according to rules or in a repetitive, stereotyped fashion, e.g. checking, counting, hand-washing. The anxiety arising from the obsessional ideas is dissipated by the associated compulsive behaviour.

Post-traumatic stress disorder

This type of anxiety state is characterized by the development of anxiety symptoms following a psychologically traumatic event. The magnitude of the event is generally outside the range of usual human experience and the effect particularly psychologically disturbing. The event is re-experienced from time to time with the resultant psychological and physiological disturbances of a severe anxiety state.

Examples of events which act as stressors in producing the above response include: natural disasters — bush fires, floods, cyclones, train crashes, ship-wrecking, multiple car crashes, bus crashes; and deliberately perpetrated acts — war, bombing, internment in prisoner of war camps, torture, rape.

Treatment

Generalized anxiety

Acute attacks of anxiety are managed with a benzodiazepine anxiolytic drug such as diazepam, oxazepam or alprazolam (see Ch. 3); the somatic symptoms are relieved also by beta- adrenergic blocking drugs such as propranolol. However, the prescription of anxiolytic medication is only a short-term measure. It is necessary to investigate the underlying causes of the person's anxiety and to assist the individual to realize the association between the symptoms and the precipitating factors. When the acute symptoms are under control, other therapeutic measures such as psychotherapy, relaxation, or meditation can be employed. Behaviour therapy may be of assistance to a minority of people, particularly the techniques of flooding, coupled with coping and anxiety-management training (Marks 1969).

Phobic disorders

Behavioural techniques, particularly desensitization — exposing the person progressively to the feared object or situation until he tolerates it and eventually overcomes his avoidance/fear response — are effective in the treatment of phobias. The concurrent use of benzodiazepine anxiolytic drugs diminishes the intensity of the symptoms of anxiety and allows the person to be amenable to treatment. Other pharmacological agents which are useful in specific situations are antidepressants: imipramine reduces the extent of panic attacks in agoraphobia (Klein 1964), and phenelzine has been found to be particularly effective in relieving agoraphobia (Tyner et al 1973).

Further more detailed description of the management of anxiety is found in Chapter 7.

PERSONALITY DISORDERS

Definition

Every individual's personality is composed of many traits formed into a combination of unique characteristics and behaviours acquired during development. The possible characteristics of a particular personality are as many and varied as the influences to which an individual is subject during the developmental process. These characteristics determine how a person behaves and how others react to him. If, during this process, personality traits are developed which are inflexible and maladaptive, a significant impairment in the individual's social or occupational functioning results, or the traits cause subjective distress. In this situation, the individual can be described as having a personality disorder.

The World Health Organization (WHO 1971) defines personality disorders as

> 'deeply ingrained maladaptive patterns of behaviour generally recognisable by the time of adolescence or earlier and continuing throughout most of adult life although often becoming less obvious in middle or old age. The personality is abnormal either in the balance of its components, their quality and expression or in its total aspect. Because of this deviation or psychopathy the patient suffers or others have to suffer and there is an adverse effect upon the individual or on society.'

A number of people suffer a change in personality which manifests as a personality disorder in someone who previously had undisturbed personality functioning. Such personality disorders are associated with brain dysfunction through trauma or neurological disease. Any disease affecting the central nervous system has the potential to cause personality disturbances, e.g. encephalitis, alcoholism, epilepsy, Alzheimer's disease, arteriosclerotic dementia, thyrotoxicosis, or multiple sclerosis.

Some of the forms of personality disorder described in DSM III include: paranoid, schizoid, histrionic, narcissistic, antisocial, borderline, avoidant, dependent, passive-aggressive. Following is a brief outline of the main characteristic features of each, extracted from the diagnositc criteria described in DSM III.

Paranoid personality disorder

A disorder which is characterized by a pervasive and unreasonable suspiciousness of other people's actions and motives, a heightened sensibility to others, and a cold, humourless affect lacking any sentimental feelings.

Schizoid personality disorder

A disorder characterized by a marked degree of aloofness, shyness and reserve. The individual is notably introspective and often socially phobic (DSM III).

'. . . there is a defect in the capacity to form social relationships, evidenced by the absence of warm, tender feelings for others and indifference to praise, criticism, and the feelings of others.'

Histrionic personality disorder

Features of this disorder are (DSM III)

'. . . overly dramatic, reactive, and intensely expressed behaviour and characteristic disturbances in interpersonal relationships. . . . Minor stimuli give rise to emotional excitability, such as irrational, angry outbursts or tantrums . . . [People with this disorder] are often quick to form friendships, but once a relationship is established they can become demanding, egocentric, and inconsiderate; manipulative suicidal threats, gestures, or attempts may be made; there may be a constant demand for reassurance because of feelings of helplessness and dependency.'

Narcissistic personality disorder

The characteristic features of this disorder are (DSM III)

'a grandiose sense of self-importance or uniqueness; preoccupation with fantasies of unlimited success; exhibitionistic need for constant attention and admiration; characteristic responses to threats to self-esteem; and characteristic disturbances in interpersonal relationships, such as feelings of entitlement, interpersonal exploitativeness, relationships that alternate between the extremes of overidealization and devaluation, and, lack of empathy.'

Antisocial personality disorder

This disorder is characterized by (DSM III)

'a history of continuous and chronic antisocial behaviour in which the rights of others are violated, persistence into adult life of a pattern of antisocial behaviour that began before the age of 15, and failure to sustain good job performance over a period of several years . . . Lying, stealing, fighting, truancy, and resisting authority are typical early childhood signs. In adolescence, unusually early or aggresive sexual behaviour, excessive drinking, and use of illicit drugs are frequent. In adulthood, these kinds of behaviour continue, with the addition of inability to sustain consistent work performance or to function as a responsible parent and failure to accept social norms with respect to lawful behaviour.'

Borderline personality disorder

A disorder in which (DSM III)

'there is instability in a variety of areas, including interpersonal behaviour, mood, and self-image. . . . Frequently there is impulsive and unpredictable behaviour that is potentially physically self-damaging. Mood is often unstable, with marked shifts from a normal mood to a dysphoric mood or with inappropriate, intense anger or lack of control of anger . . . There may be problems tolerating being alone, and chronic feelings of emptiness or boredom.'

Avoidant personality disorder

The characteristic features of this disorder are (DSM III)

'hypersensitivity to potential rejection, humiliation, or shame; an unwillingness to enter into relationships unless given unusually strong guarantees of uncritical acceptance; social withdrawal in spite of a desire for affection and acceptance; and low self-esteem.'

Dependent personality disorder

Characteristically, in dependent personality disorders (DSM III)

'the individual passively allows others to assume responsibility for major areas of his or her life because of a lack of self-confidence and an inability to function independently; the individual subordinates his or her needs to those of others on whom he or she is dependent in order to avoid any possibility of having to be self-reliant.'

Passive-aggressive personality disorder

In a passive-aggressive personality disorder (DSM III),

'there is resistance to demands for adequate performance in both occupational and social functioning; the resistance is expressed indirectly rather than directly. The consequence is pervasive and persistent social or occupational ineffectiveness, even when more self-assertive and effective behaviour is possible. The name of this disorder is based on the assumption that such individuals are passively expressing covert aggression.'

It can be seen from these descriptions that personality disorders are exaggerated traits that may be present in the personalities of a large proportion of any population. Moreover, any one personality may be composed of a number of these different traits. Similarly, an individual described as having a personality disorder can have features of a number of disorders present at one time. A significant point to consider when describing personality disorders is that predominant personality traits constitute a disorder only when the traits are 'inflexible and maladaptive and cause significant impairment in social or occupational functioning or subjective distress' (DSM III). The presence in an individual of a particular trait that other people find distasteful, unacceptable or intolerable does not necessarily warrant the diagnosis of a personality disorder.

Treatment

'Treatment' of personality disorders is notoriously difficult, and depends fundamentally on the person recognising he is 'sick' and adopting a sick role. He must realise that little can be done *to* him; he needs to be prepared to do things for himself, with the assistance of others, over a lengthy period of time. This assistance consists of two overlapping therapeutic techniques: psychotherapy, and behaviour therapy or social skills training (Argyle et al 1974). Psychotherapy examines the feeling and thinking aspects of the individual's personality formation, the process by which he perceives his environment; behaviour therapy aims at altering the way in which the individual behaves in response to his environment.

SOMATOFORM DISORDERS

This category of illnesses is included due to the probability of the presence in general medical and surgical wards of people with somatoform disorders.

Definition

Somatoform disorders are characterized by the presence of (DSM III)

'. . . physical symptoms suggesting physical disorder for which there are no demonstrable organic findings or known physiological mechanisms and for which there is positive evidence, or a strong presumption, that the symptoms are linked to psychological factors or conflicts.'

Disorders in this category include somatization disorders, psychogenic pain disorder, hypochondriasis and the relatively uncommon conversion disorder. Somatization disorders and psychogenic pain disorders are often the reason for consultations to liaison psychiatrists from physicians and surgeons, and are consequently described here.

SOMATIZATION DISORDER

Previously referred to as Briquet's syndrome, this disorder has the features of (DSM III)

'recurrent and multiple somatic complaints of several years' duration for which medical attention has been sought, but which are apparently not due to any physical disorder. The disorder begins before the age of 30 and has a chronic but fluctuating course. Complaints are often presented in a dramatic, vague, or exaggerated way, or are part of a complicated medical history in which many physical diagnoses have been considered . . . complaints invariably involve the following organ systems or types of symptoms: conversion or psuedoneurological, gastrointestinal, female reproductive, phychosexual, pain, and cardiopulmonary.'

The disorder rarely occurs in males but is prevalent in approximately 1–20% of females (Woodruff et al 1971).

PSYCHOGENIC PAIN DISORDER

DSM III describes a disorder

'in which the predominant feature is the complaint of pain, in the absence of adequate physical findings and in association with evidence of the aetiological role of psychological factors . . . The pain symptom either is inconsistent with the anatomic distribution of the nervous system or, if it mimics a known disease entity, cannot be adequately accounted for by organic pathology, after extensive diagnostic evaluation.'

The person with pain seeks treatment from many medical practitioners, often requesting, and receiving, surgical intervention, and subsequently adopts the role of an invalid. The pain experienced may allow the person to avoid situations or activities that are unpleasant to him, or gain him attention and support that otherwise would not be forthcoming.

SUBSTANCE-USE DISORDERS

The more common disorders occurring in this category are considered in detail in individual chapters of Part II. The category is noted here due to the prevalance and acceptance of the

use of many substances by individuals of most populations, and the consequent occurrence of associated disorders found among people in hospital, or presenting with illness. Most cultures use substances of various types to alter mood or change behaviour at one time or another. In our society these substances include caffeine in coffee, nicotine in cigarettes, alcohol, and other drugs both prescribed and illicit.

Definition

The category of substance-use disorders (DSM III, p. 163)

'deals with behavioural changes associated with more or less regular use of substances that affect the central nervous system. . . . Examples of such behavioural changes include impairment in social or occupational functioning as a consequence of substance use, inability to control use of or stop taking the substance, and the development of serious withdrawal symptoms after cessation of or reduction in substance use.'

REFERENCES

American Psychiatric Association 1980 Diagnosis and statistical manual of mental disorders, 3rd edn. American Psychiatric Association, Washington DC

Argyle M, Trower P, Bryant B 1974 Explorations in the treatment of personality disorders and neuroses by social skills training. British Journal of Medical Psychology 47: 63–72

Bird E D, Spokes E G, Barnes J, Mackay A V P, Iversen L, Shepherd M 1977 Increased dopamine and reduced glutamic acid decarboxylase and choline acetyl tranferase activity in schizophrenia. Lancet 2: 1157–1158

Bleuler M 1974 The long-term course of the schizophrenic psychoses. PsychologicaL Medicine 4: 244–254

Brown G W, Bone M, Dalinson B M, Wing J K 1966 Schizophrenia and social care. Maudsley Mongraph No. 17. Oxford University Press, Oxford

Brown G W, Birley J L T, Wing J K 1972 Influence of family life on the source of schizophrenic disorders: a replication. British Journal of Psychiatry 121: 241–258

Burnett F M 1981 A possible role of zinc in the pathology of dementia. Lancet 186–188

Campbell R 1981 Psychiatric dictionary, 5th edn. Oxford University Press, New York

Goldberg E M, Morrison S L 1963 Schizophrenia and social class. British Journal of Psychiatry 109:785

Gottesman I I, Shields J 1976 Critical review of recent adoption, twin and family studies. Schizophrenia Bulletin 2: 360–400

Hare E H 1967 The epidemiology of schizophrenia. In: Coppen A, Walk A (eds) Developments in schizophrenia. Headley Brothers, Ashford, Kent

Hirsch S R 1976 Interacting social and biological factors determining prognosis in the rehabilitation and management of persons with schizophrenia. In: Cancro R (ed) Annual review of the schizophrenic syndrome. Brunner/Mazel, New York

Hirsch S R, Leff J P 1975 Abnormalities in the parents of schizophrenics. Maudsley Monograph No. 22. Oxford University Press, Oxford

Hoffer A, Osmand H 1974 How to live with schizophrenia. Citadel Press, Secaucus, New Jersey

Holding T A, Kay D W K 1984 Psychiatry vol 1: General aspects. University of Tasmania, Hobart

Kety S S, Rosenthal D, Wender P H 1973 Mental illness in the biological and adoptive families of adopted individuals who have become schizophrenic. Proceedings of the American Psychopathology Association 63: 147–165

Klein D F 1964 Delineation of two drug responsive anxiety syndromes. Psychopharmacologia 5: 397–408

Klerman G L 1971 Clinical research in depression. American Journal of Psychiatry

Kreigh H, Perko J, 1979 Psychiatric and mental health nursing; commitment to care and concern. Reston Publishing Company, Virginia

Leff J P 1978 Social and psychological causes of the acute attack. In: Wing J K (ed) Schizophrenia: towards a new synthesis. Academic Press, London

Linn L 1975 Diagnosis and psychiatry: symptoms of psychiatric disorders. In: Freeman A, Kaplan M, Sadock B (eds) Comprehensive textbook of psychiatry, 2nd edn. Williams & Wilkins, Baltimore

Marks I M 1969 Fears and phobias. Heinemann, London

Pauling L 1968 Orthomolecular psychiatry. Science 160: 265–271

Price T 1968 The genetics of depressive behaviour. In: Coppen A, Walk A (eds) Recent developments in affective disorders. Headley Brothers, Ashford, Kent,

Szasz T 1970 The manufacture of madness. Paladin, London

Tyner P, Candy J, Kelly D 1973 Phenelzine in phobic anxiety: a controlled trial. Psychological Medicine 3: 120–124

Vaughn C E, Leff J P 1976 The influence of family and social factors on the course of psychiatric illness. British Journal of Psychiatry 129: 125–137

WHO 1971 Draft glossary of psychiatric disorders. World Health Organization, Geneva

Woodruff R A, Clayton P J, Guje S B 1971 Hysteria: studies of diagnosis, outcome and prevalence. Journal of American Medical Association 215: 425–428

3

Somatic therapies

The day-to-day management of ill people in any setting will, at times, involve nurses in the physical modalities of treatment utilised for alleviation of symptoms associated with mental ill-health. These physical, or somatic methods of treatment include psychopharmacology, electroconvulsive therapy, and, on rare occasions, psychosurgery. Although the latter two are specific treatments generally practised in specialist health care facilities, psychopharmacology is widely practised. It is a diverse method of treatment, encompassing a large number of drugs prescribed in many different disturbances of mental health. Consequently, nurses will find themselves almost continually in contact with drugs of this category and should be familiar with their uses, actions, desired and adverse effects, and the implication for nurses of the use of these drugs by people for whom they are responsible.

This chapter describes the characteristics, relevant to nurses, of the medications used in psychiatry, electroconvulsive therapy, and psychosurgery; it also mentions the commonly used and most recently developed diagnostic procedures and tests. Emphasis is placed on the pharmacological management of mental ill-health, particularly in relation to the nursing implications of the use of psychotropic medications.

PSYCHOTROPIC MEDICATIONS

The term 'psychotropic' is defined in Dorland's medical dictionary (1965) as 'exerting an effect upon the mind; capable of modifying mental activity.' Psychotropic medications comprise the majority of drugs used in psychiatry.

The approach to management of mental illness underwent a major change with the introduction of psychotropic drugs in the 1950s. Fewer people required incarceration in large institutions and a greater number were able to be treated on a day, out-patient or community basis, with less disruption and distress to the lives of the person and his family. Prior to the introduction of the first of the phenothiazine group of drugs in 1952, the numbers of residents in large mental hospitals had risen steadily and two out of three people admitted with a diagnosis of schizophrenia were still hospitalized after two years (Dally & Connolly 1981).

The three intervening decades have seen the closure of large institutions throughout the western world and a movement towards community-based services. Few radically different drugs have emerged since the 1960s, but knowledge of the actions of these drugs on the body and their interactions with other drugs, and the diminution of undesirable effects, as well as skill in prescribing the appropriate medication at therapeutic dosages for the requisite length of time, has vastly improved their efficacy.

The drugs included in this section constitute examples of the main groups of medications used in the management of the more common disorders of mental health (see Fig. 3.1). Non-psychiatric indications of many of these drugs are also mentioned.

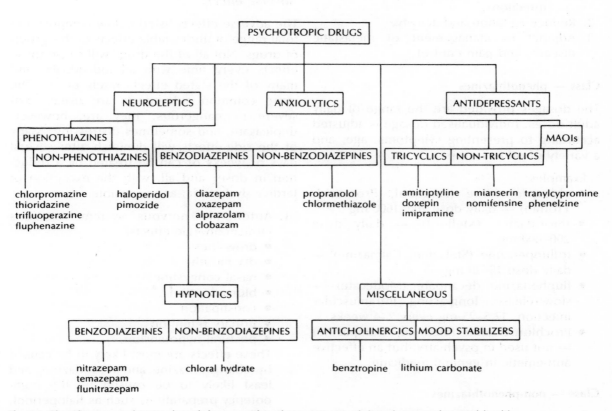

Fig. 3.1 Classification and examples of drugs used in the treatment of disturbances of mental health.

GROUP — ANTIPSYCHOTICS/NEUROLEPTICS

The term 'neuroleptic' is often used to describe drugs in this group, and is defined by Delay, the French discoverer of chlorpromazine, as having the following characteristics: inhibiting psychomotor agitation without inducing sleep; alleviating psychotic manifestations, e.g. delusions, hallucinations, mania, paranoia; and producing extrapyramidal signs with increasing dosage.

Uses

1. Diminish the intensity and duration of the manifestations of psychotic illnesses including
   (i) manic states
   (ii) schizophrenic disorders
   (iii) arteriosclerotic and organic psychoses
   (iv) states of delirium resulting from effects of alcohol and other drugs, or infections.
2. Reduce agitation and activity.
3. Adjunct to management of metastatic disease, and pain control.

Class — phenothiazines

The dosages provided are the range of daily adult doses. Individualised dosage is adjusted according to presenting symptoms, age, and a variety of other factors.

Examples:
- chlorpromazine (Largactil, Promacid, Protran) — daily dose 200–1600 mg
- thioridazine (Melleril) — daily dose 200–800 mg
- trifluoperazine (Stelazine, Calmazine) — daily dose 15–20 mg
- fluphenazine decanoate (Modecate) — slow-release, long-acting intramuscular injection, 12.5–25 mg every 2–4 weeks
- Prochlorperazine (Stemetil, Compazine) — not used in psychiatry, but an effective anti-emetic in general medicine.

Class — non-phenothiazines

Examples:

- haloperidol (Serenace, Pacedol) — daily dose 4–100 mg
- droperidol (Droleptan) — more frequently used for non-psychiatric indications
- pimozide (Orap) — daily dose 2–12 mg
- thiothixene (Navane) — daily dose 5–30 mg

Mode of action

All the antipsychotics share the same basic mode of action: blocking dopaminergic receptors, causing a decrease in dopaminergic transmission within the brain. They all have a central nervous system depressing effect.

Although similar in their action, these drugs have individual characteristics rendering some more suitable than others when a specific effect is desired or a specific adverse effect is to be avoided.

Adverse effects

The adverse effects listed below compose the total range of undesirable effects of this group of drugs. Not all of the drugs will cause these effects every time with all individuals, and many of the stated effects rarely occur. The more common side-effects are usually not severe or dangerous; they are, however, unpleasant, and sometimes distressing. Many of the side-effects will diminish after several days or weeks or can be treated by a reduction in dose; and all, with the exception of tardive dyskinesia, are reversible.

1. Autonomic nervous system reactions (anticholinergic effects)
   - drowsiness
   - dry mouth
   - nasal congestion
   - blurred vision
   - constipation
   - urinary retention
   - postural hypotension.

   These effects are most likely to be caused by chlorpromazine and thioridazine, and least likely to be caused by the high-potency preparations such as haloperidol, trifluoperazine and fluphenazine.

2. Extrapyramidal side-effects (undesirable effects on pyramidal fibres or upper motor neurones responsible for automatic movement and postural adjustment)
   (i) Parkinson-like signs
      • tremor
      • salivation
      • muscular rigidity
      • ataxia
      • shuffling gait
      • mask-like expression
   (ii) Akathesia (motor restlessness)
   (iii) Dystonic reactions
      • spasms of oropharyngeal muscles
      • spasms of limbs
      • torticollis (spasm of cervical muscles, with torsion of the neck)
      • oculogyric crisis (exaggerated, involuntary, superior movement of the eyeballs).

Parkinsonism and akathesia are the most common reactions, and the dystonic reactions are the most frightening. The high-potency neuroleptics, haloperidol, trifluoperazine, and fluphenazinne, are more likely to cause these effects. Dystonic reactions are particularly prevalent in younger individuals (Dally & Connolly 1981).

3. Endocrine changes
   • galactorrhoea
   • amenorrhoea
   • gynaecomastia
   • lactation
   • weight gain.
4. Allergic reactions
   • pruritic maculopapular rash
   • jaundice.
5. Blood dyscrasias
   • agranulocytosis
   • eosinophilia
   • thrombocytopenia
   • aplastic anaemia.
6. Cardiovascular changes
   • ECG changes such as abnormal T waves
   • ventricular tachycardia.
   These effects are particularly characteristic with use of thioridazine; drugs with low anticholinergic effects, e.g. haloperidol,

are indicated where cardiac disease is present.
7. Photosensitivity
   • extreme sensitivity of the skin to sunlight, most common with chlorpromazine.
8. Lowered seizure threshold.
9. Pigmentary retinopathy
   • major effect of thioridazine if given in doses exceeding 800 mg per day.
10. Tardive dyskinesia
   • disturbed co-ordination and motor activity, particularly of the mouth, tongue, and face, following prolonged treatment with neuroleptic drugs. The condition is irreversible and, unlike other side-effects, may become worse when the medication is ceased.

This is a comprehensive list of undesirable side-effects which could depict the neuroleptic drugs as an awesome group which appear as disturbing to people as some cytotoxic medications. In fact, serious side-effects are rare when drugs are appropriately prescribed, and less serious but distressing symptoms can be alleviated by appropriate choice of drugs. For instance, extrapyramidal effects tend to occur more frequently with haloperidol, fluphenazine, and trifluoperazine; sedation, anticholinergic effects, hypotension, allergic reactions, and seizures are more frequent with chlorpromazine and thioridazine.

Drug interactions

The neuroleptic group of drugs potentiate the effect of all other central nervous system depressants: alterations may have to be made to the doses of hypnotics, analgesics, antihistamines, barbiturates, and anaesthetics when such drugs are used concurrently with neuroleptics; alcohol should be taken with caution. These drugs also potentiate the effect of atropine and can cause a paradoxical effect of adrenaline resulting in a profound lowering of blood pressure.

The anti-emetic effect of the phenothiazine

class in particular may mask any toxic effect of other drugs, or obscure signs of an underlying organic disorder.

Interference with the treatment of Parkinson's disease with levadopa derivatives will occur due to the inhibitory effect of neuroleptics on the anti-Parkinson drugs.

Adjustment of anticonvulsant drugs will be necessitated by the neuroleptic effect of lowered seizure threshold.

Concurrent use of thiazide diuretics can produce severe hypotension. Neuroleptics can raise the plasma levels of antidepressant drugs leading to severe anticholinergic side-effects.

Heavy smokers often require larger doses of neuroleptics than do non-smokers.

Nursing implications

Over-sedation

Persons usually feel drowsy when they begin to take antipsychotic medication. This effect tends to diminish after the medication has been taken for 7–14 days. If the patient is very disturbed by the drowsiness, the nurse should notify the doctor, who may alter the dose schedule; otherwise, encouraging the person to become active early in the day will help overcome the drowsiness. Explain the side-effect to the person, and emphasize the fact that it will decrease with time.

Autonomic effects

Occurring more frequently with chlorpromazine and thioridazine, these effects are uncomfortable but not dangerous; the exception is postural hypotension, which occurs with particular frequency in the elderly, necessitating caution in cases where a sudden and marked lowering of blood pressure could have serious repercussions. The hypotension usually occurs shortly after initiating treatment and disappears 7–10 days after stabilization of dose. People should be advised to rise from sitting position slowly and instructed to report sensations of dizziness or light-headedness.

The effect is most pronounced upon first waking, thus the nurse should exhibit caution when assisting individuals out of bed. The person's blood pressure should be checked while lying and standing and a drop of more than 30 mgHg considered significant. The hypotensive effect is exaggerated by heat, therefore care should be taken when people get up and take a hot shower or stand up after having a bath.

Of the other autonomic effects, dry mucous membranes can be relieved by sucking glycerine-based cough drops or by the application of proprietory saliva-producing preparations; attention to mouth toilet to ensure adequate oral hygiene may also be necessary. Interventions should be initiated to prevent constipation, and appropriate management undertaken if it occurs. Encourage the person to report sensations of urinary hesitancy, as this can be indicative of the development of urinary retention.

Extrapyramidal side-effects

Haloperidol, fluphenazine, and trifluoperazine are more likely to cause this type of reaction in 10–15% of people receiving high doses; but it is spontaneously reversible on withdrawal of the drug. The Parkinsonian-like syndrome can be treated with drugs such as benztropine. Observe for signs of motor restlessness, muscular twitching, rigidity, tongue-rolling, chewing movements, drooling, weakness, and fatigue, as these indicate the onset of more distressing side-effects. Explain to the person these are effects of the medication and will be readily alleviated. It should be remembered that prochloperazine, although primarily an anti-emetic, is a neuroleptic drug of the phenothiazine group and is capable of producing extrapyramidal side-effects when routinely prescribed to control nausea and vomiting.

Endocrine effects

These occur due to decreased gonadotrophin liberation and may include lactation, menstrual irregularities, and decreased libido in women, and gynaecomastia, failure in ejaculation, and impotence in men. Individuals may be concerned and embarrassed by these problems. The nurse can be supportive by providing explanation and reassurance as to the temporary nature of the condition; symptoms disappear following cessation of drug administration.

Blood dyscrasias

These are rare but serious and take the form of leukopenia with the presence of an aganulocytosis. Chlorpromazine depresses the production of leukocytes, producing agranulocytosis in 1 in 5000–10 000 people. Nurses should look out for initial symptoms of sore throat, high fever, and lesions in the mouth — indications that the drug should be ceased immediately. These will occur in the first 8 weeks of treatment and necessitate a full blood examination; leukopenia will confirm the diagnosis. Other blood dyscrasias that can arise include thrombocytopenia, aplastic anaemia, and pancytopenia.

Allergic reactions

Rashes occur occasionally with antipsychotic medications — especially those of low potency. The resultant pruritic maculopapular rash usually appears on the face, neck, and chest 2–10 weeks after commencement of drug administration. Contact dermatitis can occur in those handling liquid concentrates of chlorpromazine.

Cholestatic jaundice is a rare and dangerous side-effect of chlorpromazine, evidenced by malaise, fever, nausea, and abdominal pain, followed shortly by jaundice and itching.

Photosensitivity

Chlorpromazine, in particular, is associated with this effect which causes patients to have an extreme sensitivity of the skin to sunlight. Nurses should warn individuals against exposure to direct sunlight, as even brief exposure can cause sunburn; they can also be educated in the use of appropriate clothing and protective sun barrier creams.

Hypothermia

Neuroleptic drugs affect the thermoregulatory centre in the hypothalamus. This results in body temperature variations, particularly noticeable in the evening, and characterized by the person complaining of feeling cold. This sensation of lowered body temperature can result in complications if the person overdresses in relation to the external environmental temperature. Wearing layers of warm clothing outside on a hot day could precipitate hyperthermia and heat stroke. This effect is further exaggerated if, due to the presence of extrapyramidal side-effects, the person is taking an anti-Parkinson drug such as benztropine, which has the effect of causing a cessation of the body's ability to cool itself by perspiring.

Medication compliance

Another problem related to the nursing management of people taking these drugs is that of non-compliance. Individuals and their families often have a variety of misconceptions and fears about antipsychotic drugs, resulting in a reluctance to comply with prescribed medication regimes. Some of the misconceptions are: that it is wrong or unnatural to take drugs that alter mental activity; people are also overheard discussing their dosages, believing that the higher the dose the 'crazier' they are. The sedative effect of the antipsychotic drugs is the same on mentally healthy individuals as it is for those with psychotic symptoms, and the dosage prescribed is dependent upon many variables apart from the severity of symptoms. The nurse needs to explain to people their medication regime and to encourage them to continue to take their medication regularly. Suspicious individuals may attempt to conceal their medications in hospital or not take them when at home; others may cease taking medication because they are feeling better. In both cases relapse of symptoms frequently occurs.

General medicine

The phenothiazine group of drugs will be encountered in areas of nursing not directly related to problems associated with overt disturbances of mental health. The hypothermic and anti-emetic properties were utilized, at one time, in surgical procedures; and as potentiators of narcotic analgesics and anti-emetics, this group has a place in the long-term management of pain relief. Chlorpromazine is often the drug of choice in these situations. Droperidol is indicated to produce tranquillization, and to reduce nausea and vomiting in surgical and diagnostic procedures; it also has a use in premedication, induction and as an adjunct in the maintenance of general and regional anaesthesia. Haloperidol has been used for the control of intractable hiccoughs; and chlorpromazine for the care of agitated elderly individuals, and in eclampsia and pre-eclampsia.

Other effects of this group of drugs that people find annoying include stimulation of appetite, weight gain, and oedema; however, the appetite-stimulant and weight-gaining effects are used to advantage in the treatment of anorexia nervosa where a severe loss in weight has occurred.

None of the neuroleptic drugs is addictive, and people will not develop a physical dependence on their medication, nor develop a marked tolerance to their antipsychotic effects. However, individuals often show considerable accommodation to many of their side-effects (Baldessarini 1980).

Neuroleptic drugs should not be ceased abruptly, a tapering off period being necessary. Sudden cessation of chlorpromazine or thioridazine administration may cause symptoms of nausea, vomiting and diarrhoea, and withdrawal dyskinesias may result following cessation of high-potency drugs (Appleton & Davis 1980).

Summary of nursing responsibilities

1. Observe and report any physical, emotional, or behavioural reactions of people on these medications.
2. Observe recipients' behaviour for signs of both desired effects — calmer, more in control of behaviour, more easily directed — and undesirable effects — increased anxiety, agitation, depression.
3. Watch for signs of motor restlessness, muscular twitching, rigidity, tongue-rolling, lip-smacking, chewing movements, grimacing, drooling, weakness, fatigue, drowsiness.
4. Observe person for skin changes: jaundice, dermatitis, flushing, perspiration, sunburn.
5. Ensure person lies down during and after administration of high dosage intramuscular injection.
6. Withhold medication, have person lie down, and report if blood pressure is unusually low.
7. Protect person from injury such as falling, hazardous activities, or deliberate self-harm.

Class — Mood stabilizing drugs

Example:
- lithium carbonate (Lithicarb, Camcolit, Carbolith, Priadel)

Although classified as an antipsychotic drug, lithium carbonate is not chemically related, nor does it have any of the properties or mode of action of other neuroleptic preparations.

Uses

1. Stabilization of mood in affective disorders (see Ch. 2) as both treatment and prophylaxis
   - reduces the degree and extent of manic episodes
   - modifies the depressive phase of mood cycle
   - prolongs symptom-free intervals in

recurrent bipolar and unipolar affective disorders
- may, in some cases, eliminate cycle of manic and depressive episodes.

2. Occasionally useful in disorders associated with periodicity and disturbance of mood including
   - premenstrual tension
   - alcoholism associated with depression
   - repetitious aggressive outbursts.

Mode of action

The exact mode of action is unknown, but as a naturally occurring element it closely resembles sodium and potassium and acts on cell membranes in a similar manner. The body does not metabolise lithium; it exists as an ion and is distributed evenly throughout the body, being excreted through the kidneys. Theories as to actual mode of action involved lithium in the following activities.

- Reducing the quantities of noradrenaline available to receptor sites (overproduction of noradrenaline is thought to be involved in manic episodes).
- Preventing the redistribution of intracellular sodium which occurs in affective disorders.
- Altering output of corticosteroids which in turn affects concentration and distribution of sodium and potassium in cells of muscles and nerves.
- An antiserotonin action.

Dosage

Lithium carbonate is presented in 250 mg tablets and the initial dosage is aimed at achieving high therapeutic serum levels as rapidly as is safely possible, necessitating divided doses totalling up to 1750 mg per day. Once therapeutic effect has been obtained to control the acute phase of illness, the daily dose can be adjusted to maintain a serum level within the therapeutic range sufficient to control symptomatology without producing undesirable side-effects.

Lithium is also available as a controlled release preparation (Priadel) in 400 mg tablets, administered as a single daily dose.

Adverse effects

Side-effects are dose-related. Lithium has a very narrow therapeutic range; dosage is aimed at achieving a serum concentration between 0.8 and 1.2 mmol/litre; levels above 2 mmol/litre produce toxicity.

1. Mild effects (on commencement of therapy) include:
   - nausea
   - metallic taste
   - intermittent thirst
   - fine tremor of hands
   - gastrointestinal disturbances.
2. Moderate effects (impending toxicity):
   - diarrhoea
   - polydipsia
   - polyuria
   - coarse tremor
   - muscle weakness
   - fatigue
   - acneform eruptions (pre-existing psoriasis also often becomes worse).

Severe effects (mild toxicity):
   - ataxia
   - confusion
   - stupor
   - muscle twitching.

Severe toxicity:
   - drowsiness
   - slurred speech
   - cog wheel rigidity
   - pale, grey, drawn appearance
   - myoclonic contractions
   - weakness

leading to renal failure, coma, and eventually death.

Precautions

The major risk in lithium therapy is retention of the drug, which can rapidly lead to toxicity. Prior to commencement of the drug, individuals should have baseline studies of renal, thyroid, and cardiac function, and of electrolyte levels. Frequent and regular monitoring of serum levels is necessary on commencement of therapy, and at less frequent but regular intervals (3–6 months) on maintenance doses.

Drug interactions

Neuroleptics taken concurrently with lithium may, through their anti-emetic properties, mask nausea and vomiting — symptoms indicative of lithium toxicity. Haloperidol, in particular, when taken with lithium may produce a reaction characterized by lethargy and confusion.

Diuretics, especially of the thiazide group, increase depletion of sodium and the retention of lithium, producing high serum concentration and causing toxicity.

The antihypertensive agent methyldopa causes retention and toxicity of lithium, as does the anti-inflammatory drug indomethacin.

Lithium prolongs the neuromuscular blocking action of depolarizing muscle relaxants such as suxamethonium chloride.

Aminophylline, sodium bicarbonate, and sodium chloride increase the excretion of lithium, consequently lowering serum concentration.

Nursing implications

User education

It is extremely important that people receiving lithium are adequately educated in

(i) The nature of their illness.
(ii) The nature of the drug.
(iii) The need to be compliant with their prescribed medication regime.
(iv) The early symptoms of lithium toxicity and the need to inform their doctor immediately if those symptoms occur.
(v) The importance of informing their doctor if they experience any condition that may influence fluid and electrolyte balances, e.g.
- prolonged bouts of vomiting or diarrhoea
- excessive perspiration
- physical illness.
(vi) Other factors which may influence fluid and electrolyte balance and thus serum lithium levels, e.g.
- salt-free slimming diets
- adequate fluid intake
- vigorous exercise, producing perspiration
- hot weather, or travel to areas of tropical climate or high temperature.

Nursing education

It is the nurse's responsibility to ensure that a person prescribed lithium is fully aware of the important aspects of this medication before discharge from hospital. A thorough nursing knowledge of the side-effects of lithium, the physiological processes involved, and the causes of lithium toxicity are essential. While the person is in hospital, nurses should be alert to factors that may influence fluid and electrolyte balance, e.g. concurrent use of diuretics.

Gastrointestinal disturbances

Administration of the drug with milk or food diminishes the unpleasant metallic taste of lithium tablets. Taking the drug at meal times should be encouraged, to lessen feelings of nausea, and gastrointestinal disturbances; this also facilitates compliance by establishing a routine of taking medication.

Dose omissions

As some individuals are liable to forget, or neglect, to take their lithium at the prescribed time — a problem commonly associated with any prescribed medication — they should be instructed not to attempt to counteract the deficit by doubling the next dose. Such a practice could cause a rapid elevation of serum concentrations to toxic levels.

Monitoring serum levels

Regular monitoring of the serum lithium

concentration is essential: blood specimens should be taken 1–2 times per week initially until therapeutic effect, side-effects, and serum concentration levels are stabilized; thereafter, specimens should be taken at monthly, progressing to three-monthly, intervals if all factors remain constant. To obtain accurate serum levels it is necessary for the blood sample to be taken 12 hours after the last dose of lithium; if the sample is taken following a recent dose, a false high concentration will be indicated, possibly resulting in an inadequate dose being prescribed.

Omission of the first dose in the morning usually suffices to enable an accurate measurement of serum concentration from blood obtained that morning. The nurse must ensure that this occurs, and, if necessary, have the daily dosage regime for that day readjusted to maintain the same total daily dose.

Managing side-effects

The potentially threatening side-effects indicative of lithium toxicity have been described and require immediate action to reverse the condition. There are other effects which are not indicative of toxicity, and which the person may have to endure. The nurse can initiate interventions to diminish these effects. The initial effects of nausea, vomiting, diarrhoea, weight gain, fine hand tremor, and lack of co-ordination diminish and often disappear as the individual develops tolerance to the drug. Alleviation of gastrointestinal disturbances has already been discussed. Weight gain and hand tremor may persist with maintenance therapy, as well as polyuria and polydipsia. The weight gain is associated with polydipsia, a prominent complaint in about 10% of people, who may have a fluid intake of more than 3–4 litres a day (Dally & Connolly 1981), much of which can be soft drinks containing sugar. The nurse can encourage substitution of these beverages with sugar-free fluids such as iced water, mineral water, or iced tea. Lithium's tendency to cause retention of sodium results in oedema, particularly

of the legs and face, and gives rise to the excessive thirst and resultant weight gain. Drinks containing caffeine should also be discouraged, as high levels of this substance can aggravate the agitation and insomnia of the original condition, and exaggerate hand tremor.

Hand tremor is often distressing to the person who believes it to be more obvious to others than it really is. The nurse should inform the individual's doctor if this symptom is causing distress, as it can be controlled by antihypertensive drugs such as propranolol.

GROUP — ANTIDEPRESSANTS/THYMOLEPTICS

Uses

1. To elevate mood and diminish symptoms in depressive illnesses.
2. In management of anxiety states associated with depression.

Class — tricyclics

Examples:
- amitriptyline (Laroxyl, Saroten, Tryptanol, Amitrip) — daily dose 50–150 mg
- imipramine (Tofranil, Imiprin) — daily dose 75–300 mg
- doxepin (Quitaxon, Sinequan) — daily dose 75–300 mg
- trimipramine (Surmontil) — daily dose 75–300 mg

Modes of action

Individual drugs within the group vary biochemically, but they generally act by inhibiting the uptake of various neurotransmitters, thus allowing concentration of these substances, which are thought to be depleted in depressive illnesses.

Choice of drug often depends on the individual's tolerance to particular side-effects. However, some of the tricyclics — amitriptyline and trimipramine in particular — have powerful sedative actions, whereas imipramine is a potent antidepressant but is less sedating. Through clinical experience, certain drugs have been found to be more effective than others against particular predominant symptoms, and are often chosen in preference to others on that basis; for instance, amitriptyline where agitation and insomnia are predominant, imipramine for psychomotor retardation, doxepin when anticholinergic effects are intolerable.

Adverse effects

1. Anticholinergic:
   - dry mouth
   - blurred vision
   - sweating
   - constipation
   - postural hypotension
   - urinary retention
   - sedation
   - tremor.
2. Cardiotoxic:
   - cardiac arrhythmias
   - myocardial infarction
   - tachycardia.
3. Lowered seizure threshold. Toxic serum levels (especially following overdose) produce:
   - agitation, delirium, progressing to decreasing levels of consciousness, and coma
   - seizures
   - cardiac arrhythmias.

Class — non-tricyclics

Example:
- nomifensine (Merital) — daily dose 75–200 mg divided

Mode of action

Inhibits the re-uptake of dopamine and noradrenaline potentiating neurotransmission.

Adverse effects

- insomnia

- restlessness
- headache
- dry mouth or bad taste (other anticholinergic effects occur at high doses)
- no cardiotoxic effects, even with overdosage.

Class — non-tricyclics

- mianserin (Tolvon) — daily dose 90–120 mg divided

Mode of action

Does not affect re-uptake of amines; does increase availability of noradrenaline.

Adverse effects

- drowsiness, dry mouth, headache (these symptoms are usually of short duration and experienced on commencement of therapy)
- dizziness
- weakness
- tremor
- faintness
- vertigo
- no serious cardiotoxic effects.

Class — monoamine oxidase inhibitors (MAOIs)

Examples:
- tranylcypromine (Parnate, Parstelin) — daily dose 10–30 mg divided
- phenelzine (Nardil) — daily dose 45–60 mg divided

Mode of action

Inhibit breakdown of noradrenaline by the enzyme monoamine oxidase, causing an accumulation of noradrenaline in storage site and at the synapse.

Adverse effects

1. - headache
   - dry mouth

- dizziness
- postural hypotension
- constipation
- insomnia
- mild hypomania.
2. Severe hypertension precipitated by consuming food stuffs containing the amino acid tyramine, e.g. cheese, yoghurt, yeast and meat extracts, pickled herring, paté, game, Chianti and red wines generally, home brewed beer, fermented products, broad-bean pods, banana skins, caviar, and aged samples of meat, fish, poultry, offal, packaged soups, stock cubes, cream.
3. Incompatability with a number of sympathomimetic drugs, producing severe hypertensive crisis.

Indications of an adverse drug/food or drug/drug reaction (often referred to as the 'cheese reaction') are
- sweating
- severe, pounding headache
- nausea, vomiting
- palpitations.

Drug interactions

The tricyclic antidepressants block the antihypertensive action of guanethidine or similarly acting compounds.

Adjustment of dosage of anticholinergic or sympathomimetic drugs including adrenaline is necessary as concurrent use with tricyclics may produce paralytic ileus.

The concurrent use of any other antidepressant with an MAOI is contraindicated, and a lapse of 14 days is necessary between the prescribing of these two groups of drugs.

Antidepressants potentiate the effects of alcohol, barbiturates, and other central nervous system depressants including sedatives and hypnotics.

Drugs with which the MAOIs are incompatible include

1. Sympathomimetics:
   - amphetamines
   - nasal decongestants (ephedrine, phen-

ylephrine, phenylpropanolamine, psuedoephedrine)
   - anti-obesity agents (fenfluramine, phenmetrazine)
   - anti-Parkinson drug (levodopa).
2. Anti-depressants:
   - tricyclics and non-tricyclics.
3. Analgesics:
   - morphine, pethidine.
4. Hypoglycaemic agents:
   - insulin.
5. Hypnotics, sedatives:
   - alcohol, barbiturates, and other central nervous system depressants.
6. Antihypertensives:
   - quanethidine, propranolol.
7. Anticholinergics.
8. Foodstuffs containing tyramine (as previously described).

Nursing implications

Delayed therapeutic response

Nurses and people taking antidepressants need to be aware that a therapeutic response to tricyclic antidepressant medication may not occur for up to three weeks. Depressed people will need supportive nursing care and much encouragement while waiting for the medication to reach a therapeutically effective level.

Anticholinergic side-effects

The disturbing anticholinergic side-effects experienced during the early weeks of treatment compound the problem of compliance. Many of these effects can be minimized or avoided by gradual dosage increase to the optimum or therapeutic level for the individual person. The elderly are particularly vulnerable to side-effects, especially postural hypotension; awareness of cardiovascular complications is necessary. Interventions regarding these anticholinergic effects have been discussed above in connection with neuroleptic drugs.

Monitoring blood pressure

People on antidepressants should have their blood pressure monitored routinely, with particular attention being given to those individuals receiving MAOIs. Lying and standing observations of blood pressure are necessary to elicit any postural drop. Due to the potential for hypertensive crisis with MAOIs, any incidence of persistent headache should be reported immediately, as the crisis can be accompanied by intracranial haemorrhage, hyperpyrexia, and convulsions; coma and death may occur.

Physical, emotional or behavioural reactions

The nurse should look out for and report any physical, emotional, or behavioural reactions that may occur while a person is taking these drugs. Be alert for signs of overactivity, restlessness, tremor, drowsiness, confusion or fatigue, or deepening depression. Also observe for perspiration, dehydration, constipation, and urinary retention, especially in elderly males with possible prostatic enlargement.

Suicide risk

It is important to remember that the risk of suicide is high in the early stages of recovery. As antidepressants begin to take effect, depressed individuals regain lost volition and energy, facilitating them in carrying out their suicidal intent, whereas previously the psychomotor retardation of depression had been a restraint.

Convulsions

Tricyclic antidepressants lower the seizure threshold and can precipitate epileptic seizures in individuals who have never before experienced them, or induce seizures in cases of previously controlled epilepsy. Nurses should be aware of this possibility and take appropriate precautions if a previous history of epileptic seizures is known.

Dosage reduction

Generally antidepressant medications can be gradually reduced and eventually discontinued if the person tolerates the dosage reduction without the recurrence of symptoms. Medication should not be ceased abruptly, as withdrawal reactions can occur. Individuals do not necessarily need to resign themselves to life-long medication, but should be taught the signs of a recurrence of their depressive illness so that they can seek psychiatric help promptly.

MAOI precautions

All people taking MAOIs, and particularly those being discharged from hospital on these drugs, need to be completely conversant with the dietary and other precautions required, and with the symptoms associated with the 'cheese reaction'. It is the nurse's responsibility to educate the person in these matters.

GROUP — ANXIOLYTICS

The word 'anxiolytic' means to remove anxiety. This group of drugs was formerly referred to as 'sedatives' or 'minor tranquillizers', terms which are misleading with regard to the action of these drugs.

Uses

1. Short-term relief of symptoms of anxiety.
2. Some muscle relaxant and anticonvulsant properties.

Class — benzodiazepines

Examples:
- diazepam (Valium, Ducene, Pro-Pam) — daily dose 2–30 mg, divided
- oxazepam (Serepax, Adumbran, Benzotan, Murelax) — daily dose 30–120 mg divided
- alprazolam (Xanax) — daily dose 0.5–4 mg divided
- clobazam (Frisium) — daily dose 10–30 mg divided

Benzodiazepines are now the drugs of choice in the management of anxiety and agitation, having superceded the barbiturates. Although still available and extremely effective, this latter group of drugs is no longer widely prescribed due to government restrictions on dispensing (resulting from their ability to cause physical dependence, and their potential for abuse).

Mode of action

The benzodiazepines are central nervous system depressants, thought to act on the limbic system, the reticular activating system, and the hypothalamus, decreasing serotonin turnover by antagonising adrenaline and noradrenaline.

Adverse effects

- drowsiness
- skin rashes
- impaired co-ordination
- headache
- dry mouth.

Larger doses may produce signs of intoxication similar to alcohol intoxication, including

- slurred speech
- ataxia
- blurred vision
- tremor
- lethargy
- hypotension.

They may also produce paradoxical reactions such as excitement and rage. There are no dangerous effects at toxic levels, even following large overdosage. They can lead to psychological dependence.

Class — miscellaneous

Example:
- chlormethiazole (Hemineurin)

Chlormethiazole is an anxiolytic and hypnotic with some anticonvulsant and muscle relaxant properties; one-half of its composition is vitamin B. It is used primarily in treatment of delirium tremens and other withdrawal states, and also in status epilepticus and (short-term) in agitational and confusional states in hospitalized individuals.

Dosage

192 mg capsule, and i.v. solution 0.8% in 500 ml.

(a) In withdrawal states — oral dose 2–4 capsules initially then 2 capsules hourly until sedated to a maximum of 8 g in 24 hours. Intravenous dosage should not exceed 1500 ml in 24 hours. It is prescribed in decreasing dosage over a period usually of 7 days, because of risk of dependence.
(b) As an anxiolytic — 1 capsule 3 times a day.
(c) As a hypnotic — 2–4 capsules at night.

Adverse effects

It is not generally associated with serious side-effects, but may produce

- transient nasal irritation
- conjunctivial irritation
- gastrointestinal disturbances
- moderate tachycardia
- urticaria.

Rapid intravenous infusion may cause a transient fall in blood pressure.

Class — beta-blockers

Example:
- propranolol (Inderal) — daily, dose 80–160 mg.

Propranolol is generally well tolerated. Side-effects are transient and rare but can include

- nausea
- insomnia
- severe nightmares
- depression
- confusion.

Drug interactions

The benzodiazepine group of drugs potentiate other central nervous system depressants including alcohol, hypnotics, antidepressants, and other anxiolytics. Alcohol is also considered an anxiolytic, having actions and effects similar to the benzodiazepines.

Nursing implications

Dependence

The benzodiazepine anxiolytics, if taken in large enough doses or long enough, can lead to physical and emotional dependence (Zisook & De Vaul 1977, Menuck 1980, Lader 1981). Characteristic signs of withdrawal are

- insomnia
- weakness
- muscle tremors
- anxiety
- irritability
- sweating
- anorexia
- fever
- nausea and vomiting
- headache
- restlessness and nightmares.

It is important to be aware of the signs of withdrawal and intoxication, as either can occur in a person taking these drugs.

Impaired co-ordination

People should be warned of an impaired ability to drive vehicles or operate machinery, and a general impairment of concentration, motor performance, and co-ordination.

Elderly people

Elderly people experience more side-effects, especially day-time sedation and paradoxical excitement (Zisook & De Vaul 1977). They are also more prone to toxic accumulation over time, and possible drug interaction.

Tolerance

Tolerance to benzodiazepine drugs is quickly developed, often within several days, and may cause the individual to take, or ask for, a progressively increasing dose. However, these drugs are considered not to be efficacious after four months of continuous treatment. Despite this fact, many individuals, and prescribers, continue to use these drugs on a maintenance basis over indefinite periods of time. It must be remembered that anxiolytics should be administered only for acute or short-term relief of symptoms of anxiety or tension, and cannot be used to remove these symptoms completely.

Respiratory depression

With the exception of the beta-blockers, the anxiolytics are central nervous system depressants and should be used with caution in cases of cardiorespiratory insufficiency, where respiratory depression may be aggravated. If taken in combination with other CNS depressants, observe for over-sedation and toxicity

Abuse

Anxiolytics are some of the most commonly prescribed medications; a conservative estimate based on earlier surveys (Carrington-Smith 1975, Australian Bureau of Statistics 1977–8; Engs 1980) would be that more than 4% of adult persons in Australia are currently using prescribed anxiolytics on a daily basis. Many deliberate overdoses involve one or more of these drugs, especially in conjunction with alcohol. Nurses can play a major role in educating people in the correct use of these drugs, and in the use of other forms of symptom relief (see Ch. 7).

GROUP — HYPNOTICS

These are drugs that act to induce sleep.

Uses

Treatment of sleep disturbances including

1. Initial insomnia.
2. Early morning awakening of either a psychological or organic origin.

Intended as an adjunct to short-term management of insomnia in adults.

Class — barbiturates

The original hypnotics, these drugs are now rarely used, having been replaced mainly by the benzodiazepine group of drugs.

Class — benzodiazepines

Already mentioned as anxiolytics, this group of drugs, when given in higher doses, also act as hypnotics. However, there are a number of drugs in this group that have not yet been mentioned, and which do have a specific hypnotic effect.

Examples:
- nitrazepam (Dormicum, Mogadon) — dose 5–10 mg at night
- temazepam (Euhypnos, Normison) dose 10–30 mg a half-hour before retiring at night
- flunitrazepam (Rohypnol) — dose 1–4 mg before retiring at night

Mode of action

These are CNS depressants, but act particularly on the higher cortical centres controlling consciousness and mental activity.

Class — miscellaneous

Examples:
- chloral hydrate (Chloralix, Dormel, Noctec) — dose 0.5–1 g before retiring
- chlormethiazole (Hemineurin)

Adverse effects

1. The benzodiazepine hypnotics have fewer autonomic nervous system effects than the anxiolytics, but can cause
   - ataxia

- headache
- confusion
- vertigo
- dizziness

particularly in elderly or debilitated people.
2. They interfere with rapid eye movement (REM) sleep, causing emotional disturbance and nightmares; they also produce a groggy 'hang-over' feeling next morning. Temazepam differs from others by inducing a more natural sleep and not having these undesirable effects.
3. They cause impaired psychomotor performance, extending to the morning after taking the medication. As with the anxiolytics, tolerance and dependence can develop, and addiction to chloral hydrate occurs.
4. There is a possibility of increase in frequency and/or severity of grand mal seizures with the use of temazepam in people with epilepsy.

Drug interactions

The effect of these drugs is potentiated when combined with alcohol and other CNS depressants, including barbiturates, tricyclic antidepressants, phenothiazines, morphine, pethidine, anaesthetics, and antihistamines.

Nursing implications

Sleep pattern

Sleep patterns should be observed and charted to ascertain the type and extent of sleep disturbance, if any.

User education

People should be informed of correct use of these drugs to prevent misuse and dependence.

Interventions to induce sleep

The nurse should investigate and utilize

alternative interventions to induce sleep in people, e.g.

- relaxation
- warm drinks
- daily exercise
- quite, comforting environment.

For detailed guidelines see Chapter 18.

Over-sedation

Observe for over-sedation, especially in the elderly.

Interference with natural sleep

It is important to remember that no drug can produce true physiological sleep; hypnotics interfere with the natural stages of sleep and therefore do not produce the feeling of being rested following a sleep (see Ch. 18).

Impaired motor functioning

This group of drugs are CNS depressants and consequently impair psychomotor functioning. Individuals should be warned of the hazards of operating machinery or driving a car, even on the following morning.

Short-term treatment only

Alternatives to hypnotics should always be explored, but if these drugs need to be prescribed, they should be given at a low dose, and for short periods only (2–4 weeks). Hypnotics, like anxiolytics, are efficacious for only 3–4 months of continuous treatment.

Risk of abuse

Nurses should be alert to the possibility of people abusing these drugs and ensure that medications are not being secreted or hoarded, and that they are not being given when they are not particularly indicated.

Withdrawal

People who have been taking large doses, or small doses over a long period of time, should not have the drug withdrawn abruptly. Sudden withdrawal may result in withdrawal symptoms including

- convulsion
- tremor
- abdominal and muscle cramps
- vomiting
- sweating
- nervousness and insomnia.

GROUP — ANTICHOLINERGIC/ANTI-PARKINSON DRUGS

Uses

1. Prevention and control of extrapyramidal side-effects due to neuroleptic drugs.
2. Treatment of Parkinson's disease.

Class — anticholinergics

Examples:
- benztropine (Cogentin) — dose 1–4 mg 1–2 times daily
- orphenadrine (Disipal, Orpadrex) — 150 mg per day in divided doses

Mode of action

The anticholinergic properties exert a direct inhibitory effect upon the parasympathetic nervous system, restoring the balance between the cholinergic and dopaminergic systems, by blocking the cholinergic systems.

Adverse effects

- blurred vision
- dry mouth
- constipation
- drowsiness
- dizziness
- a feeling of sedation
- tachycardia

Nursing implications

Extrapyramidal reactions

Nurses must be able to recognize the signs of extrapyramidal side-effects, and must observe people taking neuroleptic drugs for indications of the occurrence of these effects.

The anticholinergic drugs are particularly effective against the manifestations of tremor, rigidity, and the acute dystonic reactions. A statim (immediate) dose of an anti-Parkinson drug such as benztropine will quickly relieve the distressing dystonic reaction, and regular maintenance doses will prevent further symptoms.

Impaired motor ability

These drugs may impair the individual's ability to operate machinery or drive a vehicle; nurses should warn people about this restriction.

Toxic behavioural changes

Observe people for signs of tachycardia and for undue excitement and confusion. It is possible for individuals to develop behavioural toxicity associated with anticholinergic side-effects of these drugs in combination with the phenothiazines. This syndrome is characterized by disorientation, loss of immediate memory, and florid hallucinations (Davis et al 1972).

Gastrointestinal disturbances

People should be instructed to report gastrointestinal discomfort immediately, as there is a possibility of the development of paralytic ileus.

Anhydrosis and hyperthermia

The anticholinergic effects of these drugs can produce anhydrosis (cessation of perspiration). This reduction in the ability to regulate body temperature can precipitate a state of hyperthermia, especially in hot weather. This situation is further complicated when these drugs are taken concurrently with phenothiazines due to the latter group's effect on the thermoregulatory centre in the brain.

Nurses must be alert to this potential effect and initiate appropriate interventions, especially in hot weather.

CONCLUSION

It is beyond the scope of this chapter to examine alternative forms of drug treatment. However, it is necessary to mention that research has been undertaken to establish the role of vitamins and other substances in the prevention and treatment of mental illness. There is a growing number of physicians who are advocating, for instance, the use of mega doses of various vitamins of the B group and vitamin C for the management of schizophrenic disorders and mania, and zinc to diminish effects of progressive dementias. It is possible that this area of orthomolecular psychiatry and psychodietetics will in time gain more acceptance by the medical profession; but, at the moment, the use of psychotropic medication is still of greater significance in everyday management of disturbances of mental health.

In discussing drugs and mental health, it should be remembered that a large number of medications indicated in a variety of illnesses and conditions can precipitate significant disturbances of mental health. Tables 3.1–3.4 (pp. 58–59) contain lists of drugs that can produce undesirable, and frequently serious, psychiatric reactions, including depression, psychoses, hallucinations, and delirium and confusion.

ELECTROCONVULSIVE THERAPY (ECT)

The introduction of the phenothiazine group of psychotropic drugs in the 1950s was a dramatic innovation in the treatment of mental illness. However, the 1930s had seen the development of another form of physical

Table 3.1 Drugs causing depression (After Meyler 1975, 1979, Meyler & Herzheimer 1972)

Analgesics and anti-inflammatory drugs	*Anti-bacterial and anti-fungal drugs*	*Anti-neoplastic drugs*
Fenoprofen	Ampicillin	Azathioprine
Ibuprofen	Bactrim	6-azauridine
Indomethacin	Clotrimazole	1-asparaginase
Ketroprofen	Cycloserine*	Bleomycin
Opiates (morphine, etc.)	Dapsone	Mithramycin
Phenacetin	Ethionamide*	Trimethoprim
Phenylbutazone	Griseofulvin	Vincristine
Pentazocine	Metronidazole	
Benzydamine*	Nitrofurantoin	*Miscellaneous drugs*
	Nalidixic acid	Acetazolamide
Psychotropic drugs	Sulphonamides	Anticholinesterases
Butyrophenones	Streptomycin	Choline
Phenothiazines	Tetracyline	Cimetidine
Fluphenazine decanoate	Thiocarlide*	Cyproheptadine
Flupenthixol decanoate		Diphenoxylate
Prochlorperazine	*Cardiac and anti-hypertensive drugs*	Disulfiram
	Bethanidine	Lysergide
Sedatives & hypnotics	Clonidine	Methysergide
Barbiturates	Digitalis	Mebeverine
Chloral	Guanethidine	Meclozine
Chlormethiazole	Hydralazine	Metoclopramide
Clorazepate	Methyl dopa	Pizotifen
Ethanol	Prazosin	Salbutamol
Other benzodiazepines	Procainamide	
Other non-barbiturate	Propranolol	*Neurological drugs*
hypnotics and sedatives	Reserpine	Amantadine
	Veratrum*	Baclofen
Steroids and hormones	Lidocaine	Bromocriptine
ACTH	Oxprenolol	Carbamazepine
Corticosteroids	Methosperidine*	L-dopa
Danazol	*Stimulants and appetite suppressants*	Methsuximide
Oral contraceptives	Amphetamine	Phenytoin
Norethisterone	Fenfluramine	Phenindione
Prednisone	Diethylpropion	Tetrabenazine
Triamcinalone	Phenmetrazine*	

Table 3.2 Drugs causing psychosis (After Meyler 1975, 1979, Meyler & Herzheimer 1972)

Endocrines and steroids	*Anti-Parkinsonian drugs*	*Miscellaneous drugs*
ACTH	Benztropine	Atropine
Corticosteroids	Anticholinergic drugs	Aprotinin
Glucosteroids	L-dopa	Cannabis
	Amantadine	Carbimazole
Antidepressants	Trihexyphenidyl*	Chloroquine
Amitriptyline		Dextromethorphan
Desipramine	*Anticonvulsant drugs*	Diphenhydramine
Imipramine	Carbamazepine	Disulfiram
MAOI drugs	Ethosuximide	Hyoscine
	Methsuximide	Lysergide
Stimulants and appetite suppressants		Methysergide
Amphetamine	*Sedative hand anti-anxiety drugs*	Pentazocine
Cocaine	Barbiturates	Phenylbutazone
Diethylpropion	Bromides	Propranolol
Fenfluramine	Mandrax	
Ephedrine	Benzactyzine*	*Anti-bacterial drugs*
Methylphenidate		Clotrimazole
Phenmetrazine*		Cycloserine*
Phentermine		Dapsone
		Ethtinamide*
		Isoniazid
		Mepacrine*
		Nitrofuran
		Para-amino-salicylic acid*

* Not available in Australia.

Table 3.3 Drugs causing hallucinations (After Meyler 1975, 1979, Meyler & Herzheimer 1972)

Anti-Parkinsonian	*CNS stimulants*	*Other drugs*
Amantadine	Amphetamine	Benzodiazepines
Anticholinergic drugs	Bemegride*	Baclofen
Bromocriptine	Methylphenidates	Vitamin D
L-dopa		Nalidixic acid
Stramonium*	*Narcotic analgesis*	Nitridazole*
	Dextromoramide	
Antidepressants	Morphine	*Cardiac and antihypertensive drugs*
Amitriptyline	Pentazocine	Beta-adrenergic receptor
Imipramine		blocking drugs
Maprotiline*	*Analgesics/anti-inflammatory*	Digitalis
	drugs	Procainamide
Antihistamines	Phenacetin	Lidocaine
Diphenhydramine	Indomethacin	Mecamylamine
Pheniramine	Phenylbutazone	
Cyclizine	Salicylates	
Tripelennamine*	Benzydamine*	

* Not available in Australia.

Table 3.4 Drugs causing delirium and confusion (Afer Meyler 1975, 1979, Meyler & Herzheimer 1972)

Cardiovascular and antihypertensive drugs	*Anti-psychotic drugs and antidepressants*
Digitalis	Droperidol
Mecamylamine	Protriptyline
Mexiletine	Lithium
	Nomifensine
Antihistamines	*Anti-Parkinsonian drugs*
Promethazine	Orphenadrine
Cimetidine	Amantadine
	L-dopa
	Benzhexol
Sedatives and hypnotics	*Miscellaneous drugs*
Barbiturates	Aprotinin
Bromisoval*	Boric acid
Carbromal	Chloroquine
Ethanol	Chliquinol
Methaqualone	Coumarin
Benzodiazepines	Flurothyl*
	Ketamine
	Meclof enamic acid*
	Metrizamide
	Niridazole*
	Sodium valproate
	Vitamin A

* Not available in Australia

treatment which also played a significant part in modern psychiatry. This form of treatment, electroconvulsive therapy, which also at times has been referred to as 'electroplexy', 'electrocerebral stimulation therapy', and 'shock treatment', still holds an invaluable place in the management of mental illness. ECT is an electrically induced, modified grand mal seizure for therapeutic purposes.

History

Convulsive treatment originated in 1933 when a Hungarian physican, Dr von Meduna, observed that schizophrenics were never epileptic, while epileptics were similarly free of schizophrenia. From this observation he postulated that there might be some mutually antagonistic effect between epileptic fits and the development of schizophrenic illness. The attempt to treat a person's schizophrenia by the artificial induction of epilepsy was the next logical step taken by Dr von Meduna. His hypothesis has since been disproved, but convulsive therapy continued to be tested as a practical treatment.

Dr von Meduna's original method of inducing a grand mal seizure was to inject camphor oil intramuscularly; this was later changed to intravenous cardiazol. In 1938, two Italians, Cerletti and Bini, introduced electrically produced fits to replace the previous unreliable, frightening, and dangerous procedure. At this time the treatment was given to conscious and aware individuals, but was soon developed to include the introduction, in late 1940s, of general anaesthetics and muscle relaxants prior to inducing a convulsion, to reduce the possibility of fractures. The only other change in this form of treatment was the introduction in 1958 of unilateral ECT. This method employed the technique of producing a generalized convulsion by applying the electrodes to the non-dominant cerebral hemisphere of the brain. Although there was no significant difference in the degree of clinical improvement following the original bilateral or new unilateral procedures, unilateral ECT caused less memory loss (Lancaster et al 1958). Dr von Meduna's original hypothesis was quickly disproved, but it was observed that his treatment was effective in improving the depressed mood of schizophrenic individuals, albeit having no effect on their schizophrenic symptoms. This observation has been verified through clinical practice and has led to ECT now being used consistently in depressive illness, and not so commonly under other circumstances.

Indications

ECT is considered to be the treatment of choice for distraught, agitated, depressed people, especially when life is at risk from the physiological consequences of their depressive illness or from suicidal intentions. There is substantial and incontrovertible evidence that ECT is an effective treatment in severe depressive states (Royal college of Psychiatrists 1977, Weeks et al 1980) but, as Freeman (1979) has pointed out, 'ECT is not a treatment for unhappiness. It cannot mend marriages, or restore to the bereaved their relatives.' Manic states proving unresponsive to antipsychotic drugs will respond to ECT, and this treatment is still occasionally needed to control mania.

In current practice, the only other conditions under which ECT is indicated and performed are in schizophrenic disorders where there is a strong component of depressed mood, or where catatonic stupor is present and rapid alleviation is a life-saving necessity.

Contraindications

ECT is one of the safest forms of somatic treatment and has relatively few contraindications. Generally speaking, if a person is able to have the general anaesthetic, there is little risk from ECT. The exceptions to this generalization are cases of a recent myocardial infarction, the presence of a space-occupying lesion in the brain, raised intracranial pressure, existing fractures or severe osteoarthritis, peptic ulceration, and any atherosclerotic condition. When any of these conditions exist, an assessment of the individual's fitness for treatment by a physician/surgeon and an anaesthetist is required. Old-age or pregnancy are not necessarily contraindications for ECT.

Procedures

The doctor must explain the treatment to the person and obtain a written consent to the anaesthetic and course of treatment. The person is fasted for at least 4 hours prior to the treatment, having previously been declared fit for anaesthesia by an anaesthetist. Premedication is not necessarily routine, but if ordered may be a prescription for atropine and/or an anxiolytic (such as scopolamine or diazepam). False-teeth, tight clothing, and jewellery should be removed, and the bladder emptied immediately before treatment.

The nurse's responsibilities prior to treatment are to ensure that the person receives nothing orally and to remain with the person to offer support and alleviate apprehension and anxiety. On rare occasions when anaesthetic complications could be possible, the treatment may be performed in theatre. This being the case, it is beneficial and reassuring to the person if a nurse familiar to him is in attendance during transfer to theatre and on recovery from the treatment.

A short-acting general anaesthetic, either methohexitone sodium (Brietal) or thiopentone sodium (Pentothal, Intraval) is administered and followed, via the same needle, by a muscle relaxant such as suxamethonium chloride (Scoline, Anectine). The person is thoroughly ventilated with oxygen before the current is applied. Following cleansing of the skin at the site of placement of the electrodes, two electrodes are placed on the head in the positions relating to the type of treatment favoured by the psychiatrist: using the bilateral technique the electrodes are placed on the temporal lobes so that the current is passed across the anterior portions of the cerebral hemispheres; with the unilateral method the non-dominant hemisphere is selected, one electrode placed on that temporal lobe and the other approximately 8 cm away on the same side of the head.

The machine delivering the current is preset to deliver the desired intensity (in milliamps) for a predetermined number of seconds in either a continuous or pulsating current. In practical terms the current and voltage used (90–260 volts) would cause a household light-bulb to flicker momentarily.

Gauze pads soaked in a normal saline solution are placed between the electrodes and the skin to enhance conductivity and prevent electrical burns; Electrogel can also be used.

On application of the current the person exhibits a tonic muscle spasm followed almost immediately by a generalized clonic phase of a grand mal seizure. However, as a muscle relaxant has been administered, a 'modified' response takes place, the only evidence of convulsion being a flickering or fanning of the toes. For this reason, it is necessary for the nurse to ensure that the individual's feet are exposed prior to administering the current.

The .anaesthetist then oxygenates the person until spontaneous breathing is restored (within a few minutes), at which time the person is transferred to the recovery area. During recovery the nurse must observe the person's colour, maintain a patent airway, and take observations of vital signs. Within 20 minutes the person should be fully awake, and if observations are stable, can return to bed for a period of time to sleep off the effects of the anaesthetic.

People receive a course of ECT, consisting of a number of treatments, at intervals of 2–3 days. There is no predetermined number of treatments in a course; however, an average of 6–9 treatments produces an alleviation of symptoms in the majority of people. If an effective response is not achieved following this number, ECT is discontinued. A clinical response is evident after 2 or 3 treatments, but if the course ends too soon a relapse can occur within 1–2 weeks.

Side-effects

On waking, the person may be confused and complain of disturbances of memory, particularly loss of short-term memory, and a frontal headache. These effects are transient, usually diminishing during the course of the day. Agitation and excitement may sometimes be seen in people during recovery. In some cases the mood is elated or euphoric, but soon reverts to a less excited state within a few hours.

Mechanism of action

Electroconvulsive therapy is an empirical treatment, its exact mechanism of action being unknown. Several psychoanalytic theories have been suggested as to why ECT alters mood states, but more convincing hypotheses have arisen from studies by neurobiologists (Essman 1974, Colman 1971, Kety 1974). Such studies indicate that ECT causes changes in levels of various brain chemicals, producing increased dopamine levels, a sustained increase in synthesis and utilization of norepinephrine, and a short-acting inhibition of brain protein synthesis. These alterations presumably promote synaptic activity in depressed individuals, in whom such activity is usually diminished (Kety 1974).

The significance of the findings of the neurobiologists is expressed by Carl Salzman (1978): 'Biochemical amine hypotheses seem most plausible, since alterations in catecholamine function are increasingly thought to influence affective illness.'

ECT is usually performed in a specialized unit. However, nurses may have contact outside such a unit with individuals who have received this treatment in the past or are soon to receive it. The latter may be in a medical ward because of physical debilitation resulting from an existing serious depressive illness for which ECT is indicated. These people may turn to the nurse for details regarding the treatment, for reassurance as to its need, or to express doubts, fears, and anxieties. Consequently, nurses need to have a knowledge and understanding of the treatment to be able to meet their responsibilities confidently, and to demystify a useful treatment which has attracted much negative comment.

PSYCHOSURGERY

This form of physical treatment is not commonly used and is considereed as a treatment of last resort. It has, however, held a place in the treatment of mental health disturbances and nurses should at least be aware of some basic facts regarding the practice. The procedure involves destruction of healthy brain tissue, including nerve tracts, in order to relieve severe symptoms of mental illness, or alter subjectively debilitating behaviour.

Indications

Neurosurgical intervention is indicated in certain disturbances of mental health in which the individual has suffered severely disabling symptoms continuously over several years, and which have proved resistant to all other forms of treatment. Those prolonged intractable, disabling symptoms which respond best to surgery are tension, severe anxiety, chronic depression, and obsessional symptoms (Ingram et al 1981, Dally & Connolly 1981).

Techniques

The original neurosurgical procedure of standard leucotomy was performed 'blind' through burr-holes created in the temporal lobes. Present-day procedures utilize stereotactic techniques in which precision placement of instruments allows individual nerve tracts to be severed. These procedures aim to produce limited lesions in the limbic system or its connections. The limbic system is considered to be involved in feelings and emotions, and it is dysfunctions within this intricate system that give rise to disturbances of mood and some behaviour.

Performing the operation does not necessarily rid the individual of symptoms, but does produce a response to other treatments which had previously failed. Careful selection of people to ascertain suitability for treatment and likelihood of favourable response is imperative. Adequate follow-up and rehabilitation subsequent to the operation ensure assessment of response to further treatment, and observation of any other effects of surgery, such as personality changes, epilepsy, or persistence of original symptoms.

PHYSICAL DIAGNOSTIC INVESTIGATIONS

Compared with other branches of medicine, and other systems of the body, there are very few tests available to assist in diagnosing or assessing the effects of treatment in disturbances of mental health. The most common investigations in this area are primarily used either to exclude, or assess the degree of involvement of, physical illness as a causative agent. Non-invasive investigations in this category include computerized tomographic scanning (CT scans), X-rays, brain scans, and electroencephalography, and the recently developed techniques of nuclear magnetic resonance imaging (NMR) and positron emission tomography (PET). PET allows identification and location of metabolic changes in the brain in mental illness, and particularly organically induced changes. Readers should refer to other texts for details of these investigations. Routine blood examinations are also necessary to ensure that any disturbance of mental health is not the result of, or associated with, physical illness. Included in these routine tests are determination of the levels of electrolytes, creatinine, urea, vitamin B_{12} and folate, as well as a full blood examination. More specific tests often requested are liver function tests, blood glucose tests, thyroid function tests, drug screens, VDRL (to screen for the presence of venereal disease), and tests for the therapeutic serum levels of lithium carbonate and tricyclic antidepressant drugs.

Dexamethasone suppression test (DST)

One laboratory test that has been developed in recent years as a specific diagnostic aid in affective disorders is the dexamethasone suppression test. This test has resulted from knowledge gained in the study of links between neuroendocrine function and human behaviour (Carroll 1980, Langer 1979, Schlesser 1980).

In mentally healthy individuals and in those who have disturbances of mental health other than depression, the hypothalamus and portions of the limbic system produce corticotrophin releasing factor which stimulates the pituitary gland to release adrenocorticotropic hormone (ACTH). This then causes the adrenal cortex to release cortisol. High cortisol levels then inhibit the further release of ACTH. Synthetic glucocorticoids, of which dexamethasone is one, will also suppress production of ACTH and cortisol. In certain individuals with depressive illnesses, dexamethasone does not cause this suppression, there being instead a hypersecretion of cortisol with failure of the normal system of inhibition (Brown 1979, Brown & Shuey 1980, Carroll 1980).

Blood samples, to establish serum cortisol levels 17 and 24 hours after an oral dose of dexamethasone, reveal whether or not the individal is suppressing the release of cortisol. A positive test result (high cortisol levels) is 96% accurate in the diagnosis of a depressive illness; a negative result is non-significant and does not exclude the presence of a depressive illness. Various factors can produce a false-positive or false-negative result: high dose oestrogens, Cushing's syndrome, severe weight loss, hepatic enzyme induction, uncontrolled diabetes mellitus, major physical trauma, and fever will cause an increase in serum cortisol levels and produce false-positive results; false-negative results can be obtained in the presence of Addison's disease, corticosteroid therapy, hypopituitarism, and high dose benzodiazepine medications.

The clinical uses of this test are two-fold. Firstly, it facilitates the diagnosis of depression in individuals who are not displaying the typical symptoms of depressed mood — agitation or retardation, insomnia, weight loss, decreased appetite, fatigue, feelings of worthlessness, and thoughts of self-harm. Secondly, the test can be used to monitor recovery from depression and indicate when doses of antidepressant drugs can be reduced or ceased without fear of relapse of symptoms (Goldberg 1980). Some people may show clinical signs of recovery, but relapse quickly when the antidepressant therapy is reduced. A positive DST in these individuals would indicate the need to maintain antidepressant therapy, despite clinical signs of recovery, until normal cortisol levels were achieved.

REFERENCES

Appleton W S, Davis J M 1980 Practical clinical psychopharmacology, 2nd edn. Williams & Wilkins, Baltimore

Australian Bureau of Statistics 1977–1978 Australian health survey

Baldessarini R J 1980 Chemotherapy in psychiatry. In: Nicholi A (ed) The Harvard guide to modern psychiatry. Harvard University Press, Massachusetts

Brown A 1979 The 24-hour dexamethasone suppression tests in a clinical setting: relationship to diagnosis, symptoms, and response to treatment. American Journal of Psychiatry 136: 543–547

Brown W A, Shuey I 1980 Response to dexamethasone and subtype of depression. Archives of General Psychiatry 37: 747–751

Carrington-Smith D 1975 Do women need drugs to cope

with life? Women's health in a changing society. Commonwealth Department of Health 3: 240–3

Carroll B J 1980 Clinical application of neuroendocrine research in depression. In: Van Praag M (ed) Handbook of biological psychiatry, Vol 3. Dekker, New York

Cotman C W, Barker G Z, Zernetyer S F, McGaugh J L 1971 Electroshock effects on brain protein synthesis. Science 173: 454–456

Dally P, Connolly J 1981 An introduction to physical methods of treatment in psychiatry, 6th edn. Churchill Livingstone, Edinburgh

Davis J M, El-Yousef M K, Janowsky D S, Sekerke H J 1972 Treatment of benztropine toxicity with physostigmine. Fifth International Congress on Pharmacology 5:52

Engs R 1980 Drug use patterns of helping profession students in Brisbane, Australia. Drug and Alcohol Dependence 6: 231–246

Essman W B 1974 Effects of electroconvulsive shock on cerebral protein synthesis. In: Fink M, Kety S, McGaugh J, Tilliams T A (eds) Psychobiology of convulsive therapy. Winston, Washington DC

Freeman C P L 1979 Electroconvulsive therapy: its current clinical use. British Journal of Hospital Medicine 21: 281–292

Goldberg I K 1980 Dexamethasone suppression test as indicator of safe withdrawal of antidepressant therapy. Lancet No. 8164:376

Ingram I M, Timbury G C, Mowbray R M 1981 Notes on psychiatry, 5th edn. Churchill Livingstone, Edinburgh

Kety S S 1974 Biochemical and neurochemical effects of electroconvulsive shock. In: Fink M, Kety S S, McGaugh J, Williams T A (eds) Psychobiology of convulsive therapy. Winston, Washington DC

Kiloh L G 1983 Non-pharmacological treatments of psychiatric patients. Australian and New Zealand Journal of Psychiatry 17: 215–225

Kolb L C, Brodie H K 1982 Modern clinical psychiatry, 10th Edn. Saunders, Philadelphia

Lader M 1981 Benzodiazepines panacea or poison. Australian and New Zealand Journal of Psychiatry 15: 1–9

Lancaster N, Steinert R, Frost I 1958 Unilateral electroconvulsive therapy. Journal of Medical Science 221:104

Langer G 1979 Hyperactivity of hypothalamic-pituitary-adrenal axis in endogenous depression. Lancet No. 7985:524

Menuck M 1980 Unwanted effects of benzodiazepines tranquillisers. Modern Medicine of Australia 23 (12): 27–31

Meyler L 1975 Side effects of drugs, Vol 8. Excerpta Medica, Amsterdam

Meyler L 1979 In: Dukes M N G (ed) Side effects of drugs annual (1977–79). Excerpta Medica, Amsterdam

Meyler L, Herzheimer A 1972 Side effects of drugs, Vol 7. Excerpta Medica, Amsterdam

Roberts R (ed) 1984 Mims annual (Australian edition). IMS Publishing, Crows Nest

Royal College of Psychiatrists 1977 Memorandum on the use of electroconvulsive therapy. British Journal of Psychiatry 131:161

Schlesser N A 1980 Hypothalamic-pituitary-adrenal axis activity in depressive illness, its relationship to classification. Archives of General Psychiatry 37: 737–743

Weeks D, Freeman C P L, Kendell R E 1980 ECT III: Enduring cognitive deficits? British Journal of Psychiatry 137:16

Zisook S, De Vaul R A 1977 Adverse behavioural effects of benzodiazepines. Journal of Family Practice 5(6): 963–966

To live is to grow. All manner of life grows physically. And yet humans are more. They may grow intellectually. They may grow emotionally. They may put it all 'together' — physically, emotionally and intellectually — and find fulfilment in themselves and others. Or they may not.

Carkhuff, 1977

4

Interpersonal skills

THERAPEUTIC RELATIONSHIPS

One of the most important aspects of effective nursing care is the relationship between the nurse and the care-receiver. This is a special relationship, in no way casual, differing from simply making acquaintances as we would at a party or with our nursing peers. It is a therapeutic relationship in which the nurse, in the role of helper, attempts to assist the helpee towards, or in the maintenance of, optimal health.

This concept is neither as naive nor as simple as it at first seems. The role of helper is often construed as an acceptance of responsibility for the well-being of another. The nurse in this role makes decisions for the person in much the same way as a parent directs and controls a child. In fact, all too often the whole process of hospitalization is directed towards defining and maintaining this parent-child relationship. On admission the individual is in an alien environment, with little external control, and constantly receives directions that reinforce helplessness. Climbing into night attire and the hospital bed under orders is a re-enactment of the sick child role with which most of us are familiar and often willingly adopt. The nurse takes on the role of surrogate parent in carrying out basic activities such as bathing, powdering, providing food and reducing temperature for a passive care-receiver, all with rigid time-schedules that reduce personal decision-making. In a psychodynamic sense the 'patient role' involves an act of regression to helplessness.

This parent role exists as a part of all of us and is learned from our early experiences with parental figures (Harris 1969). It is not hard to understand how the parental role becomes integrated into the nursing role and supported by a health-care system that is largely institutional in nature. Similarly, helpless child behaviour is a part of the psychological repertoire into which we slip given the appropriate cues, such as being sick. One of the features of this relationship is that the responsibility for self is removed from the ill person and shifted to the nurse. In some cases this may be appropriate; but in most cases we should be looking towards shifting the responsibility for health back to the individual and fostering independence, along with decision-making, for self-care.

In the role of health catalyst the nurse adopts a more collegiate attitude, with the emphasis on being aware of the total individuality of each person. In the process of helping those with psychological problems, effectiveness depends very much on developing a therapeutic relationship.

Therapeutic aims

In very general terms the therapeutic aims of caring for people with psychological problems fit into two broad categories. These are

1. To assist the person in effectively changing aspects of self or life circumstances.
2. To maximize whatever potential exists, within certain physical, psychological or sociological constraints.

The person who is anxious or depressed may need to learn new life strategies to reduce tension or depression, or to confront an issue through to resolution. For such people, learning to be more assertive, reducing daily stress, and working through grief reactions are examples of therapeutic measures which attempt to achieve the aims arising from category 1. It may also be possible to achieve these aims with people suffering from more severe illnesses such as schizophrenia or affective psychosis, with strategies such as social skills training and reality-testing. With people who have some degree of dementia these aims may be unattainable. Considering the physical problems involved, the most that can be achieved might be to maintain a lower level of performance but at maximum potential, as in category 2. This may mean reinstating or maintaining good hygiene habits and an awareness of events in the immediate environment. In both cases the goal is to improve the individual's quality of life. Perls (1969) claims that, 'Everything is founded on awareness which is . . . the only basis of knowledge communication . . ... Awareness is the means to growth — the ability to function more completely and more effectively. The therapeutic relationship is directed towards helping others develop awareness of self, of those with whom they interact, and of the environment, and hence to grow.

One of the deficiencies in medical models of health and many problem-oriented health care models, is the emphasis on the individual's illness behaviour. Strategies of care can also be directed towards the development of whatever strengths the person may have. This is highly pertinent to the area of psychological growth, where it may be difficult to cure dementia, depression, self-destructive behaviour or alcoholism, but where other aspects of the person could be strengthened.

A question of terminology

Counselling and helping

The word 'counsellor' is normally used to describe a particular role such as staff counsellor, marriage guidance counsellor, or drug and alcohol counsellor. People who perform these functions usually have specific skills and knowledge related to their particular role. These usually include the ability to use various special therapeutic techniques that may be described as belonging to the rather broad field of psychotherapy. The word 'counselling', however, may be taken to mean 'creating a situation where the client's own resources can be mobilized where she can be enabled to make a decision and to take any necessary action herself' (Nurse 1975). Counsellors may also be described as being 'concerned with encouraging their clients to examine their attitudes and values and consider how these might be changed' (Venables 1971). The extent to which a person carries out these functions depends on individual skills. In fact, being aware of personal limitations enables the counsellor to be aware of the problems that are beyond his or her capabilities to manage.

Some writers such as Egan (1975) pefer to use the term 'helping' to describe what is essentially a therapeutic counselling process. 'Helping' is perhaps more descriptive than 'counselling', and certainly less dependent on role-definition.

Our initial description of nurse-helpee relationships involved the notion of their therapeutic nature. In the context of nursing those people with psychological problems, helping and counselling may be seen as synonymous. In the context of nursing as an overall concept, helping occurs by degree. Effective communication can be seen as the fundamental skill at any level of helping.

Patients, clients, and people

We have chosen not to use the words 'patient' or 'client' in this book to describe someone who is receiving help. This decision is based on a belief that the word 'patient' is usually taken to mean those people who have given up, for any number of reasons, their independence in terms of decision-making and responsibility for their return to health. In an attempt to avoid this nuance of passivity, we prefer 'person' or 'individual'.

The word 'client' refers to those people who seek out help but retain responsibility for their problem or situation (Nurse 1975) and who pay for services rendered. 'Client' is perhaps not inclusive enough to describe all those who receive help from others.

COMMUNICATION

The achievement of a therapeutic relationship and the realization of therapeutic aims depends on effective communication. This is true whatever the role of the nurse; from a simple supportive one to the rather more complex role of counsellor. Although we do a great deal of communicating, it should not be assumed that we are necessarily good at it all the time. Miscommunication among people is a common problem. In our everyday lives we make choices about the extent and content of our interaction with others. There is some semblance of control. In addition, most of us are aware of the style and form of communication that is appropriate in certain situations. This is something we learn from our past experience in interacting with others (Argyle 1978). In normal circumstances we do not evaluate our communication techniques in any depth, at least not at a conscious level, unless we become aware of problems or deficiencies.

In a therapeutic relationship a rather different view needs to be taken since, as helper, the nurse often takes the initiative in establishing effective communication in order to achieve certain therapeutic goals. The nurse cannot rely on automatic communication in its social sense, but has to be more cognizant of miscommunication and non-communication with the helpee. Nursing demands the special skills required to be effective in the area of human relations. According to Egan (1975), research indicates that people in helping professions are not necessarily skilled helpers in the area of human relations. These skills often need to be learned.

A communication model

There are three aspects of communication on which it is useful to concentrate: the process, the message, and influencing factors. A model which incorporates these facets is shown in Figure 4.1 and is adapted from a number of sources (Egan 1975, Taylor et al 1977, Argyle 1978, Berlo 1960).

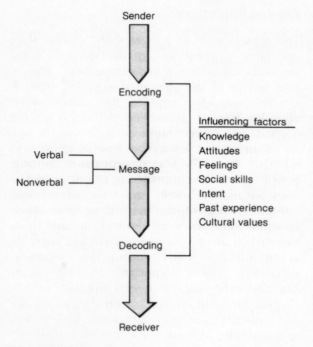

Fig. 4.1 Components of communication.

The Process

'Encoding' refers to the cognitive processes which occur in the mind of the sender of the message. There is usually intent in the communication, which may be to achieve a particular goal or need. On transmission of a message the receiver in turn relies on his cognitive processes to decode what he sees and hears. From the point of view of communication in general, and more particularly in helping, there are a number of possible ways in which miscommunication can occur. Specifically, these are in the encoding and decoding stages or in the actual transmission of the intended message.

The message

There are two principal ways in which we transmit messages to other people: by verbal, and by non-verbal means. 'Verbal communication' refers to our use of speech and its content. While words are a vital aspect of getting a message across, it appears that

60–80% of the actual meaning in speech is conveyed through non-verbal communication (Taylor et al 1977).

In its simplest sense, 'non-verbal communication' refers to body language involving such features as body posture, gestures, facial expression, eye gaze, non-linguistic aspects of speech like tone, pitch and rate, and bodily contact. Other important aspects are appearance, physical proximity, our physical orientation, and utterances (Argyle 1978). It is not difficult to appreciate the extent to which we communicate non-verbally. Emotions such as anger, fear, sorrow, and joy are often expressed much more powerfully through facial expression, body posture, or silence, than by speech, which often fails to express what is really being felt. Most of our first impressions of what people are like and what mood they are in are obtained through simple observation. The way we approach other people and our responses to them are guided by these impressions in an attempt to transmit an appropriate message. As such the process of communication is very much a learned skill of which there are varying levels of effectiveness. Most of us can think of times when we have misjudged what a person is feeling and have responded quite inappropriately.

Being aware of non-verbal behaviour and its implications can be of enormous value in helping. First, this awareness can help us to be more aware of distress signals others are giving out and generally more sensitive to their needs. Secondly, it is possible to approach others more appropriately, being aware of what they are 'saying' non-verbally. Thirdly, the helper can control personal non-verbal behaviour and communicate a more open, accepting, helpful and non-judgemental attitude. In achieving this attitude the helper is opening the communication door by becoming approachable and reducing threat.

Verbal effectiveness can be measured by both content and style. What the communicator says can turn the other person away or draw him or her closer. Style involves the way in which a person presents verbally. Communication is adversely affected by mumbling, not finishing sentences, speaking too softly or loudly, pronounced accents that are difficult to understand, rapid or slow speech, and excessive domination of actual speaking time. It is useful for helpers to evaluate their verbal presentation from time to time. This can be achieved in a number of ways: by peers, video playback techniques, or by engaging in communication sessions that enable feedback to be obtained.

Influencing factors

There are a great number of factors that influence the effectiveness of communication, and some of these are shown in Figure 4.1. In the position of helper the nurse can make best use of the effects of these influences and hence facilitate effective two-way transactions.

Table 4.1 summarizes a number of potential barriers to effective communication. The lifting of these barriers is important at any level of the helping relationship between nurse and helpee: the same communication skills apply whether we are taking someone's temperature, bathing them, or helping the dying. However, in helping those with

Table 4.1 Barriers to communication

The nurse (helper)	The person (helpee)	The environment
Pre-judgement of the person	Lack of trust in helper	Other people
Attitude to the person	Attitude to the helper	Noise (distraction)
Inappropriate mood	Excessive emotional distress	Tension
Excessive stress or anxiety	Physical discomfort	Alien environment
Indifference	Misunderstanding of helper's role	Interruptions
Fatigue	'Patient' role	
Preoccupation with other matters (either emotional or practical)	Lack of knowledge about condition or circumstances	
Physical discomfort		

psychological problems, the consequences of poor communication and poor helping (in a psychological sense) are of even greater potential import.

HELPING SKILLS

In the following discussion we shall identify some of the skills that can be used by the nurse to facilitate communication with others. Their application will be explored in the context of helping or counselling those with psychological problems.

The art of listening

Attending

Attending refers to the skill of being able to convey a sense of being with or being open to another person. Carkhuff (1977) identifies attending with freeing the other person to express himself or herself. It is an act of openness on the part of the helper that contributes to establishing trust on the part of the helpee, without which a relationship will not be formed. Although the helper may be consciously manipulating the communication process, attending is in no way artificial nor does it involve pretence. It is vital to be actually interested and eager to listen, both of which may be subsumed under the label 'caring' as described earlier in this chapter.

Non-verbal components of listening

The helper should face the other person squarely and maintain an open posture. In contrast, non-verbal messages of indifference, anxiety, or being guarded, are given by folding the arms across the chest (this is also an aggressive sign), or adopting a position that appears temporary — as if the helper is ready to escape. Desks, bed tables, or other similar physical barriers do not facilitate openness. Although many nursing administrators still frown on the practice, sitting on the person's bed is most appropriate; but if this is not possible, sitting on a chair is the next best thing. Sitting down suggests availability and creates an optimum 'climate' for communication to take place. This attitude may be compared to standing at a distance, watching the clock, and looking around as if much too busy to listen carefully.

It is also important not to sit too close or too far away from the person. Being too close may create tension by violating normally accepted social standards of physical proximity. Excessive closeness is associated with intimacy and aggression (Argyle 1972), both of which may cause anxiety. Leaning slightly forward is a listening posture that displays interest. As Carkhuff (1977) puts it, 'when we posture ourselves for others, we tend to think of others. When we posture ourselves for our own comfort and convenience, we tend to think of ourselves.'

If the nurse wishes to maintain the power of position, this will be communicated by standing or sitting higher than the helpee, folding arms, and being obviously temporarily involved. To be open is to abandon the position of power and to allow a partnership and interaction to develop.

The use of eye contact is a major component in effecting and maintaining interpersonal interaction. A listener tends to look at a speaker when interested in what is being said. The speaker looks from time to time at the listener to confirm that the listener is in fact listening, and gives slight pauses that offer the opportunity for the listener to react. This reaction is either affirmatory or confirmatory. Good listening involves good eye contact. Active listening gestures such as appropriate nods and utterances are similarly important.

The helper should be relaxed. This excludes fidgeting, breaking of eye contact, nervous laughter, clearing the throat, and a closed posture. Relaxation should not be confused, however, with informality.

Non-verbal effectiveness depends very much on awareness of oneself and overcoming barriers that may be a part of our normal interpersonal repertoire. As Egan

(1975) states, 'The high level helper knows, at least instinctively, what he is doing with his body. He knows that his body has impact value on the relationship. He is aware that his body does communicate, and he uses it to communicate . . .'

Reflective listening

There are three goals involved in skilled reflective listening. These are

1. To let the person know the helper is listening.
2. To ensure that the helper transmits an understanding of the helpee's message.
3. To encourage further self-disclosure and self-explanation on the part of the helpee.

Expressing an understanding of what is being said is achieved by simply asking the person for clarification, 'Are you saying that . . .?' or making an accurate statement such as, 'You are saying that . . .'. Paraphrasing also may provide both the speaker and listener with the opportunity to reflect on what has been said. In some respects this skill is similar to summarizing a book or article in which the principal points are identified. Another advantage with paraphrasing is that it can bring the person back from a tangent to an important point or issue. Clarification and paraphrasing are sometimes described as 'reflective listening'.

A willingness to listen further is transmitted by the helper saying, 'Please go on', and asking appropriate questions for clarification. People often feel as if they are being a nuisance or inconsiderate by talking so much and burdening the helper with their worries. This is particularly true of people in hospital who think they are taking up too much of the nurse's time. Encouraging further self-disclosure will help negate this and facilitate the development of a trusting relationship.

If the helper's responses are to be effective in generating self-exploration and awareness they need to be based on what the helper is hearing from and seeing in the person.

Responding to cues

It is an interesting, but understandable, feature of human communication that we do not always say exactly what we mean. This is particularly true when an element of risk is involved in exposing the real self to someone in whom total trust has not been developed. A statement of feeling anxious, for example, may be construed as weakness and hence leave the person open to ridicule. Another fear is that of rejection after having taken the risk of self-disclosure. In addition it is sometimes uncomfortable to talk about feelings since it brings the helpee even closer to awareness, and we often avoid this, preferring to talk in more concrete or abstract terms.

Current distress, the anticipation of distress, or a particular worry may not be openly referred to by a person. Instead of saying, 'I'm really frightened about this heart attack and what are my chances?', a person might provide a cue to this distress by laughingly asking, 'I suppose that wavy line on that machine means I'm alive?' In another example, someone who is wanting the results of a pathology test for cancer may keep asking when the result will be available, perhaps demonstrating a degree of anxiety. These cues could easily be dismissed by a nurse as simple factual questions and an opportunity to discuss the individual's real concerns lost. It is also quite possible that a particular nurse will be singled out by a person as someone with whom it might be safe to share feelings. In failing to hear what is really being said, an opportunity may be lost for ever in the fast-moving environment of a general hospital.

Porritt (1984) calls this 'listening for the music of the message, not just the content'. If the music is heard, then an appropriate response such as 'You sound a bit worried about . . .' or 'How do you feel about . . .' can be made. The non-verbal behaviour of the person usually aids interpretation of a verbal cue. If the nurse is not at first accurate, this will soon be discovered, and nothing will be lost; it is more likely that much will be gained. Many other verbal and behavioural cues of distress are discussed in the second part of this book.

Empathy

Empathy involves understanding the other person's experience — to '. . . get inside the other person', and to '. . . look at the world through the perspective or frame of reference of the other person, and get a feeling for what the other's world is like' (Egan 1975). More simply put, it is feeling *with* the other person, and may be contrasted with sympathy, which is feeling *for* another or being '. . . simultaneously affected with the same feeling' (Nurse 1975). This is an important distinction, since empathy is an effort to understand the other person, while sympathy is an expression of the sympathizer's feelings. As Porritt (1984) suggests, a sympathetic reaction involves the breaking down of personal boundaries and being '. . . swamped in another person's reality and experience.' Sympathy debilitates the helper in a number of ways:

- Making the helper so aware of his or her own feelings that understanding of the helpee is prevented.
- Interfering with the objectivity that may be required to truly help someone else.
- Creating stress in the helper which may accumulate over time, resulting in a personal stress reaction. It is possible that 'helper burnout', in which the nurse becomes personally detached from others, may be a mechanism of self-protection from excessive emotional involvement — an effect of oversympathizing. (This is not to say that nurses should, or indeed could, remain emotionally involved. Rather it is a question of being able to deal effectively with our own feelings in a helping role.)·

Empathy is much more helpful to others. Carkhuff (1977) suggests that, having heard what has been said, the helper should ask self the question, 'If I were this person and were doing and saying these things, how would I feel?' Having done this, the feeling should then be translated into a mutually understandable expression and then the accuracy of the observation checked. For example

Helper: 'You seem to feel angry that such a thing should have happened.'

Helpee: 'Yes, I do feel angry. Really angry at what's happened since I've been here.'

The helper is not only demonstrating good listening and developing a more trusting and open relationship, but also facilitating self-exploration through emphasizing the feeling state of the person, bringing it out into the open.

A common misconception regarding empathy is that it is necessary to actually have undergone the same experience as someone in order to empathize. This is not true: it is a matter of understanding *how* a person feels rather than having a qualitative or quantitative knowledge of the actual feeling itself. So when someone says, 'You don't know how I feel', it is reasonable and empathic to say, 'Not exactly, no. But I can understand why you feel the way you do.'

Respect

Showing respect involves demonstrating concern and caring for the person who is troubled. Components of respect include being warm, accepting, non-judgemental, fully attentive, and not jumping to conclusions too readily, or giving quick, largely inappropriate solutions to problems. Respect involves seeing the other person as important and his perspective and choice of problem-solving alternative as worthwhile.

Warmth is displayed by touch, physical proximity, and facial expression. Its antithesis is best described as aloofness and lack of concern. Non-verbal signs of wanting to leave and get on with something else are a trap into which many nurses fall in busy hospital wards. Attempting to show helpful concern for what someone is saying is incongruent with the image of the busy nurse. Too often the person

in hospital is heard to say, 'Yes, it was important. But the poor nurses were too busy, I didn't want to bother them.' Hospitals are often seen as sterile places and individuals learn all too quickly that there is no place for the expression of feelings or posing apparently unsolvable problems.

Suspending judgement is sometimes difficult when the other person has values and beliefs that differ from our own. Similarly, positive judgements may quickly be made when we find personal similarities. Approval and disapproval may inhibit growth and self-exploration on the part of the person seeking help. The helper should accept him as personally worthwhile without being clouded by judgements, particularly those hastily made.

Another common mistake, when confronted with a distressed person or someone who has decided to talk about a problem, is to try to find quick, easy solutions. This usually consists of the helper making some sort of interpretation of the cause of the problem and providing the answer. The person verbalizes agreement, 'I guess you might be right' and, sensing the helper is in a hurry, withdraws with a smile. Not only are the interpretation and solution probably wrong but there has been no internalization or exploration on the helpee's part, simply because there was no opportunity. Respect involves helping the other person make causal relationships and take responsibility for making decisions regarding self. The effective helper does not act for the helpee but mobilizes the person's resources for self action (Egan 1975).

When the helpee makes some sort of constructive move the helper can reinforce this behaviour by being genuinely positive. Similarly, negative behaviours should not be judged or simply accepted by a helper, but explored. For example:

Helpee: 'My wife visited last night but I didn't mention my worries about our finances like I was going to.'

The inappropriate response would be, 'Well, that's alright. Maybe tonight.', since it condones avoidance. More appropriate would be, 'How do you feel about that?' or 'Did you find mentioning the problem too difficult?' These responses enable greater exploration by looking at reasons and feelings.

Being constructively open

Openness requires the helper to give of self and to engage in a two-way communication with the other person: the helper does not hide behind the role of nurse or counsellor and is sincere and non-defensive. This requires a degree of self-awareness and security in the helper; removing barriers to self and being open is usually restricted in our society to close relationships. It is interesting that over the last ten to twenty years psychologists and others have turned their attention to providing the public with tools for living more fulfilling lives. Most of them resemble the skills required for effective helping. This has prompted some writers to describe them as 'interpersonal skills' (Egan 1975), since they affect daily living rather than just the helping process.

To be open, the helper shows real concern rather than just going through the motions of helping as if it were a duty. Reactions to the speaker must be honest so that there is no risk of incongruity.

A most powerful technique is for the helper to report his or her own relevant experiences and feelings to the helpee. The important point here is to take care not to take the focus away from the helpee and in effect to change roles. This disclosing of oneself is an important strategy in developing trust; it cements the relationship further and enables the helpee to compare his feelings with someone else's, and to reflect on the comparison. A more equal relationship is facilitated in this way, with both parties accepting each other on the same communication level.

Concreteness

Statements made by the helpee are concrete if they are specific rather than vague. Specificity applies to feelings, situations, and to behavioural reactions. The skill of the helper lies in enhancing self-exploration (our goal) by assisting the helpee to examine vague statements more deeply.

'I don't feel well', is a vague statement. Asking the person to be more specific may lead to concrete descriptions of feelings such as, 'I feel really anxious'. Further exploration may lead to situational concreteness. 'It tends to happen when I'm not in control of situations.' A concrete statement of behavioural reaction might reveal, 'When I feel like this I tend to get aggressive with people.'

These concrete statements reveal quite a iot of information on which to base further self-exploration and action. It would then be possible to be more specific about feeling anxious, to explore situatioins in which loss of control is experienced, and to look at actual situations in which aggressiveness has occurred.

Confronting

One of the side-effects of self-exploration is coming across knowledge about ourselves which makes us uncomfortable or anxious; it is often easier to avoid confronting the knowledge by evasion or by blocking it out in some way. Vagueness, contradictions, discrepancies, incongruity between verbal and non-verbal expressions, and talking around something are examples of evasion.

The helper can confront the helpee constructively by gently pointing out these tactics and attempting to bring the subject out into the open. Confrontation can be very destructive if approached in an attacking, judgemental way that fails to acknowledge how the helpee is likely to feel. Similarly, attempting to provide what amount to explanations for the other person's behaviour is not helpful. In these cases the helpee will become defensive, close up, and lose confidence in the relationship. Below are two examples of fairly simple confronting.

1. 'You say you feel fine but you don't look very happy when you say it.'

2. 'If I recall correctly, earlier on you said you didn't mind if your husband left you and now you say you'll do something desperate if he does. What does this mean?'

It can be seen from these examples that confrontation may quickly open doors and enable action. Since confrontation may lead to emotional responses, the helper must be prepared to help the person deal with his feelings and explore the issue through to resolution.

Encouraging action

The principal function of self-exploration is to facilitate behaviour change that in some way improves the quality of life. In the process of helping, the role of the helper is to encourage decision-making on the part of the helpee and to support the application of decisions in the real-life situation.

The first step in encouraging action is to enable the helpee to determine achieveable goals. Many people who seek help are in conflict, and the actual problem is a failure to decide on a course of action. In these cases reaching this stage may occur only after considerable self-exploration and perhaps emotional pain. A good example of this type of situation is marital breakdown. Frequently one or both partners wish the marriage to end but find making this decision very difficult due to guilt, insecurity, and fear of the unknown. The desire to end the relationship remains unconscious and unhappiness with the situation becomes symptomatic, resulting in such activities as extra-marital affairs, working late, drinking, or in illness such as anxiety or depression. Helping the client to decide what he really wants is not achieved quickly. In other cases a person may seek help with a goal in mind, (such as being more assertive), or wanting to deal with a particular situation.

The value in stating goals is that both the helpee and helper will know what they are aiming for, and can explore change that will achieve the goal. Both will also be able to identify when they have achieved that goal.

Action requires going further than goal-setting and involves specifying particular behaviours that will achieve goals. These behaviours should be achievable by the individual and where possible should begin by utilizing existing strengths. Success is positively reinforcing and initial steps should be small rather than large. An example may help to demonstrate this point.

Let us suppose a person with a stress-related illness realises that he has been working too hard; this has resulted in deteriorating family relationships, and a certain amount of guilt on his part. He acknowledges that he is a chronic over-achiever and would like to change. A goal here might be for him to talk his problem over with his family in much the same way as he has with the helper. His family is his strength, and by obtaining their support he will be operating from strength. If he thinks that too much self-exposure might be too threatening, he can start by discussing how stress has contributed to his illness. The next step could be to explain how he would like to work less and spend more time at home. Finally, an expression of responsibility might be risked.

Once this has been achieved he can make some decisions about how to reduce his workload. This should include exploring the effects of such a decision on lifestyle, and identifying alternatives to work. The achievement of decisions such as changing jobs or discussing the problem with the boss, for example, can be discussed in terms of their effect on the individual. Reinforcement should come from improved relationships within the family, assuming this was the cause for breakdown, but the helper provides reinforcement by pointing out how goals have been achieved.

In some cases it may be appropriate to set time-limits for achieving certain goals. Assertiveness training programmes frequently consist of practising certain skills within set time-frames and evaluating success at their completion.

POTENTIAL PROBLEMS IN HELPING

Rescuing

One of the potential traps for helpers is that of searching out people to help. This usually involves making the assumption that someone with a problem needs help and then acting by confronting the person as a helper. People with problems do not always require help, and if they do will chose who they want to consult. The helper is better occupied fostering a relationship which allows the other person the opportunity to seek help and the freedom to decide when.

Advice

Advice involves providing solutions to problems and has the problem of not involving any growth on the part of the helpee, as well as shifting responsibility for decisions to the helper. If the solution fails, as it might, the person may blame the helper. The object of helping, so far as we see it, should be to enable the helpee to make decisions and take responsibility for them.

Advice is all too easy to give when time is short and often is given when the nurse is in a hurry to find a solution to a problem. There is no place for quick solutions in counselling situations, and the helpee should reach conclusions without pressure from the helper. Another point worth noting is that the helper's solutions come from a personally different perspective of the world and hence are unlikely to be helpful. People are also more likely to act in a determined way if a decision is one of their own choosing.

Transference

This very important emotional reaction is usually mentioned in relation to psychotherapy and, more particularly, psychoanalysis. Transference involves shifting of feelings that the helpee has towards significant people in his life toward the helper. Very strong transferences can lead to reactions such as overdependence or infatuation on the part of the helpee. A mildly positive transference of course will facilitate the relationship. A negative transference involves reactions such as antagonism or even open hostility towards the helper. In psychotherapy the therapist may sometimes confront the individual with the transference. If the nurse suspects that a strong transference is occurring he or she should seek guidance from an experienced therapist on how to manage the situation.

Counter-transference occurs when the helper develops strong attitudes or feelings to the helpee. Rather than being potentially useful, counter-transference interferes with the therapeutic relationship on which the helping process is based.

Over-identification

Like counter-transference, over-identification involves the feelings of the helper and is commonly seen in nursing staff. We are said to identify with another person when we can see personal likenesses in values, behaviour, or attitudes. Young people are more likely to identify with each other than with an older person. It is also possible to identify with the emotional reactions of other people, e.g. the sadness related to the loss of someone close.

Over-identification is excessive identification in which the helper's judgement is impaired by closely mimicking the values or emotions of another. In the process of over-identifying, a helper may actually interfere with the treatment programme by identifying with non-compliance or suicidal desires, for example, and reinforce these behaviours.

UNDERSTANDING SELF

One of the most important things that a person contributes to the helping relationship is self. The ability to use the skills we have mentioned here depends a great deal on less tangible attributes such as sensitivity and self-confidence. The ability to relate freely and to allow oneself to be open to others are life skills not always easily obtained. Helpers need to grow and it is important to take opportunities to develop awareness when they arise. This can be done by reading, attending courses, and listening and watching other more experienced therapists at their work, as well as by self-reflection.

Behavioural change is always a slow process; but the more we want to grow, and the more we take notice of ourselves and of others, the greater the likelihood that change will occur.

REFERENCES

Argyle M 1978 The psychology of interpersonal behaviour. Penguin, Harmondsworth

Berlo D 1960 The process of communication. Holt Rhinehart & Winston, New York

Carkhuff R R 1977 The art of helping III. Human Resource Development Press, Amherst

Egan G 1975 The skilled helper. Brooks Cole, California

Harris T A 1969 I'm OK, you're OK. Pan Books, Sydney

Nurse G 1975 Counselling and the nurse. H M & M, Aylesbury

Perls F J 1969 Gestalt therapy verbatim. Real People Press, Moab

Porritt L 1984 Communication: choices for nurses. Churchill Livingstone, Melbourne

Taylor A, Rosegrant T, Meyer A, Samples B T 1977 Communicating. Prentice Hall, Englewood Cliffs

Venables E 1971 Counselling. National Marriage Guidance Council, London

Once at 3000 feet, standing outside the plane on a platform the size of a licence plate, hands permanently affixed to the strut, the organism applied one more last ditched effort to deal with this prolonged, over taxing state of strain. I became totally immobile. I could not jump and I could not go back into the plane. My instructor gave me a push and after a momentary confusion of lines and fabric flapping, I looked up and saw the parachute open wide and full above me. This had to be a true dynamic equilibrium. I floated totally relaxed and isolated, alone with myself and the beauty of the air and the view, for approximately four minutes. The silence was extraordinary; my senses were very acute. I landed without much difficulty and that day made a sincere and lifelong promise to myself: never jump out of a perfectly good airplane.

Baldwin, 1980

5
Stress

ADAPTATION

One of the most important characteristics of the human body, as in all living organisms, is the ability to respond to changing internal and external stimuli. As a stimulus changes it acts as a cue (monitored by the nervous and endocrine systems) for a response which will maintain body homeostatis. Sensitivity to change is an important property, because cellular damage or death will quickly ensue if the organism's delicate structural or functional balance is disturbed beyond certain limits. For example, fluctuations in the external environmental temperature result in physiological responses that keep internal body temperature within an optimal range. A sudden bright light causes the pupils to constrict and we may turn our head to protect the retina.

Not all stimulus-response relations involve simple automatic physiological mechanisms. Conscious and unconscious psychological factors complicate this issue by becoming cues for a physiological response. A simple example would be the decision to go for a jog, which once acted upon causes a multitude of physiological changes. Similarly, decisions to relax, smoke cigarettes, or act purposefully in any way, affect us in myriad ways. Less obvious are unconscious drives, the nature of which is still the matter of some controversy (described in more detail in Chapter 1). Taking one model as an example, we might consider the needs for affiliation, positive self-esteem, love, and self-actualization (Maslow 1970) as normal psychological drives.

The prediction of likely responses to certain stimuli is a challenge that confronts both physiologists and psychologists alike; a host of factors, tending to vary from individual to individual, results in variable responses. These factors include: physical attributes, health status and status and resistance to disease, the immediate environment, mental abilities, mental state, knowledge, experience, and social conditioning. Understanding individual variation is an aspect of understanding people and, as we have seen in Chapter 1, it is important in the effective delivery of health care.

There is never a moment in our lives when demand is not placed on our bodies; the absence of demand signifies death. 'Stress' is the name given to the body's response to demand as it attempts to adapt to changing stimuli. This response is '. . . manifested by a specific syndrome which consists of all the non-specifically induced changes within a biologic system' (Selye 1976). As we shall see, these changes involve a varying degree of automatic and endocrine activity, producing a number of observable, and subjectively felt effects. Stimuli which cause this response are known as 'stressors'

A useful way of conceptualizing stress is as a continuum (Fig. 5.1), ranging in intensity and related to a number of states.

Some stress is obviously beneficial; short bursts of moderate stress energize the body, and a high stress response may be life-saving. It is towards excessive and prolonged stress that doctors, nurses, psychologists and others have turned their attention in recent years, so that it is now seen as a major pathophysiological agent. It is of particular relevance to

nurses because of their potential role in stress prevention and management, both at the bedside and in the community. In addition, there is the need for nurses to understand the stress inherent in their own profession and to take steps to reduce its deleterious effects.

A REVIEW OF THE PHYSIOLOGY OF STRESS

Most of us are familiar with a sudden external threat to our physical safety.

> The urgent, strident shock wave of a car horn shakes you out of your day-dream a yard off the kerb. The heart pounds in the chest and throat, the mouth goes dry, a pallor accompanies a sense of blood draining away, the stomach lurches and the breath comes quickly. Despite these uncomfortable sensations, the almost reflexive leap back onto the pavement saves you as the car screeches past.

This phenomenon is known universally as the 'fight or flight' response and occurs automatically in the face of an external threat to provide energy for muscular effort. The threat will either be avoided or met head on to force it away. Cognitive input is demonstrated by the fact that we realize it is important to avoid fast moving vehicles rather than to confront them physically.

Awareness of a threat results in the hypothalamus stimulating both the sympathetic nervous system and the release of hormones such as antidiuretic hormone (ADH) and adrenocorticotrophic hormone (ACTH) from the pituitary gland. These sympathetic and hormone responses are summarized in Table 5.1.

This homeostatic mechanism is designed to release glucose in a useable form, to provide oxygen, and to direct both in large quantities to cardiac and skeletal muscle. At a cellular level oxygen is used in the aerobic stage of glucolysis (oxidative phosphorylation) to release the large amounts of energy essential for sudden action.

From the point of view of maintaining body integrity the 'fight or flight' response is essential for survival. There are other causes of what Selye (1976) has called the 'alarm reaction', such as sustained physical

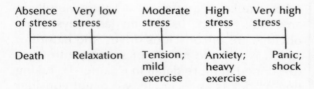

Absence of stress	Very low stress	Moderate stress	High stress	Very high stress
Death	Relaxation	Tension; mild exercise	Anxiety; heavy exercise	Panic; shock

Fig. 5.1 The stress continuum.

Table 5.1 The alarm reaction

Response	Effect	Sensation or sign
Increased heart rate Increased stroke volume	Increase in cardiac output to circulate O_2 and glucose to cells	Feeling of heart pounding in chest and throat; raised blood pressure
Coronary blood vessels dilate	Increase O_2 to heart as its workload increases	—
Peripheral vasoconstriction	Diverts blood to vital organs; indirectly raised blood pressure	Palor; increased blood pressure
Musculoskeletal vasodilation	Increases blood supply to muscles	—
Gastrointestinal shutdown	Diverts blood to vital organs	'Butterflies' or feeling of stomach contracting.
Decreased secretions	Parasympathetic nervous system response is over-ridden by sympathetic nervous system	Dry mouth
Bronchodilation and hyperpnoea	Increase O_2 intake	Increased respirations
Increased blood flow to the brain	Increase mental alertness for quick decision-making	Increased sensory awareness
Dilation of pupils	Increased visual activity	Dilated pupils
Adrenaline release	Is a sympathomimetic and releases glucose stores; increases mental altertness	A feeilng of tension and being hyperalert
Cortisol secretion	Increased fat metabolism to realise energy; anti-flammatory response.	—
Decreased renal blood flow	Divert blood to vital organs and retain water; stimulates renin production	Increased blood pressure
Increased renin production	Raises blood pressure	Increased blood pressure
Sweating; contraction of bladder and bowels and relaxation of spincters	Parasympathetic activity increased	Frequency of micturition; need to defaecate

demand on the body in illness, strenuous exercise, and psychological stressors. Remember the last time you sat an examination or had a personal confrontation. The feelings were probably very much the same as when you had a fright. These are examples of psychological stressors that result in the same physiological reaction described above. Important in this is the relationship between cortical activity and the more primitive limbic centres such as the hypothalamus. If psychological factors can produce a stress response, then it can be argued that psychological factors can reduce it through cognitive effort. Relaxation training is an example of this mechanism (Benson 1975, Meares 1969).

The physiological reactions described above form the basis of the syndrome which is the stress response. In many cases the process subsides once the threat disappears or is removed and the body returns to normal. It is when the process is sustained that problems seem to occur, and it is with these effects that the next section is concerned.

STRESS AND ILL-HEALTH

Prolonged or intense stress has long been known as a significant factor in both physical and mental ill-health. The gastric ulcer was for many years the traditional stress disorder and part of the image of the go-ahead achiever. Greater interest and research into the pathophysiology of stress has shown it to play a rather broader role in ill-health (Seyle &

Garfield 1979, Wilson-Barnett 1979). Seyle has attempted to account for this relationship by describing what he calls the 'general adaptation syndrome', which consists of three stages.

1. *The alarm reaction.* An increase in hormone levels and an enlargement of the adrenal cortex and lymphatic system (see Table 5.2).
2. *Stage of resistance.* Prolonged demand results in various derangements of a number of hormones, and faulty adaptation. The most significant feature of this stage is the release of corticoids under the control of ACTH; these may either be anti-inflammatory or pro-inflammatory hormones which are normally functional in body defence. Cortisol, an anti-inflammatory hormone, tends to suppress the immune response, making the body more prone to the effects of antigens. Pro-inflammatory hormones cause general irritation of tissues, thereby encouraging disease.
3. *Stage of exhaustion.* This stage occurs because of the inability of the body to continue adapting to prolonged stress.

An understanding of the physiology of stress provides relatively simple explanations of the pathophysiology of disease. Table 5.2 is not intended to be exhaustive but does provide a picture of the possible links between stress and disease.

It is not difficult to see how, coupled with other causative agents, stress can contribute to disease. Examples are given below.

The middle-aged man whose father died early of myocardial infarction, who smokes twenty cigarettes a day, is obese, and who is under prolonged moderate stress is a strong candidate for heart disease.

A young woman who has fair skin but sunbathes regularly, to the extent of getting burnt, over a period of twelve months, loses a child due to cot death, and separates from her husband. She develops a malignant melanoma on her shoulder.

An elderly lady is placed unwillingly in a nursing home by her well-meaning family. Previously mentally well, she becomes confused, disoriented and depressed over a period of three months; eventually she is persistently incontinent and bedridden.

A young man at a routine medical check up is found to have a significantly high blood pressure. Follow-up shows he is suffering from a severe anxiety state following the death of his mother twelve months previously. Excessive drinking is compounding his blood pressure problem. Over a period of two years he develops renal disease and cardiac myopathy; his anxiety state fails to subside, as does his drinking.

A young Chinese student develops an acute psychotic reaction with profound thought disorder and bizarre hallucinations. It is discovered that he is about to sit university examinations and has been studying almost around the clock for two months. Following treatment, and after passing the exams, this is the only episode of overt mental illness he ever develops. The need to succeed as a culturally determined phenomenon, and lack of sleep and adequate nutrition worked together to cause him to succumb.

The interesting feature of stress-related disorders, highlighted by the cases outlined above, is their idiosyncratic nature. Certain disorders will affect certain people, depending on a host of individual factors which may be physical, psychological, or social. In addition, the degree of reaction to a particular stressful situation is variable: a baby's crying may induce only mild irritation in some mothers, and passive calm in others, yet in the occasional case it results in impulsive violence against the child. Bereavement will cause some degree of stress in all of us, but for some it will lead to severe depression or anxiety that is not easily resolved. A more easily understood example is the way in which some people are able to resist severe illness and survive, yet another person lacks the physical or mental attributes to fight off a far less dangerous disease.

With this in mind, we now turn to the notion of stressors, the causes of stress.

Table 5.2 Stress and disease

Response to stress	Disease state
Cortisol secretion	Decreased immune response results in ability to combat antigens hence susceptibility to infection and neoplasia
Increased blood clotting and increased circulating fat	Thrombosis
Increased cardiac workload	Cardiac problems
Increased fibrillatory threshold	Cardiac arrythmias
Increased stroke volume, vasoconstriction and renin production	Hypertension
Pro-inflammatory response	Allergies, gastrointentinal disorders
Increased blood sugar	Diabetes mellitus
Decreased potassium	Cardiac arrhythmias
Increased sodium retention	Fluid retention
Central nervous system stimulation	Psychotic and neurotic symptoms. Impulse behaviours, personality change, mental strain

Stressors

Awareness of the problem of stress and being able to identify our personal stressors is perhaps the most important element in preventing its ill effects. It is a matter of being able to take measures towards prevention if you know that the potential for a problem exists. These measures will be even more successful if identification occurs before the presentation of unwanted responses. This approach has popularized the awareness of stressors far beyond the medical field to the pages of popular magazines. This indicates an increasing community awareness about health and disease as well as a tendency on the part of health workers to demystify their work.

Stressors may be categorized into two broad groups: physical and psychological.

Physical stressors

Acute illness may create a stress reaction as the demand on the body increases and the fight to restore balance intensifies. The classic example of this phenomenon is the development of Curling's ulcer, which may occur only a few hours after prolonged insult to the body as in the case of severe burns.

Physical illness may also result in any number of psychological reactions. It is not uncommon for elderly people who sustain fractures and are hospitalized to develop confusion, disorientation, or depression in the absence of other causes such as fat embolism.

Excessive physical activity in conjunction with factors such as being ill-prepared, or not having sufficient rest, is also a stressor. The body needs time to adjust itself to exercise and also needs time to recuperate. Grandmother's warnings of the dangers of 'burning the candle at both ends' are not far wide of the mark. Perhaps the reader can remember a time when too many late nights and early mornings eventually resulted in tonsillitis, a cold sore, or an attack of the common cold.

Psychological stressors

We have already discussed the relationship between the cerebral cortex and the hypothalamus. It would seem that a psychological threat will also precipitate the general adaptation syndrome and eventual ill-health.

The most obvious stressors involve some danger to our general understanding of ourselves or the world around us. Self-esteem, prestige, self-image, control, and sense of affiliation are examples of components of our psyche that may be endangered by life events. The perceived intensity of particular threats varies among individuals. Of the subconscious stessors, guilt is a very powerful learned stimulus for conflict and resulting stress.

Stressors can involve, however, any factor that causes change in our lives. Any change, positive or negative, results in a demand. Decisions to change jobs or buy a new house are usually conscious efforts to improve our lives and would be described by most as being good changes. It has been suggested, however, that a significant amount of stress will still be generated (Benson 1975). Personally threatening changes, such as separation or divorce, are quite clear stressors to our self-esteem; but few people would realize that marriage is similarly stressful, although for other reasons. Benson (1975) states that a stressor involves conditions that require some behavioural adjustment. In this sense, as creatures of habit, uncertainty is a very powerful stressor for many of us. Some people are in a constant state of anticipatory anxiety, the body and mind in a continuously energized condition.

Another important feature of stressors is that we may be able to withstand change from time to time, but that several changes occurring together may have a cumulative effect. The Holmes & Rahe 'social readjustment scale' (1967) gives examples of stressful life events and an outline for assessment of their cumulative effect (Table 5.3). Each life event is given a score, and it is postulated that the higher the score in any one year, the more likely it is that an individual will succumb to an overwhelming stress reaction. Scores were obtained from the self-evaluation of 394 people.

Hospitalization, apart from the effects of the illness itself, is a significant stressor for most people. Loss of independence, break in normal relationships, the formal relationships of hospital life, strange equipment and noises, and the personal indignities involved in care are some general features of hospitalization that produce stress (Chilver 1978, Keane 1978, Dossett 1978). Wilson-Barnett & Carrigy (1978) identified five groups of people likely to develop anxiety and depression. These are

1. Those with characteristically high levels of anxiety and depression-proneness.
2. Females under 40 years of age.
3. Those not having been previously hospitalized.
4. Those admitted for a series of special tests.
5. Those with a 'neoplastic', 'infective' or 'undiagnosed' illness.

Tables 5.3 The social readjustment rating scale (After Holmes & Rahe 1967)

Event	Scale
Death of spouse	100
Divorce	73
Marital separation	65
Jail term	63
Death of family member	67
Personal injury or illness	53
Marriage	50
Fired at work	47
Marital reconciliation	45
Retirement	45
Change in health of family member	44
Pregnancy	40
Sex difficulties	39
Gain of new family member	39
Business readjustment	39
Change in financial state	38
Death of close friend	37
Change to different line of work	36
Change in number of arguments with spouse	35
Mortgage over $10 000	31
Foreclosure of mortgage or loan	30
Change in responsibilities at work	29
Son or daughter leaving home	29
Trouble with in-laws	29
Outstanding personal achievement	28
Wife begins or stops work	26
Begin or end school	26
Change in living conditions	25
Revision of personal habits	24
Trouble with boss	23
Change in work hours or conditions	20
Change in residence	20
Change in schools	20
Change in recreation	19
Change in church activities	19
Change in social activities	18
Mortgage or loan less than $10 000	17
Change in sleeping habits	16
Change in number of family get-togethers	15
Change in eating habits	15
Vacation	13
Christmas	12
Minor violation of the law	11

More obvious stressors include surgery, bereavement, intensive-care environments, dialysis, and death (Wilson-Barnett 1979).

The nurse too is a victim of stressors. In a day the nurse may: experience angry reactions from colleagues and those who he or she is helping; comfort the dying and the bereaved relatives; clear away the excretion of the incontinent; respond to a cardiac arrest; change dressings on delicate plastic surgery, the success of which depends on his or her skill; bathe the comotose; quietly explain to a cancer victim the consequences of chemotherapy; and write reports that may come under professional and legal scrutiny.

Before moving on to discuss the nursing care involved in stress management it is important to mention the role of the nurse in regard to stress control. The nurse must make every effort to reduce the stressors due to hospitalization. Nurses should attempt to identify, as part of their daily routine, ways of maintaining independence, self-esteem, and control in those who are ill. Information regarding the illness and treatment is vital in reducing the perception of threat (Wilson-Barnett 1984). A warm empathic approach by the nurse may be no substitute for the person's normal relationships, but it does provide the opportunity for openness on the part of the individual. There are also a number of ways in which people can maintain control over their own lives. Not least of these is full involvement in planning and evaluating self-care.

THE ROLE OF THE NURSE IN STRESS MANAGEMENT

The nurse's role in stress management involves the subjective and objective identification of stress; stress-reducing interventions; and maintenance of a state of reduced stress.

Assessment

Successful control and management of stress and its ill-effects depends almost entirely on obtaining appropriate and complete information. The medical examination and diagnosis, past history, and laboratory tests are good sources for evaluating the possible role of stress in the person's life. Best of all, however, is what the individual and those close to him can tell the nurse regarding stressors, general lifestyle, and known coping mechanisms. The problems most likely to be identified here will usually relate to a lack of understanding regarding stressors, stress and

their effects. Poor coping mechanisms and unhealthy living may also be readily identified. A sound interviewing technique that provides a comfortable forum for people to express themselves is vital if a useful complete history is to be obtained.

In assessing the degree of stress and its effect on the person, there are two important categories of information. The first of these, subjective data, involves what the person feels and what he says is wrong. Secondly there is objective data, which is what the nurse observes. Below we give a list of common subjective and objective information that may lead to a diagnosis of excessive stress and the identification of specific patient problems.

Subjective. Lack of energy, feeling tense, forgetfulness, inability to concentrate, errors in judgement, difficulty in sleeping, disturbed sleep, feeling of being overwhelmed by life, inability to cope, somatic symptoms (headaches), palpitations, chest pains, gastrointestinal disturbances, irregular menstrual cycle, loss of sexual interest, depression, loss of weight and anorexia, increased substance abuse, overeating.

Objective. Nervousness, inability to keep still, accelerated speech, fluctuating mood, anxious looks, indifference and withdrawal, irritability and aggressive outbursts, hypochondriasis, care-eliciting behaviour, hypertension, tachycardia,. increased susceptibility to illness, increased ability to empathize, decreased tolerence towards other people, confusion.

Another important aspect of assessment involves discovering the degree of resistance the person normally has to stress. Factors that tend to create resistance include those things we normally would consider as contributing to a healthy lifestyle: frequent strenuous aerobic exercise; good nutrition; non-smoking; low alcohol intake; frequent periods of relaxation; and a generally good health status. An absence of one or more of these may indicate that the person is more susceptible to stress. In addition, there may have been a recent change in these factors, perhaps due to illness, hospitalization, family circumstances, opportunity, or simply lack of forethought.

Throughout this assessment constant clarification must be sought from the person to ensure that both he and the nurse are identifying the same problems. It is not uncommon for the nurse to misinterpret information or make a misjudgement and evolve invalid treatment programmes. Similarly, poor insight on the part of the individual may be a problem in itself that must be overcome before other problems can be confronted.

Nursing treatment

The stressed person and the nurse together should attempt to formulate realistic and attainable goals of care on the basis of the identified problems. Some examples of long-term goals might be: reduction of the number of stressors in the person's life; a greater understanding of stress and its effects; an increase in resistance to excessive stress; the replacement of poor coping mechanisms with better ones; and a change in attitude to life.

In many cases it will be important to attain some short-term goals before moving on to the long-term. Alleviation of symptoms, for example, is an important short-term goal, since symptoms are often the most personally upsetting aspects of excessive stress.

The first step in any good stress management programme should be to provide a sound understanding of the mechanism, causes, and effects of stress. As a guide, a great deal of what has been covered in this chapter would be appropriate knowledge for most people, excluding perhaps some of the more complicated physiology. There is no room here to discuss teaching, but every nurse should acquire the basic skills and art, since it is, in our opinion, such a vital nursing role.

At this stage we refer the student to Part Two of this book, since it is there that we discuss in depth most of the nursing manage-

ment of stress-related problems already mentioned in this chapter. Relaxation is a vital treatment method for many stress-related problems. It reduces the effects of stressors, and provides a degree of resistance. It provides symptomatic relief, can be used as a means of combating sleep disturbance, and has the benefit of having no ill-effects.

We have already discussed hospitalization as involving a large number of potential stressors. It should be clear that increasing stress will delay healing and every effort should be made to provide as stress-free an environment as possible. Keeping the person informed, reducing the noise and general activity around the individual, maintaining a sense of independence, stepping down from the formal nurse role which in transactional analytic terms encourages a parent-child relationship, and providing a forum for the expression of fears are general measures which reduce hospital-caused stress.

Observation is vital in identifying resolution of problems, or development of new ones. It is important to remember that there is both a subjective (what the person says) and an objective (what the nurse sees) approach to observation and evaluation of care. Frequently, significant others are a source of evaluation — they will often notice improvement or deterioration.

Identification of the person's stressors and discussion of ways of dealing with them provides the centre of nursing care. Joint problem-solving between the individual and nurse, with the client making the majority of decisions, requires an application of the skills outlined in Chapter 4. Sometimes the person's problems may be too difficult or extensive for the nurse to manage. In these cases referral through the medical officer is the appropriate course of action. Long-term or involved psychotherapy can be provided by a psychiatric nurse therapist, clinical psychologist, psychiatrist, or qualified counsellor. In most circumstances, however, effective symptomatic relief and short-term help and education may be all that are required.

RELAXATION SCHEDULE

Preparation

One of the advantages of learning relaxation techniques in a controlled way is that with practice they can eventually be used in almost any situation to reduce a stressful experience or to 'recharge the batteries'. Many people can relax sitting at a desk, at a meeting, while driving, or even when walking.

However, to learn the technique it is best to utilize optimum conditions. Relaxation exercises should be carried out in a quiet place, preferably dimly lit (not dark), and the person should be lying down or sitting in a comfortable chair. Sensory stimuli should be reduced to a minimum. About 20–30 minutes are needed.

Loosen tight clothing and remove shoes; a pillow may be used. The legs should be uncrossed and the arms resting loosely by the side, not touching the body or any other distracting objects. Stretch the body, wriggle about a little then lie still with eyes closed.

Progressive Muscle Relaxation

Muscular relaxation is facilitated by progressive tensing and relaxing of major muscle groups. It is helpful to concentrate on comparing the relatively different sensations of muscular contraction (increased tension) and muscular relaxation (reduced tension).

Clench your fists as tightly as possible and feel the tension. Hold for about five seconds and then relax. Repeat. This procedure is repeated in turn for arm muscles, lower legs, upper legs, abdomen, neck and face.

Breathing

Relaxation should now be deepened by use of controlled breathing.

Take a deep breath, hold it briefly and then exhale slowly. Repeat.

Now imagine that every time you breathe *out* the air leaving your body is tension. Say to yourself, 'Relax' every time you breathe out. Help your concentration by imagining the word 'relax' in your mind as you say it to yourself. See the word 'relax'. Each time you breathe out you will relax more and more.

If your thoughts wander just bring your mind back to seeing the word 'relax'.

Feel your body becoming heavier and heavier, relaxing more and more with each exhalation. Continue for 3–5 minutes.

Images

Now imagine you are in the shower and have just turned off the taps. The warm water is dripping off your body onto the floor. Imagine the water flowing down your arms, off your fingers, and away from your body. The water is tension flowing away from you. Now imagine the water flowing off your legs and trunk. Let the water (tension) leave you . . . flowing away. Tension is leaving your body with the water and you relax as it flows away.

Now concentrate on the breathing exercise again by imaging the word 'relax' as you breathe out.

A useful exercise is to spend the last few minutes imagining a favourite peaceful scene.

REFERENCES

Baldwin J E 1980 Never jump out of a perfectly good airplane. American Journal of Nursing, May

Benson H 1975 The relaxation response. William Morrow, New York

Chilver W L C 1978 On being a patient in an intensive therapy unit. Nursing Mirror, April 6

Clarke M 1984 Stress and coping: constructs for nursing. Journal of Advanced Nursing 9

Dossett S M 1975 The patient in the intensive therapy unit. Nursing Times, May 25

Holmes T H, Rahe R H 1967 The social readjustment rating scale. Journal of Psychosomatic Research 11: 213–218

Keane B 1978 The management of the anxious patient in the general hospital ward. Australian Nurses Journal 7:9

Maslow A 1970 Motivation and personality, 2nd edn. Harper & Rowe, New York

Meares A 1969 Relief without drugs. Collins, Glasgow

Perls F 1969 Gestalt therapy verbatim. Real People Press, Utah

Randolph G L 1984 Therapeutic and physical touch:

physiological response. Nursing Research 33:1
Richter J M, Sloan R 1979 A relaxation technique. American Journal of Nursing, November
Selye M 1976 The stress of life. McGraw-Hill, New York
Selye M, Garfield C (eds) 1979 Stress and survival. Mosby, St Louis
Wilson-Barnett J 1979 Stress in hospital. Churchill Livingstone, Edinburgh

Wilson-Barnett J 1984 Alleviating stress for hospitalized patients. International Review of Applied Psychology 33: 493–503
Wilson-Barnett J, Carrigy A 1978 Factors influencing patient's emotional reactions to hospitalization. Journal of Advanced Nursing 3: 221–229

6

Nursing practice and psychological care

THE THERAPEUTIC FUNCTION OF THE NURSE

The medical disease model (involving diagnosis, treatment, and cure) has asserted an important influence on nursing practice. As a result, nursing care has tended to be directed by the doctor's orders, with the nurse participating minimally in decision-making within the health-care system. Nursing curricula, nursing texts, and nursing care have revolved around symptomatology and disease, with an emphasis on the internal processes occurring within the 'patient'. Boylan (1982) states that this has led to standard recipes of care based on a given medical diagnosis. The role of the nurse has been very much that of hand-maiden to the doctor, and has involved carrying out tasks that no-one else wants (Tiffany 1981). Another important and related aspect of this subservient role of the nurse has been its basis in the hospital setting, with regimented, militaristic, and institutional routines (Henderson 1982). Nursing has tended to be task oriented, and decision-making has not been in the hands of the nurse at the bedside; rather, it has rested with those who have greater perceived power. It has been suggested that the traditional role of the nurse can be explained socially by the politics of power where women take a secondary role to men, have little say in decision-making, are submissive, and hence are powerless (Hase 1984).

In defining the '. . . unique function of the nurse . . .', Henderson (1966) identifies a basis for the development of an independent role of the nurse and the delivery of care. The use of the word 'unique' is not accidental. It reflects the struggle for power (Partridge 1984) and professionalism (Hase 1983), and the values of the feminist movement (Hase 1984, Partridge 1984). Whatever the causes, this drive for an independent nursing role has been the most significant impetus for change in nursing in recent years. It is this change in thinking that has enabled us to describe nursing activity in terms of nursing, rather than medical models. This suggests that nurses have a significant contribution to make in the provision of health care in any setting.

The attempt to attain an independent role, however, is based on more than the quest for power and professionalism. As Jenkins (1982) has pointed out, 'The history of nursing is replete with examples of struggles by nurses, to continually improve the quality of nursing practice and provide services that meet the health needs of the diverse groups which form the society.'

The area of specific focus in this book is the role of the nurse in caring for those with psychological problems, and the maintenance of psychological health. Of all those professions involved in health care, the relationship between the nurse and the person under his or her care is unique by virtue of length of exposure time, and in the very nature of the functions of the nurse. The potential for the nurse to accurately assess psychological needs and problems, address problems as they arise and when distress is most intense, and to intervene, is very great indeed. In addition the sheer numbers of people who experience the psychological problems discussed in this book places the nurse in a unique position to provide immediate and consistent care.

This potential has received an increasing amount of attention in recent years, especially in regard to highly sensitive areas such as grieving, with nurses accepting that there is a need for special skills if effective help is to be provided. Some nurses have specialized towards areas such as stoma care and mastectomy counselling, for example, which require high order interpersonal skills and a knowledge of the special problems involved. Nurse education programmes, both basic and post-basic, have increased their emphasis on the behavioural sciences, and in particular offer courses that provide interpersonal and helping skills. The breadth of techniques available to nurses, such as relaxation training, assertiveness training and stress management skills, has increased. Peplau (Fitzpatrick et al 1982) has suggested that such diverse areas as interpersonal and systems theories, crisis theory, and rhythm theory have contributed to the expanded role of the nurse in mental health. In the United Kingdom, for example, specialist nurses are trained as behaviour therapy practitioners. In order to increase and expand their expertise, nurses are gaining qualifications in areas such as psychology and sociology, to be applied in diverse ways — for example, in research aimed at increasing the understanding of the psychological effects of ill-health, hospitalization, surgery, and stress.

The therapeutic role of the nurse includes assisting others to maintain or obtain a state of physical and mental well-being through a process of growth. In this process nurses are agents who can bring a wide range of skills to therapeutic relationships and utilize them by virtue of their unique role in the health care environment.

PEOPLE AND HEALTH

One of the most important changes in recent years regarding our concepts of health-care delivery has been the acceptance of a holistic view of people. The notion that biological, psychological, social and spiritual factors interact and influence who we are and how we respond to our environment is central to many nursing theories and conceptual models.

A holistic view of the individual enables us to consider how, for example, a change in biological state will affect the individual psychologically, sociologically, and spiritually.

This has broad implications in terms of provision of nursing care, since we go beyond simply focusing on biological needs or problems. Similarly, holistic nursing care implies that the nurse takes into account how psychological factors may influence susceptibility, response, and outcome of biological disease states. Psychological stress provides a good example of how this interaction can be conceptualized. The traditional medical model has tended to consider only the biological factors in health and ill-health, with a principal interest in symptomatology, treatment, and outcome. It is interesting to note that some nursing models, such as Henderson's, take a principally biological stance with little consideration for the psychological or sociological nature of the individual.

Another way of looking at biological, psychological, sociological, and spiritual factors is as dynamic forces that account for the uniqueness of the individual. The idea that we are all unique may seem fundamental, but it is only in recent years that nursing has recognized its importance and turned towards individualized care. Uniqueness implies that people will respond differently to life's circumstances. In regard to ill-health, each person's problems are unique both quantitatively and qualitatively. Individuals will vary in the way in which they overcome problems, adapt, and grow from the experience.

In the context of psychological health and behaviour individual variation is enormous. An implication of this is that each person requires a special understanding that can best be achieved by a close therapeutic relationship. Along with many contemporary nursing theorists, we believe that nursing needs to be individualized and directed at a person's uniqueness.

Another belief we hold about people, and on which most of our nursing care is based, is that we all have the potential for growth and self-realization: the individual has the potential for making the most of his or her attributes, maximising potential, obtaining contentment, and making sense of the world. This is essentially a humanistic view and has

been used in nursing theory development (Paterson & Zderad 1976) and as a framework for nursing care delivery (Atkinson & Murray 1983, Keane 1981, Jones 1978). A major part of this potential for growth is the ability to make decisions and to be responsible for them. This is an existential rather than a deterministic view of man and implies that individuals are capable of shaping their own world and can change it within the context of their biological, psychological, sociological, and spiritual attributes.

One way in which people can be helped to achieve potential is through education, by providing the knowledge to enable action. For example, it is difficult for someone to manage stress without having an understanding of the stress response and the skills required to reduce its effects. Education is a means of providing the power to make decisions and a vehicle for accepting responsibility for oneself. Orem's model of self-care (Orem 1980) has a central theme of assisting those she calls 'patients' to achieve a state of self-care, in the process of which the nurse accepts a significant educative function. Much of the nursing care described in this book involves providing people with information of either an educational or confrontational nature that offers the opportunity for cognitive development and action.

METHODOLOGY FOR NURSING PRACTICE

One of the most important developments to affect nursing practice has been the adoption of what is popularly known as the 'nursing process'. In many respects this is an unfortunate term, since the method is not unique to nursing (Hase 1983, Henderson 1982) but is rather the application of a universally used problem-solving approach to nursing. The reader is urged to consider that its components, borrowed from philosophy, can be applied to all manner of decision-making situations, such as management, counselling, mending a fuse, or retrieving a kite from high up in a tree.

However, the universality of the problem-solving approach doesn't detract from its application to nursing care as the 'nursing process'. This section deals with the particular application of the nursing process to psychological care.

THE NURSING PROCESS

The steps of the nursing process can be simplified into four primary components, as shown in Figure 6.1.

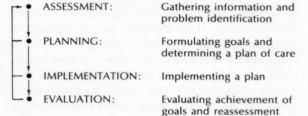

ASSESSMENT:	Gathering information and problem identification
PLANNING:	Formulating goals and determining a plan of care
IMPLEMENTATION:	Implementing a plan
EVALUATION:	Evaluating achievement of goals and reassessment

Fig. 6.1 The nursing process. (After Atkinson & Murray, 1983.)

The arrows linking the four stages indicate their logical sequence, as well as their dynamic nature; evaluation allows modification at any level. If a goal is not achieved or only partially achieved, reassessment culminates in a new goal or plan. New information gained at a later stage may also modify the nursing care plan.

Utilization of the nursing process facilitates individualized care by specifying each person's particular problems on the basis of a unique assessment, and by the development of an appropriate care plan. Methodologically the nursing process is scientific (Darcy 1980) in providing a rational basis for care. Other advantages have been described, such as enabling people to participate in planning their own care and goals, and facilitating continuity of care and improved quality of care (Atkinson & Murray 1983). Stanton et al (1980) also relate the nursing process to the interpersonal nature of nursing and a holistic view of the person. One of the driving forces for the development of the nursing process has been the search for an independent role

for nurses in the making of decisions about the delivery of nursing treatment (Henderson 1982). Hence its important place in the application of nursing models.

The individual's problems confronting the nurse, rather than being couched in terms of medical diagnosis, can be related directly to rational nursing activities which can be evaluated as to their effectiveness. In terms of psychological care the nursing process enables us to avoid all-encompassing labels such as 'schizophrenia' or 'dementia'. Instead, more specific individual problems can be addressed that are within the scope of nursing expertise and involvement. A diagnosis of dementia or schizophrenia may indeed be given by a psychiatrist, but people with these conditions all have quite different specific problems quantitatively and qualitatively, requiring different goals and strategies of care. In addition it may be a mistake to assume that the individual will accept the care that the nurse considers appropriate (Ward 1985). Many individuals may choose to refuse the sick role and the psychiatric label that is provided by diagnosis. As with other aspects of nursing care, the person can and should be consulted regarding psychological health goals and the ways in which they can be achieved.

THE NURSING PROCESS AND NURSING THEORIES

It is important to note, before going on to discuss the steps of the nursing process in relation to psychological care, its relationship to nursing theory. Although many writers allude to the nursing process as a philosophy (Ward 1985), it is principally a systematic method of thinking and doing. The nursing process is applied within the framework of a nursing theory that guides the way in which the problem-solving approach will be used. Some theories, such as Henderson's (1966) for example, stress the nursing process within a philosophy of individualized care and holism. Other theorists such as Peplau use a problem-solving approach somewhat different from the nursing process both formatively and conceptually (Belcher & Fish 1980). It is, however, safe to say that most modern theories use the nursing process in some way or another in describing nursing activity.

Theories, however, guide the use of the nursing process in different ways. For example, Roy's adaptation model stresses assessment and implementation in terms of a goal which promotes adaptation of the person in four modes: physiological needs, self-concept, role function, and interdependence (Tiedman 1983). Orem (1980) identifies problems in terms of self-care deficits, whereas Rogers' nursing diagnoses reflect the principle of haemodynamics (Falco & Lobo 1980).

Our particular approach has been to use the notion of problems rather than needs, self-care deficits, or diagnoses, although any of these may be applicable within an appropriate theoretical framework.

Assessment

Assessment involves a process of data collection, data analysis, and the identification of the individual's problems.

Information should be collected from all available sources, including

- the person
- the person's significant others
- past records
- the nurse's examination and interview
- medical examination, diagnosis, and treatment
- other paranursing assessments
- psychiatric or psychological assessment.

Information obtained from the person is best described as belonging to two categories. On the one hand there is subjective data consisting of what the individual actuallyy says. For example, 'I feel nervous', 'My heart is pounding', 'The voices tell me I'm going to die', are all examples of subjective information. These can be documented in parentheses with the person's actual words to facilitate evaluation and communication with colleagues. On the other hand there is objective data arising from the nurse's observation and examination. Objective information might include: looking worried, restlessness, systolic blood pressure of 160 mmHg, dishevelled appearance, staring into space, and uncommunicativeness.

Information from the person may be obtained from either a formal or informal interview depending on circumstances and the likely response from the individual. As Keane (1981) points out, the most effective way of obtaining information is through the development of a good relationship in which the person feels confident and safe. Right from the beginning the individual can be involved in a collegiate fashion with the nurse in guiding his own care. Where this is not achieved quickly or easily, information gathering will involve more than one interaction and perhaps many. It is usual to expect that further information may be obtained up to days after admission and then used to modify the care plan. Assessment is also ongoing so that new problems can be identified as they arise or as circumstances change.

In crisis situations both the assessment and intervention are combined in one interaction with an immediate short-term goal of lessening the impact of a problem on the person. A more complete assessment can be obtained at a later, more opportune moment. In other cases the time may just not be right for a full assessment, and the nurse will need to proceed slowly so as not to threaten the individual.

There are many ways of documenting data, a predesigned nursing history sheet being perhaps the most popular method. Another method is to use simple guidelines and a blank sheet of paper on which the information is recorded. In either case it is useful to decide on a number of categories into which information may be grouped: for example

- psychological
- physical
- sociological
- spiritual
- activities of daily living.

When information has been gathered, the nurse's skill and knowledge enables conclusions to be made about what the information means. It is from this analysis that the person's problems are identified and may then be discussed with him to ensure their validity. At the same time the problems can be prioritized, with the nurse assisting the individual to identify the most important problems and those which are of a secondary nature. Ward (1985) suggests that no longer than 24 hours should be allowed for the establishment of an initial nursing diagnosis after the assessment, since the situation can change quite quickly and dramatically.

The following example illustrates a nursing assessment centred around a psychological problem for a person in a general hospital setting.

NURSING ASSESSMENT

Name: Mr Y.
Age: 36 years

Psychological

Mr Y. says, 'I've been feeling anxious for weeks now and being admitted to hospital has just about been the last straw. I just can't cope with all this.'

Throughout the interview he states that he has been under considerable stress lately. Looks worried and depressed although denies the latter. Very agitated and easily distracted by sudden noise. Preoccupied with symptoms and health.

Demonstrates very little understanding about physical diagnosis and is irritated by the suddenness of events.

He says, 'I can't concentrate on anything except my problems and what will happen to me.'

Dr C. has diagnosed an acute anxiety state and ordered oxazepam 15 mg t.d.s.

Mr Y. has had no previous history of psychological problems or admissions to hospital.

Physical

Lesion removed from left side of neck one week ago and found to be a malignant melanoma. Wide excision and graft tomorrow. Three sutures in situ at site of removal of lesion. Suture line is slightly inflamed and painful.

Smokes 15 cigarettes per day and drinks approximately 40 grams of ethanol per day.

T36^8 P90 R18 BP 140/85.

Complains of occasional bouts of palpitations and states, 'My heart sometimes feels like it will jump out of my chest at any moment.' Physical examination shows no other problems. Dr C. has not identified any cardiovascular problems.

Sociological

Mr Y. is married with two children: a girl aged 6 and a boy aged 3. Separated from family two months ago after mutual decision that 'Things were not going so well'. Children are with his wife. Mrs Y. is fully aware of Mr Y.'s admission. He has his own business selling computer software but his partner will be able to manage for at least two weeks with little problem.

Lives alone in flat for time-being and a friend will take care of this until after discharge.

Mr Y. feels that pressure of work restricts his social life to business lunches.

Activities of Daily Living

Sleeps poorly, especially has trouble getting off to sleep. 'My mind goes around and around with all sorts of ideas and business problems.'

Exercises rarely due to work but occasionally plays a game of squash.

Eats out, usually business lunches. Does not eat breakfast. Showers twice daily. Normal bowel habits. Friend will take care of laundry while in hospital.

Problem list

Anxiety due to multiple stressors:

— knowledge deficit regarding melanoma, operation, and prognosis
— family conflict
— overwork
— poor methods of stress reduction, especially exercise, recreation, relaxation, smoking and drinking habits
— difficulty in sleeping
— painful suture line
— episodes of palpitation.

Another group of 'problems' that needs to be considered are those that may arise given the specific risk factors identified during assessment. These are known as 'potential problems'. For example, a depressed individual may not be suicidal at the time of assessment but there may be evidence that there is a future risk of suicidal ideation. There are obviously innumerable potential problems that a person could develop, so the quantification of risk is an important consideration requiring considerable nursing skill. A person who experiences persecutory hallucinations and paranoid delusions is much more likely to behave impulsively than is a moderately anxious alcoholic, for example.

Planning

Effective planning of care involves an analysis of problems that: prioritizes them in terms of their relative effect on the individual's well-being (Atkinson & Murray 1983); identifies attainable and measurable goals or objectives; determines appropriate care strategies to attain goals; and takes into consideration the potential for change.

A goal indicates what the person will be able to do, or what his condition will be, if the care is successful (Ashworth 1980). It is essential that the individual be involved in goal-setting whenever possible. Goals may be short- or long-term, depending on the type of problems that confront the individual. Short-term goals can sometimes be more readily achievable stages towards some long-term goal. The setting of goals underlines the rational basis of the nursing process and makes provision for the evaluation of care-effectiveness.

Goals should also be realistically attainable, measurable, precise, and have a time-frame attached (Ward 1985). Goals should also be easy to understand by those other than the writer. For Mr Y. the goals of care might be as shown in Table 6.1 (p. 94).

The next logical step in planning is to determine the nursing activities and the behaviours in which the individual can engage that will contribute to the achievement of the goals. Documentation takes the form of a nursing care plan which sets out the problems, goals, and nursing activities. Some plans also include a section for evaluation, although the nursing notes are arguably the best place to carry out this final stage. It is also important to date the problems to facilitate accurate review. The care plan should be discussed with the individual and, where appropriate, significant others who may be involved in the person's care. The care plan for Mr Y. shown in Table 6.1 includes notes on implementation.

Implementation

This stage involves the actual delivery of care as described by the nursing care plan. Part two of this book deals with implementation in regard to psychological care. However, it is worthwhile noting that elements of assessment, planning, and evaluation are also included during this interaction with the individual. Nursing is an interpersonal activity and is the realization of nursing skill. Implementation really begins in the planning stage with the identification of appropriate nursing actions and ends with an understanding of the consequences of the care given for the individual.

Evaluation

Evaluation involves a measure of the extent to which the individual has changed towards the goals determined in the plan of care. This is an ongoing process that will necessitate reassessment of problems, goals, and implementation, carried out by collection of information in much the same way as in the initial stage of assessment. Evaluation provides the rational basis for the nursing process by enabling the nurse to identify success and failure.

The outcome of evaluation may be the identification of new problems, an alteration in effective care, the elimination of a problem, a change in a goal, or the recognition that progress is being satisfactorily made towards achievement of a goal. Failure to resolve a

Table 6.1 Nursing care plan

Problem	Date	Goal	Nursing implementation
1. Painful suture line, left neck.	7/8/85	1. To minimize pain and discomfort preoperatively.	1. Analgesia as required. Reduction in movement and posture for comfort. Observe for signs of infection.
2. Difficulty in sleeping.	7/8/85	2. To ensure a minimum of 6 hours sleep preoperatively. To establish a pattern of 7 hours sleep per night by discharge.	2. Hypnotics nightly preoperatively. Teach progressive relaxation schedule when recovered postoperatively. Monitor sleeping pattern on sleep chart. Do not disturb between 23:30 and 07:00.
3. Anxiety due to multiple stressors a. Knowledge deficit regarding melanoma, operation and prognosis. b. Family conflict. c. Overwork. d. Poor methods of stress-reducation especially exercise, recreation, relaxation, smoking and drinking	7/8/85	3. To provide immediate symptomatic relief. To decrease knowledge deficit regarding illness, treatment and postoperative recovery prior to surgery. To decrease impact of family conflict by discharge. To provide a programme of stress reducing strategies by discharge.	3. Anxiolytics as ordered until anxiety reduced then decrease use. Arrange for Dr C. to discuss melanoma and treatment with Mr Y. this afternoon. Discuss postoperative recovery and arrange preoperative visit by theatre staff. Encourage exploration of reasons for anxiety and help develop an understanding of feelings being experienced. Support and encourage Mr Y.'s expression of emotion. Facilitate in resolution of family conflict and work stressors. Support and encourage Mr Y.'s expression of emotionn. Facilitate in resolution of family conflict and work stressors. Progressive relaxation practice twice daily and when anxious. Discuss with Mr Y. possible changes in lifestyle, especially work, relaxation, exercise, smoking and drinking habits.
4. Episodes of palpitation.	7/8/85	4. To establish cause or precipitating factors and reduce incidence.	4. Mr Y. to record when palpitations occur and any identifiable behavioural, environmental or cognitive precipitant. Instruct Mr Y. to call for nurse and initiate anxiety-reducing techniques.

problem may have resulted from errors in assessment, planning, or evaluation, so it is important to evaluate each step of the nursing process. Success is also important other than for the obvious benefit for the individual — it provides an opportunity to add to nursing knowledge, especially where new techniques have been used.

The evaluation is usually carried out between the person and the nurse, although it may be appropriate to include significant others. The nurse can reassess the subjective experiences of the individual and also feed back objective information. In Mr Y.'s case it would be most appropriate to state that he no longer looks anxious, his blood pressure is down, he looks rested, and does not appear preoccupied with his bodily symptoms as much as previously. Mr Y. can then clarify whether or not this objective appraisal is accurate. One difficulty to be considered in evaluating the achievement of behavioural outcomes is the stability of the behaviour. In this respect judgements need to be made with considerable care and skill.

The documentation of evaluation is best carried out in the nursing progress notes or nurse's report. This provides a meaningful and rational basis for making notes by using the care plan and an ongoing history of the person's behaviour. Progress notes can be written with the individual under care.

A sample from Mr Y.'s notes is given below.

Progress Notes

25/7/85 22:00	At 18:00 Mr Y. complained of a 'very sore' suture line on left neck. Whole of suture line red and inflamed. He appeared very anxious and stated he was 'in a bad mood'. Panadol II was given at 18:15 and Mr Y. was discouraged from moving neck. Pain subsided by 18:45 except for discomfort on sudden movement. A brief discussion regarding the reason for the inflammation, and about his feelings regarding being in hospital appeared to assist in reducing his anxiety. Dr C. fully discussed the problem of the

melanoma, treatment, and postoperative consequences with Mr Y. who now states he feels much less worried about the forthcoming operation.

Mr Y., however, still appears moderately anxious and feels that his life is getting a bit out of control with so many things happening to him. He will need considerable emotional support in the pre-operative period to reduce his anxiety.

S. Hase RN

CONCLUDING COMMENT

The nursing process is a relevant problem-solving approach to nursing that suits a philosophy that values the individualistic and holistic nature of people. It also provides an opportunity for the consumer of health-care to participate actively in goal-directed behaviour and maximises the nurse's accountability for action. However, it is important to apply the nursing process within the framework of a theory or conceptual model that provides direction as to how the sequential steps are to be carried out. In the ensuing chapters we have attempted to provide an appropriate data base and nursing guidelines for a number of psychological problems within a problem-solving framework.

REFERENCES

Atkinson L D, Murray M E 1983 Understanding the nursing process. Macmillan, New York
Ashworth P A 1980 A way to better care. Nursing Mirror, August 28
Belcher J R, Fish L J B 1980 Hildegard E Peplau. In: The Nursing Theories Conference Group Nursing theories: the base for professional nursing practice. Prentice-Hall, Englewood Cliffs
Boylan A 1982 The nursing process and the role of the registered nurse. Nursing Times, August 25
Darcy P T 1980 The nursing process — a base for all nursing developments, Nursing Times, March 20
Falco S M, Lobo M L 1980 Martha E Rogers. In: The Nursing Theories Conference Group. Nursing

theories: the base for professional nursing practice. Prentice-Hall, Englewood Cliffs
Fitzpatrick J J, Whall A L, Johnston R L, Floyd J A 1982 Nursing Models and their psychiatric mental health applications. Brady, Maryland
Hase S 1983 The nursing process — is it idol worship? Australian Nurses' Journal, July
Hase S 1984 Assertiveness through communication. Australian Nurses' Journal, September
Henderson V 1966 The nature of nursing. Macmillan London
Henderson V 1982 The nursing process — is the title right? Journal of Advanced Nursing 7
Jenkins E 1982 In: Jenkins E, King B, Gray G (eds) Issues

in Australasian nursing. Churchill Livingstone, Melbourne

Jones P D 1978 An adaptation model for nursing practice. American Journal of Nursing, November

Keane B 1981 The nursing process in a psychiatric context. Nursing Times, July 8

Norton D 1981 The quiet revolution: Introduction of the nursing process in a region. Nursing Times, June 17

Orem D E 1980 Nursing: concepts of practice. McGraw Hill, New York

Partridge B 1984 The swinging pendulum of nurse-doctor relationships. Australian Nurses Journal, February

Paterson J G, Zderad L T 1976 Humanistic nursing. Wiley, New York

Silverton A 1979 Nursing care plans: a vital tool. The Canadian Nurse, March

Stanton M, Charlotte P, Reeves J S 1980 An overview of the nursing process. In: The Nursing Theories Conference Group. Nursing theories: the base for professional nursing practice. Prentice-Hall, Englewood Cliffs

Tiedman M E 1983 The Roy adaptation model. In: Fitzpatrick J J, Whall A L (eds) Conceptual models of nursing: analysis and application. Brady, Maryland

Tiffany R 1981 Striving to be more than Cinderellas. Nursing Mirror, December 16

Ward M F 1985 The nursing process in psychiatry. Churchill Livingstone, Edinburgh

PART | # TWO

Approaching People

Slowly, he sat up. Now the torments were coming again; now he was condemned to lie hour upon hour; anguish and dread in his heart, alone, suffering useless pangs, thinking useless thoughts, fretting over useless cares. Out of the nightmares that had awakened him crawled greasy, hulking feelings, disgust and horror, surfeit, self-contempt.
Herman Hesse, 1979

7

The anxious person

DEFINING ANXIETY

One of the most useful ways of conceptualizing anxiety is to compare it with the more familiar sensation, fear. In everyday language we tend to use the words interchangeably. Greater precision in use, however, will highlight the similarities and differences, allowing a meaningful definition of anxiety.

We have already discussed the alarm reaction (fight or flight response) in Chapter 5. This reaction occurs in the face of a threat and is designed to prepare the body for action. Both 'fear' and 'anxiety' describe the feelings that result from this 'energized' state, and they may subjectively be quite similar.

Fear is an appropriate response to an obvious external threat that usually involves our physical well-being. An important feature of fear is that it passes as the threat passes. By comparison, anxiety generally is unrelated to any obvious external threat, or the threat is disproportionate to the emotion it evokes. Energy is not required to 'fight or flee' yet the body is still 'energized' and can remain so despite the absence of any recognizable threat, and with the individual being unaware of the reasons for the consequent feeling state.

In more descriptive terms, anxiety is an unpleasant emotion (Keane 1978). It is portrayed in rather vivid terms in the quote at the beginning of this chapter. The individual Hesse describes is suffering something more than fear; its origins are in inner conflict and torment. Although we might describe anxiety in general terms as involving apprehension, tension, uneasiness, and a sense of danger, the actual sensations and behavioural sequence tend to be idiosyncratic. One or more bodily sensations may be pin-pointed by an individual: palpitations and tachycardia may be reported, for example; yet for another person fatigue and the inability to concentrate may be the most distressing feelings. Some people react to anxiety with aggressive behaviour, while others may withdraw, becoming passive and compliant.

A useful model depicting the processes involved in anxiety has been proposed by Lader (1975): all individuals continually process internal and external stimuli, assessing any threat. If the individual perceives a threat, the fight or flight response ensues and the consequent reported feeling state is fear when the threat is objective and consciously experienced, or anxiety when the appraisal of threat is subconscious.

Anxiety is a prominent feature of mental disorders such as depression and schizophrenia, and particularly of those classified as neurotic, including phobic disorders, obsessional states, and hysterical syndromes (see Ch. 2). The symptom of anxiety is present also in a number of physical illnesses, including: thyrotoxicosis, paroxysmal tachycardia, hypoglycaemia, phaeochromocytoma and toxic confusional states. In addition, anxiety is, in its own right, a significant manifestation of acute, transient, or sustained mental ill-health.

UNDERSTANDING A PERSON'S ANXIETY

In the light of the definitions of anxiety given above, it follows that we should look for its origins in the psychological processes of the person who is experiencing the emotion. While fear arises from some objective external threat, anxiety results from something happening within the individual. In Chapter 1 the problems associated with determining what this 'something' might be were discussed.

The plethora of theoretical positions and the absence of any single explanation for a psychological phenomenon such as anxiety makes understanding very difficult. Although theoretically cowardly, it is our intention here to take an eclectic position and give the reader as broad a view as possible of this important aspect of mental ill-health. More detailed explanations, complete with arguments for and against the theories, may be found in the references for this chapter.

Psychological conflict

One of the most obvious ways of explaining the existence of an internal threat is in terms of psychological conflict. A state of conflict can occur when the individual experiences thoughts or feelings which he perceives as being unacceptable. For some people, feeling intense anger towards someone they are supposed to love, a parent for example, produces conflict. This is particularly true if they have learned, from lifelong parental messages, that such a feeling is wrong. Instead of issuing forth, the anger is held back or, in Freudian terms 'repressed' (Davison & Neale 1978). The result is a state of anxiety, since there is a danger of the anger actually being expressed outwardly.

Conflict may also arise when a person feels trapped in a situation from which he would like to escape but is unable to do so because of his obligations. We might see here a husband who no longer loves his wife but cannot make the decision to leave. The reason may lie in his obligation to the children; the belief that marriage is for life; the fear of being alone; or simply his not wishing to take the responsibility of having his behaviour affect others. Whatever the case, conflict arises and anxiety may ensue as the need for decision becomes stronger.

Guilt

In many conflict situations it is the feeling of guilt that creates anxiety through the fear of social disapproval. Freud called this 'moral anxiety' (Rouhani 1978), and although he saw sexuality as the principal cause of moral anxiety, it is possible to think in broader terms. Dyer (1976), suggests that we have a guilt-producing culture in which we learn to punish ourselves internally for thoughts, feelings, and behaviours which we have learned to believe are unacceptable. In many ways guilt is a powerful socializing agent; it acts as an internal 'policeman' to make us conform to the wishes of others. For some, guilt may be so overwhelming that the threat of being punished results in anxiety. Some important points to remember here are that it is sometimes difficult to understand how a person can feel so guilty when we compare them with ourselves — something we should avoid doing; that people are often unaware of the origins of their guilt or that guilt is a cause of their anxiety; and that we learn guilt from others.

The person in hospital may experience guilt because he has left his family to manage without him, or may perceive the illness as his own fault. An over-stressed partner, the wife, left with the children, may not help the situation by reacting with anxiety or anger at visiting times. The anxiety associated with dying may not just be due to facing the unknown. Cary (cited by Kubler-Ross 1975) found that two-thirds of the dying people in his study experienced extreme anxiety due to the possibility of being a burden to others.

Threatened self concept

A somewhat related cause of anxiety involves threat to our self-esteem. Failure, or the threat of failure, exemplifies this idea, and one only has to remember sitting an examination to conceptualize this cause of anxiety.

Some writers (Rouhani 1978) describe the motivational aspects of anxiety, seeing it as normal; others, for instance educationalists (Lefrancois 1982), describe the motivation in terms of arousal. This idea is based on the belief that fear of failure, as when sitting an examination, is a learned behaviour; the threat is internal, and a maladaptive response,

in the form of anxiety, is the result. However, there is no reason to suggest that feeling confident and non-anxious results in poorer performance. Perhaps other motivational factors may be learned, such as the desire to achieve or self-actualize (Maslow 1970). This need to develop one's full potential is considered by Maslow to be a motivation behind all human behaviour — an innate constant drive. The continuous desire to develop this potential, or the inability to achieve it, often results in anxiety, despite the absence of any threat to the self. Whatever the case, some individuals become so anxious prior to examination that they become totally immobilized on the day, or cannot concentrate on study and are consequently insufficiently prepared for the examination.

There are many aspects of illness and hospitalization that threaten self concept. Most people have a certain degree of control over their lives in the normal situation and generally make choices that suit their needs and wants. These are usually directed towards most good for oneself and least threat. We do not generally attempt to do things which involve certain failure or loss of control. Illness removes a great deal of choice, forcing immobilization and sometimes even a permanently changed self-image, as in paralysis and amputation. Hospitalization takes away the sense of independence and choice, requiring the acceptance of a new role in what Donnelly (1980) has described as an 'anxious play'. The hospital's needs can, and often do, supercede those of the individual, who develops a sense of anonymity beneath one of many identical quilts on identical beds. Wilson-Barnett & Carrigy (1978) report feelings of helplessness and ignorance in people on admission to hospital. Above all, the fear of death, often associated with illness and hospitalization, is the most widely acknowledged threat to an individual's self concept.

Hospitalization also results in disrupted interpersonal relationships, a sense of violation, and withdrawal of love through separation. These factors have been identified by some psychoanalysts as being responsible for anxiety (Henderson & Nite 1975). In addition there is the problem of the unknown which leads to feelings of insecurity and helplessness. As creatures of habit, humans are careful to structure their lives so as to maintain control and reduce anxiety. But in the case of illness, the death of a spouse, or changed relationships (such as a breakdown of marriage), loss of control is often felt.

Problem avoidance

A more concrete example of how anxiety can occur in some cases is 'problem avoidance'. Very minor financial problems, for example, if not resolved, can compound themselves until they become a tremendous burden. Anxiety results, as coping strategies, such as indifference, become less effective and vulnerability becomes evident. In this case the feeling of being overwhelmed with the complexity of a problem has resulted from avoidance, which is a distinguishing feature of some people's personality.

Learned behaviour

That anxiety will occur in one person and not in another, given the same or similar circumstances, is an interesting problem that has not been resolved by any psychoanalytic theory. Some psychologists have attempted through a more scientific and experimental approach, to explain anxiety as being a learned behaviour (Davison & Neale 1978) established through the process of classical conditioning (see Ch. 1). Wolpe (1958) has also suggested a stimulus-response explanation of anxiety upon which is based his famous treatment method — systematic desensitization. Bandura (1971) explains the acquisition of fears through the process of modelling or vicarious learning: we see another person respond with anxiety to a particualr stimulus or situation and so learn the behaviour.

Another way of explaining the idiosyncratic nature of anxiety is in terms of social competence. Wolpe & Lazarus (1966) describe the anxiety that can be promoted by a person's inadequacy in social encounters, and in particular they describe lack of assertiveness as an example. The relationship between mental ill-health and social skills is outlined in Chapter 1 and may be related readily to the problem of anxiety. Similarly, Ellis' theory of psychological disturbance as resulting from irrational thinking. is described in Chapter 1, and has particular application to anxiety in the hospital setting where change and loss of control are intrinsic to the 'patient' role.

Mental defence mechanisms

In much the same way as physiological processes exist in the body to maintain homeostasis or balance, it would seem that we are able to call on psychological mechanisms in an attempt to prevent anxiety. This is not surprising in view of the rather unpleasant nature of the emotion and the internal threat. These preventive measures are called 'mental defence mechanisms', or 'ego defence mechanisms', and prevent unacceptable thoughts and feelings from entering consciousness (Sainsbury 1980). Most people use these mechanisms from time to time, but when they are over used growth is prevented, problems are not solved, and immobilization may result. A number of the more common defences are described here, since their occurrence will be an important feature in determining appropriate nursing intervention. It is important to point out that these mechanisms occur quite unconsciously, outside the person's awareness.

1. *Denial*. This is avoidance of psychological material that threatens to overwhelm the person, by refusal to acknowledge it and ignoring its existence. A good example involves someone who has been told he is dying. In the face of such a threat the person may simply deny the information to the extent that he believes he has never been told (Kubler-Ross 1969).

2. *Regression*. The threat is avoided by a retreat to immature behaviour characteristic of an earlier stage of development. The development of bed-wetting in a previously trained

child in the face of a threat such as changing schools is a classic example. Childish and immature acts in adults may indicate regression if excessive stress threatens to become overwhelming.

3. *Rationalization.* This is the presentation of apparently logical reasons for a feeling, thought, or action that is otherwise unacceptable to the individual. The nurse may be reprimanded for failing to carry out some aspect of nursing care and rationalize her failure as due to some negative attribute of the hospitalized person or the working environment. We might blame our failure in an examination on the poor choice of questions, inadequate lecturers, or the text-book.

4. *Displacement.* This involves shifting an emotion from the object toward which it was intended to another object or person. Anger is usually involved here, since it will often be a source of conflict for the individual. It is perhaps injudicious to express anger towards authority figures, for example; instead the anger might be displaced onto the cat or children.

5. *Repression.* This is the unconscious removal of disagreeable thoughts, conflicts, memories, or feelings from consciousness. It is thought that these feelings and ideas still operate at an unconscious level and give rise to neurotic symptoms, irrational attitudes, and dreams (Sainsbury 1980). From the psycho-analytic point of view repression is seen as a key factor in neurotic anxiety (Davison & Neale 1978).

6. *Conversion.* This is a severe form of defence in which overwhelming conflict or a repressed idea becomes manifest as a physical symptom. A soldier in a combat zone could be so fearful (yet be unable to run away due to his sense of duty) that he develops a paralysis, deafness, or some other dysfunction. The disorder is very real to the person and is not simply a case of malingering. The same type of response is possible in people about to undergo surgery or some other necessary, but frightening, treatment.

7. *Projection.* This involves attributing unacceptable thoughts, feelings, or urges involving oneself to others. The workman blaming his tools for shoddy work, or criticism of others for weaknesses that are our own, are examples of projection. At a more complex level, a person may ascribe his own hostility as emanating from others, or his sexual urges as the distorted attitudes of someone else.

8. *Reaction formation.* This is the display of an emotion that is the opposite to the person's true feelings, which are felt to be unacceptable and hence threatening. A person may be extremely fearful of hospitalization or his illness, but responds with apparent calm and indifference. Sexual feelings towards a relative, for example, may be so threatening that hostility towards that person results.

9. *Sublimation.* This occurs when an unacceptable drive is directed towards a more socially acceptable activity. Most sports require a degree of aggressiveness and as such allow people to redirect hostility or aggression in a socially sanctioned activity. People with long-term or debilitating illnesses may sublimate their drives into extremely useful projects or valuable self-education. Sublimation is considered to be a most healthy mechanism.

10. *Compensation.* This is the overemphasis of a positive personal attribute due to the perception of some other deficiency in self. A person may compensate for physical deficiencies by being highly competitive in business, but with aggression and a tendency towards over-control.

11. *Withdrawal.* This may be a conscious or unconscious process of simply moving away from a situation that threatens to overwhelm. When withdrawal is unconsciously mediated it may involve distortion of reality.

12. *Suppression.* This is a conscious process which involves quite deliberately postponing the expression of an emotion until a later date. Temporary relief from anxiety may be obtained by pushing the feeling away and diverting attention to some activity requiring concentration and effort.

The discussion so far has been directed towards obtaining some idea of how anxiety can be conceptualized. This has not been an exhaustive treatment, however, and the student nurse should be aware of the potential for a much wider appreciation of anxiety as a mental health problem by reading further on the subject. We may now turn to the actual nursing activity involved in caring for anxious people.

NURSING CARE

CASE ILLUSTRATION

Mr A. N., a 45-year-old company executive, is recovering from a myocardial infarction in the coronary care unit of a general hospital. Despite having made a full recovery, Mr A. N.'s blood pressure remains elevated and he is tachycardic. He presses the call buzzer frequently, requesting attention by nurses for minor matters, and does not appear at ease unless someone is near him almost all of the time. Continually seeking reassurance as to his condition, Mr A. N. appears apprehensive and states repeatedly that he feels something drastic is going to happen to him. He is tremulous, perspires constantly, and is unable to concentrate on other people's conversation. His own speech is pressured, frequently returning to his feelings of distress, and his sentences are often left incomplete. He is unable to rest during the day and at night he sleeps fitfully, awakened by disturbing nightmares. Concerned that Mr A. N.'s agitation will prolong his period of recovery and hospitalization, nursing staff talk with him about his feelings and their possible causes and endeavour to diminish his state of anxiety.

This case is typical of the anxiety experienced by people recovering from potentially life-threatening illness.

ASSESSMENT

As with a great number of manifestations of mental ill health, one of the dilemmas associated with identifying anxiety in a person is that it is not always obvious to the nurse and sometimes not even to the individuals themselves. That people may not know they are anxious may seem a little strange. The point is that certain feelings may be obvious but that the person may not attribute them to anxiety. Somatic (bodily) symptoms are an example of this problem. In the initial assessment it is important to avoid confronting a person with the prospect that his feelings are due to anxiety, since this may impose further threat and interfere with the process of building a therapeutic relationship. Clarifying with the individual statements of feeling is important, however, as it facilitates an accurate assessment of problems. In most cases the expression of anxiety will be obvious and, when allowed to, people will freely admit how they feel and identify in themselves either fear or anxiety.

Subjective experiences

Tension

The most obvious sensation felt by the anxious person is one of tension, which may be described by a large number of pseudonyms such as: being on edge; feeling jittery; nervousness; worried; apprehension; or, more directly, anxiety. A feeling that something terrible is about to happen is a common manifestation of anxiety. A useful technique when confronted with pseudonyms is to ask the individual to explain exactly what is meant by asking for a description of the sensation in concrete terms.

Somatic complaints

Somatic complaints are the most frequently noted features of anxiety. Having the same basis as the alarm reaction described in Chapter 4, these complaints may take a variety of forms, some of which are listed in Table 7.1.

Any or all these complaints may be interpreted as indicating some physical disorder and may frequently be the reason for someone seeking help in the first place. Assuming that a diagnosis of physical abnormality has been eliminated, anxiety may be considered as a possible cause. It is also true that the actual physical sensations or dysfunctions themselves will create even more anxiety, since they constitute a further threat to self.

Table 7.1 Somatic symptoms of anxiety

Palpitations
Hyperventilation
Dyspnoea (globus hystericus)
Sweating (particularly the palms of the hands)
Gastrointestinal upsets (diarrhoea, nausea, vomiting, constipation, and anorexia)
Dry mouth
Headaches
Chest pains (usually non-radiating)
Vague aches and pains
Dysmenorrhoea, menorrhagia, or cessation of menstruation
Dizziness
Fatigue and/or weakness
Disturbance of sexual function (impotence, premature ejaculation, inability to achieve orgasm, loss of libido, or dyspareunia)

Altered sleeping habits

A very common result of anxiety is some disturbance in sleeping habits, a topic which will be discussed in detail in Chapter 18. The usual complaint is of an inability to get off to sleep, or a sudden waking after a short time and inability to drift off again. This may be associated with dreams and waking in a panic, with the heart thumping and an overwhelming sense of danger. While lying awake the person will be both physically and mentally restless as thoughts keep flooding through the mind over and over again.

Behavioural changes

The amount of energy expended in being anxious, a preoccupation with feelings and thoughts, and a general psychological dysfunction, lead to a number of possible complaints, depending on the level of anxiety and insight. Poor concentration, errors in judgement, memory lapses, decreased work performance and drive, disrupted interpersonal relationships, and loss of sympathy or empathy with others may occur. This latter feature is seen in nurses suffering what has been described as 'burnout' (Storlie 1979). Some individuals may also say they feel depressed, which is understandable when anxiety has been fairly longstanding. Feelings towards others may also become blunted, and a sense of loss of love for a spouse or offspring may be very disturbing.

Detachment

Another distressing sensation sometimes encountered is a feeling of detachment from events and the environment — a feeling of unreality and of being not quite in touch, and out of control.

It is not unusual for those affected to say, 'I feel as if I'm going mad', particularly when symptoms are severe. They feel as if they are just one step away from losing reality altogether. The most common reason for believing this is the apparent unrelatedness of the symptoms and signs to any objective cause, except perhaps in the case of phobias.

Objective assessment

Like many mental health problems, anxiety — an internal psychological event — in most cases produces a number of observable behavioural, emotional, and physical phenomena. It is often obvious that is overlooked in evaluating problems, especially in this age of high technology and the desire to obtain truly objective measures. Where subjective assessment involves listening to what the person says, objective criteria are obtained by observation.

The anxious person looks anxious. This statement is not as tautologous as it sounds since the measure involves comparing what we understand as normal with what is being observed. Most people with an average repertoire of social skills are able to judge behaviour and emotions that deviate from the expected. In Chapter 5 we discussed one of the basic features of human interaction, involving an almost automatic evaluation of other people's non-verbal messages. In normal circumstances we just as automatically respond to these messages to facilitate a successful personal outcome. What is required in evaluating the emotional state of others is to bring these features into a condition of conscious awareness.

Manifestations of anxiety include a worried appearance with frowning, forced smiles, strained features, and a certain tension apparent around the eyes and mouth. Anxiety is the antithesis of a relaxed state: the person fidgets, cannot keep still, tends to startle easily, may be tremulous, and has difficulty in keeping eye contact, while looking furtively about. Speech tends to be accelerated, as do most actions, including eating and toiletry for example. Anxious people often appear to be preoccupied, and engaging them in conversation involves changing topics frequently in order to avoid long silences. The picture is one of restlessness and can be understood in terms of a state of being energized, ready for danger and action.

In very severe states of anxiety — panic attacks — the person may on the one hand become immobile or on the other become so active that remaining still is impossible; the body trembles and there is the appearance of uncontrollable fear. Attacks of panic invariably include tachycardia, raised blood pressure, sweating (particularly on the palms of the hands), and perhaps even incontinence. Blood pressure and pulse rate are not necessarily good signs of anxiety, apart from in panic attacks, since they may be only moderately raised. A pulse rate of 90, for example, may be normal for some people and due to simple causes (other than disease).

As the ' . . . Marcel Marceau of emotions' (Keane 1978), anxiety may often be well disguised. This may occur as a defence against the unpleasant feeling, as in ego defence mechanisms, or due to a reluctance on the part of the person to display his feelings to others. Fortunately, in most cases it is not necessary to carry out some sort of deep psychotherapy to identify anxiety behind a disguise. The exception is of course when the ego defence mechanisms are being used with such effectiveness that no anxiety is apparent, but only the defence itself (denial, for example).

Aggression

Aggressive behaviour is a common way of expressing, and alleviating to some degree, anxiety. In everyday life, driving the car too fast, kicking the cat, arguing with a partner or children, smashing things, and finding fault with others are examples of this type of behaviour. In hospital setting aggressiveness may involve being nasty to the nursing staff, and complaining about the care, or the food, or the general attitude of anyone involved with helping. It is important to note that anger can have other causes (see Ch. 9), and it may be quite justified; but it certainly can be caused be anxiety. In this way others become convenient scapegoats for otherwise unpleasant feelings. Some writers (Alchin & Weatherhead 1976) suggest that in small doses these behaviours may be appropriate, but they do have the disadvantage of interfering severely with interpersonal relationships. As anything other than in infrequent coping mechanism, aggressiveness, in our view, is maladaptive.

Care-eliciting behaviour

Demands for attention often signify some degree of anxiety. Frequent 'buzzer' ringing and an apparent reluctance to let the nurse leave the room may be important messages from the person that there is something worrying him. Requests for attention to multiple trivial details is a common behaviour signifying anxiety, as is the almost apologetic request for something just as the nurse is leaving. Unfortunately these individuals are often labelled as 'difficult' rather than as insecure, or anxious. Another misused term is that of 'attention-seeking'. If someone is seeking attention then that is what they need and should get, as a general rule.

Withdrawal

Some people may cope with anxiety by withdrawing. This is discussed in Chapter 12, and involves shutting out other people, self-isolation, and non-communication. Anxiety is frequently a component of depression and should always be considered when the latter is seen. In antithesis, garrulousness may also signify anxiety and in some cases the person may talk of nothing else but what is bothering him. In particular a preoccupation with bodily complaints (hyperchondriasis), despite reassurance, is a common manifestation.

Significant others

The significant others in a person's life may provide valuable information in two ways. First, they will be able to give their own account of how they believe the anxious person has changed and perhaps confirm the nurse's diagnosis of anxiety. They may indicate for example whether a behaviour is a 'normal' condition or reaction, or is rather out of character. Secondly, the interaction between the individual and significant others may indicate the presence of anxiety. Aggressive outbursts, nagging, insecurity, crying, and other related behaviours may become obvious only when the person is in the company of those with whom he or she feels safe.

Clarification may have to be postponed when anxiety is disguised by other behaviours, emotions, or beliefs, since early confrontation may cause an increase in anxiety. It is sufficient at the early stage of assessment to identify problem behaviours and to attempt to deal with these.

GOALS OF CARE

The principal goals of the nursing care of the anxious person are to

1. Alleviate the unpleasant and debilitating effects of anxiety.
2. Enable him to recognise anxiety, discover the cause, and take effective action to deal with it.
3. Provide the opportunity for growth through awareness and the development of strength in order to prevent anxiety in the future.

These broad goals provide an overall framework on which to base the treatment plan. More specific goals depend upon the actual problems identified by the nursing assess-

Table 7.2 Some examples of problems and goals of care for the anxious person

Problem	Goal
Difficulty in sleeping	Minimum of six hours sleep per night by the fifth night and subsequent nights
Preoccupation with heart rate	Diminish sensitivity to heart action within ten days
Difficulty in discussing recent amputation of leg without severe anxiety	*Short term*. Discuss some aspect of condition for ten minutes per day for 1 week *Long term*. Freely discuss amputation and its problems without anxiety.
Overdependency on nursing staff	Recover ability to take responsibility for self and make independent decisions and actions

ment. Some examples are given in Table 7.2.

Prioritizing goals is of particular importance. The very unpleasant somatic complaints, expecially in the case of panic or near panic, usually need to be dealt with before more substantive help can be initiated (i.e. long-term attitudinal or behavioural change). Sometimes the development of strength to cope with these feelings may be sufficient. Exceptions to this rule of course do exist. A decision on the part of the person in the solving of a problem may alleviate the anxiety altogether.

NURSING ACTION

Early care

Suppression of the sense of anxiety is usually achieved in the early stages by the administration of minor tranquillizers and hypnotics ordered by the medical officer (see Ch. 2). Most of these medications over the short-term are very effective in reducing symptomatology, but it is vital to realize that they are not usually curative. Other forms of psychological treatment are facilitated by the reduction of the level of anxiety caused by anxiolytics and should be implemented.

Long-term use of tranquillizers for the relief of anxiety in our view constitutes abuse and simply prevents the person from coming to terms with the cause. The fact that medication makes a person feel better should not lead the nurse to assume that a cure has been effected. On the other hand, assiduous attention to drug regimes is an important nursing function.

Before discussing the actual delivery of nursing care it is important to repeat what we stated in Chapter 6. In some cases the nurse will encounter people who require more help than can be given, due to time constraints, lack of skills, or the difficulty of the problem. In this case the appropriate nursing action is referral through the medical officer in charge. Psychologists, psychiatrists, social workers, liaison psychiatric nurses and chaplains exist for just this function. As the ill person's advocate the nurse should ensure that proper attention is given to the individual and prescriptions for tranquillizers and hypnotics should not be accepted as satisfactory. Very often the nurse is most aware of the real anxiety these people are feeling, and is the one with whom the person chooses to discuss intimate problems.

Panic attacks

Attacks of blind panic may occur quite spontaneously, as in free-floating anxiety, or as a result of a phobia. The person becomes very distressed, with racing heart, palpitations, shortness of breath, paraesthesia, dizziness or faintness, a sensation of impending death, chest pains, dissociation, and may feel as if he is going crazy.

The most immediate nursing action is to identify the cause, if possible, and eliminate it by removing the stimulus from the person or vice versa. The nurse should attempt to stay calm and not become over-concerned with the symptoms displayed, otherwise the panic may increase or take longer to subside. Attention can sometimes be drawn to the fact that the person has had these attacks before and it eventually went away with no lasting ill-effects. Asking the person what he thinks will help may provide useful clues to management as well as helping him to see his way through

what is happening. Some people like to feel someone close during an attack; holding a hand or arm can be helpful, as is putting an arm around the waist. The nurse should stay with the person, providing reassurance until the attack passes, thereby reinforcing support and the knowledge that it will pass.

Some people find it helpful to talk about the symptoms as if dissipating their effect through speech. The nurse should be empathic, listen, and perhaps even show an awareness of what is causing the distress. If possible, ask the individual what he thinks is causing the attack and pursue this if the person seems prepared.

The basic techniques of relaxation which involve taking control again of the body can be very effective (see Ch. 5). Lying still may be very difficult, but many of the basic relaxation techniques can be used while the person is sitting or even walking around, especially deep breathing and muscle stretching. Other cognitive methods include getting the person to tell the feeling to go away, or to stop, and to concentrate intently on diminishing sensations.

In the long-term these people should be referred for psychotherapy, particularly in the case of phobias, and initial treatment with appropriate medication may be necessary (see Ch. 2). Relaxation skills training for regular use and in the event of panic attacks is a valuable therapeutic tool that the nurse could employ if another therapist is not providing treatment. In addition the techniques described above can be taught to the person as a rational way of dealing with the problem. Talking about the person's anxieties and their possible causes is of course important and is described below under general management. Assuming that other causes of the symptoms have been eliminated (e.g. paroxysmal atrial tachycardia, thyrotoxicosis, phaeochromotcytoma) it is important to convince the person that there is no underlying pathophysiological cause that is likely to cause death during an attack. Once this is established some people learn to 'live with' the phenomenon and manage quite effectively when an attack occurs.

General management of anxiety

The most effective means of dealing with anxiety is through a process of self-growth facilitated by self-awareness and understanding. The degree of growth may range from simple decision-making and problem-solving, to major changes in lifestyle or personality. The nurse's role with anxious people is to assist this growth through self-exploration and education. Most of the skills explaining how the nurse can effectively carry out this process are described in Chapter 5 and this should be read prior to the specific details involving anxiety which follow.

Sometimes the cause of the anxiety is easily established and the individual can be encouraged to take effective action. An empathic response and good listening skills on the part of the nurse may be all that is required to solve a problem or relieve anxiety. The verbalization of anxiety or a problem seems to make it more visible and hence more approachable. The important skill on the part of the nurse is the ability to recognize when a person is ready to talk, to provide a cue, and then to listen. Sometimes the discourse needs to be guided by the nurse through paraphrasing, clarification, concreteness, and redirecting the emphasis.

Resolution of conflicts may be more difficult, but a basic problem-solving approach that attempts to enable the development of insight on the part of the individual is a valuable strategy. This process involves helping in the recognition of anxiety and its possible causes, and then discussion of ways of resolving the conflict. Confrontation is usually a threatening situation for people to go through, since it involves facing up to reality rather than avoiding or defending against it. An emotional catharsis may precede resolution as awareness is developed. An example of confrontation might be the awareness of loss after a period of denial. This may occur in impending death, amputation, paraplegia, loss of love, or the expectation of long-term hospitalization. If the opportunity arises for the nurse to lead the person into confronting

a problem, it should be done gently and she should be prepared to provide a great deal of support afterwards. A stage of personal rebuilding is often necessary after catharsis.

Preoccupation with bodily symptoms may occur with some individuals and after the initial assessment should not be reinforced. The person's conversation should be diverted to the causes of his anxiety, or his attention to more useful activity. In general, diversional activities are a valuable means of directing attention and energy away from unpleasant feelings and thoughts.

If past methods of coping with anxiety can be identified the person can be encouraged to utilize them. Other methods of reducing stress may also be explored as well as talking out problems. These include putting worries aside until later, fixing 15-minute worry sessions daily, avoiding anxiety-producing situations, and, where possible, taking exercise. It is very important to help these people avoid further worries and situations that are likely to increase stress. When anxiety is due to some situation that will obviously be resolved in the future, helping the person to 'see through' to the end may help.

Relaxation skills training (see Ch. 5) is an enormously valuable learning experience for anxious individuals. It is both palliative and preventive if practised frequently — diminishing symptoms, facilitating sleep, and enabling the person to participate in more constructive self-exploration. In the long-term relaxation may provide a substitute for tranquillizers and hypnotics. One intuitively appealing feature of the ability to consciously relax is the sense of regaining control.

An important feature of the hospitalization of already anxious people or those prone to become anxious should be the reduction of stressors. Wilson-Barnett & Carrigy (1978) report in an interesting study that many people experience feelings of helplessness and ignorance when hospitalized. At-risk individuals included those who had not been in hospital before, those undergoing special tests, and those with neoplastic, infective or undiagnosed illness. Nurse-'patient' relationships (or health worker-'patient' relationships) that foster a submissive 'patient' role and a parenting nurse role tend to maintain ignorance and helplessness. Encouraging hospitalized people to accept responsibility for their own care by involving them in decision-making about treatment should be the nurse's aim. It is really a matter of shifting the focus of control from nurse to care receiver. Clear explanations and health education will reduce anxiety as well as facilitating interpersonal communication.

Most acute general hospital wards almost burst at the seams with tension during a normal day's work. The frantic hustle and bustle is stressful enough for staff, and individuals who are not desensitized may quickly become anxious. A useful nursing measure is to give some thought to the bed placement of anxious or at-risk individuals. The best place is in a quiet multiple (4 or 6) bed ward. The worst places are near extremely ill people, near the nurses' station, or in single rooms. As one writer points out, what is required is awareness, sensitivity, clear communication, and respect for the individual's needs (Donnelly 1980).

REFERENCES

Alchin S, Weatherhead R 1976 Psychiatric nursing: a practical approach. McGraw-Hill, Sydney

Bandura A 1971 Psychotherapy based upon modelling principles. In: Bergin A E, Garfield S L (eds) Handbook of psychotherapy and behaviour change. Wiley, New York

Davison C D, Neale J M 1978 Abnormal psychotherapy: an experimental clinical approach. Wiley, New York

Donnelly J A 1980 The patient in hospital: actors in an anxious play. Australian Nurses' Journal, June

Dyer W 1976 Your erroneous zones, Avon, New York

Henderson V, Nite G 1978 Principles and practice of nursing 6th edn. Macmillan, New York

Hesse H 1979 Klingsor's last summer. Picador, Suffolk

Keane B 1978 The management of the anxious patient in the general hospital ward. Australian Nurses Journal, April

Kubler-Ross E 1969 On death and dying. Macmillan, New York

Kubler-Ross E 1975 Death: the final stage of growth. Prentice Hall, Englewood Cliffs

Lader M H 1975 Psychophysiological aspects of anxiety. Medicine 2nd ser 10: 429–432

Lefrancois G 1975 Psychology for teaching. Wadsworth, Belmont

Maslow A 1970 Motivation and personality. Harper & Row, New York

Rouhani G C 1978 Understanding anxiety. Nursing Mirror, March 9

Sainsbury J 1980 Key to psychiatry. Australia & New Zealand Book Company, Sydney

Storlie F J 1979 Burnout, the elaboration of a concept. American Journal of Nursing, December

Wilson-Barnett J, Carrigy A 1978 Factors influencing patient's emotional reactions to hospitalization. Journal of Advanced Nursing 3

Wolpe J 1958 Psychotherapy by reciprocal inhibition. Stanford University Press, Stanford

Wolpe J, Lazarus A A 1966 Behaviour therapy techniques: a guide to the treatment of neuroses. Pergamon Press, Elmsford

In sooth, I know not why I am so sad;
It wearies me; you say it wearies you;
But how I caught it, found it, or came by it,
What stuff 'tis made of, whereof it is born,
I am to learn;
And such a want-wit sadness makes of me
That I have much ado to know myself.
              The Merchant of Venice, Shakespeare

8

The person who is depressed

UNDERSTANDING DEPRESSION

Like anxiety, depression is a mental state that most people have, or will experience, at some time or another in their lives. Its severity may range from a feeling of sadness to a state of total withdrawal in which the individual may not have the motivation to even end his miserable existence. In between these two extremes are those who: commit acts of self-harm; take alcohol or drugs to ease the pain; struggle just to exist; or simply live at a sub-optimal level with no growth at all. Its widespread occurrence has prompted the statement that it is 'the common cold of mental illness' (Miller & Seligman 1973). As such, and because of the circumstances surrounding illness or hospitalization, the nurse will encounter many people experiencing transient or prolonged depression at any level of severity.

DEFINITION

One of the problems associated with using the word 'depression' is that it is used in everyday language and can have differing meanings or interpretations for different people. Depression can describe a normal variation of mood (unhappiness), a morbid and sustained lowering of mood (a symptom), and an illness state (or syndrome). Although it is important to know the diagnostic labels used to define the illness state, nursing intervention does not depend on a diagnosis. It is with the specific behaviours with which the individual presents, and his experiences, that the nurse is concerned. This means that the nurse will act whether the person is simply tearful over some issue or suffering from many emotional and behavioural problems. 'Depression' then is a poor descriptive word, and great care should be taken in its use. It certainly has no place on a nursing care plan or in the nursing notes unless referring to a medical diagnosis based on the DSM III categorization (see Ch. 2).

CAUSES OF DEPRESSIVE BEHAVIOUR

Most people experience transient sadness or melancholy at some time in their life and we do not consider these states to be at all abnormal unless they become increasingly severe or persist for a long time. These feelings do not usually interfere to a great extent with daily responsibilities, routines, and activities, although they may make functioning at an optimum level more difficult.

Loss

Loss is usually a precipitating factor in the development of a depressed feeling state. However, in many severe depressive illnesses with psychotic features (see Ch. 2) it is difficult to identify a loss as a precipitating factor; or, if such a factor is evident, the resulting illness response is disproportionate in its intensity to any precipitant. The grieving process, which nearly all of us will experience at some time in our lives with the death of someone close, is a commonly recognised response to loss and is characterized by sadness or even depression.

It is important to note that grief, or the grieving process, and depression are not the same entity. Some writers such as Kubler-Ross (1969) suggest that depression is a part of grieving. Raphael (1975b) refers to the 'extreme sadness' that occurs at the loss of someone close, and states that 'grief is a complex amalgam of sadness, anger, guilt, despair.' Depression may of course result from poorly resolved loss. The nursing care of the grieving person is dealt with in more detail in Chapter 11.

A sense of loss may also result from the loss of 'limb, strength, health, independence and many other things' (Raphael 1975a). It is not surprising then that many hospitalized people experience sadness or even overt depression. Hospitalization is a significant stressor to which the person may respond with depressive behaviour, hand-in-hand with anxiety. There are, of course, many other stressors to which individuals may respond by becoming sad or depressed.

Change to self-image

Significant stressors that could result in depression are illnesses such as carcinoma, and extensive surgery which may be quite mutilating (Robinson 1977). Amputation, mastectomy, and colon resection with a colostomy involve drastic changes to the person's self-image. Some surgery may also involve radical dissection of the face and neck. People with burns frequently become depressed as a result of disfigurement, grafting, and long-term hospitalization. Similarly affected are quadraplegics, paraplegics, and those having had cerebrovascular accidents in which there is an alteration in self-image.

As well as adjusting to a changed self-image these people need to cope with a vastly altered lifestyle that has suddenly been forced upon them. Many who become paraplegics or quadraplegics are young, usually fit individuals, not uncommonly active sports people, who, without preparation, have to come to grips with being suddenly changed. The loss of a breast is important because of the importance usually attached to breasts as sex organs; they are a traditional measure of desirability and attractiveness.

Chronic illness

Chronic illness may cause similar problems,

for example with arthritis, heart ailments, or pulmonary disease. Diminished function also accompanies ageing, an awareness of change occurring during the menopause, and retirement.

The reaction to these conditions is one of grieving, but when feelings of anger and sadness are unresolved, depression may follow. The nurse can do much to help prevent psychopathology from occurring by managing the grieving process appropriately. Such is the importance of early intervention, that special counselling is usually made available to those preparing for mutilating surgery and those who have become paralyzed.

PSYCHOANALYTIC INTERPRETATION

That a depression is a reaction to loss, the loss being real, perceived, or fantasized, is a psychoanalytic interpretation that also takes into account the notion of inwardly turned anger, a common feature of depression. It suggests that when loss occurs that individual regresses to a state of helplessness due to the trauma in childhood of losing mother's affection. Freud theorized that depressed individuals tend to be excessively dependent on other people for maintenance of their self-esteem (Davison & Neale 1978). Regression occurs when external approval diminishes. Anger towards oneself represents the feelings towards the affect of loss, which are introjected or turned in on oneself.

Behavioural and cognitive models

Positive reinforcement

Lewinsohn (1974) explains depression in terms of the reduced availability of positive reinforcers to the individual's behaviour. Reduced activity results in depressive behaviour which may, in the end, become positively reinforced by others showing concern and sympathy, for example. Positive reinforcement depends on a number of variables such as the potential for the environment to provide reinforcers, and

the ability of the individual to obtain reinforcement through his social skills. In very simple terms this model suggests that feeling good about ourselves depends on the ability to obtain, and the availability of, positive reinforcement (appreciation) of our behaviour.

Learned helplessness

Another model of depression proposes that depression results from a state of learned helplessness (Seligman 1975). Learned helplessness involves a sense of an inability to control life events and reduced capacity to formulate coping mechanisms in the face of stress.

Negative views

Another cognitive model suggests that depression consists of: a negative view of the world, a negative view of self, and a negative view of the future (Beck 1967, Rehm 1977). These negative views are maintained by distorted thinking or mental schema of which there are four modes.

1. *Arbitrary inference*, which involves drawing unwarranted conclusions from the available information. A person may decide, for example, that he is useless or worthless because there is a power failure in the middle of preparing dinner for a party of guests.
2. *Selective abstraction* occurs when the individual focuses on one small detail and ignores all others in a multi-faceted situation. A nurse might blame himself/herself for an individual's poor response to therapy when in fact many people are involved.
3. *Overgeneralization* involves making a sweeping evaluation of self based on one incident. For example, a nurse may come to the conclusion he or she is worthless on the basis of a single event such as forgetting to provide a particular aspect of nursing care.
4. *Magnification and minimization*, in which the person shows gross inaccuracy in

judging the significance of an event. A mistake is blown completely out of proportion in the person's own mind (magnification), and a success results in no increase in self-esteem and continued feelings of worthlessness (minimization).

These distorted schema are thought to develop in early childhood, and when faced with stress the individual is more likely to respond with depressive behaviours.

Rehm (1977) has described a paradigm which describes depression as a process in which the person engages in

1. Poor self-monitoring, in which negative events are attended to, and immediate rather than delayed outcomes are the focus.
2. Poor self-evaluation, where there is a failure to see responsibility for a positive event, and there is a high degree of self-blame for poor outcomes or behaviour. This evaluation may be based on too stringent standards and poor judgement about behaviour.
3. A low level of positive reinforcement and excessive self-punishment either overtly or covertly.

BIOCHEMICAL FACTOR THEORY

Some forms of depression, particularly profound psychotic depressive illnesses, seem to be linked to genetic factors and biochemical abnormalities (Kiloh 1984). These illnesses tend to be rather more severe than other episodes and may involve delusions, auditory hallucinations, total withdrawal, severe agitation and dangerous suicidal ideation. Biochemical theories point to the possibility of low levels of neurotransmitters such as norepinephrine and seretonin, decreasing neurological function.

This brief résumé of some of the theoretical formulations of depressive behaviour highlights the fact that there are still large deficiencies in our understanding of the condition. The more modern behavioural and cognitive theories, however, do seem to have some appeal in that they provide what appears to be a reasonable and logical basis for helping. In its very simplest sense we can approach the 'depressed' person with a view to positive action on his part, since management involves a reformulation of thinking about self and the environment. Management may involve social skills training; finding methods to achieve positive reinforcement; reducing stress; relaxation; exercise; decision-making regarding aspects of living; or altering the way in which the person believes the world to be.

NURSING CARE

ASSESSMENT

The term 'depression' should be used with care. Many people in hospital may exhibit sadness or some aspect of depressive behaviour without actually deserving the label 'depression'. In assessing the person then, we may find what is a normal reaction to some external event. On the other hand a severe depressive illness may be apparent, requiring psychiatric management and very special nursing intervention. With this in mind we will look at a wide range of subjective and objective criteria that may indicate a problem.

The following case illustration describes a person who has many problems indicative of a major depressive illness.

CASE ILLUSTRATION

Mrs P. D., a 56-year-old married mother of three adult children had been admitted to hospital for investigation of anorexia, lethargy, and complaints of generalized aches and pains. She had a history of abdominal surgery, including a hysterectomy six months previously, but had shown a good postoperative recovery. Investigative findings on admission were essentially negative, except for indications of recent weight loss, constipation, and mild dehydration, none of which were considered to be direct sequelae of her previous surgery.

Mrs P. D. spent most of her time lying in bed, moaning quietly, or sitting on the chair beside her bed wringing her hands and weeping frequently. Her slumped posture and dejected facial expression gave her the appearance of a much older woman. If nursing staff did not encourage her continually she would not eat, or pay any attention to her personal appearance and hygiene.

Although fatigued, she slept very little, always waking in the early hours of the morning. Mrs P. D. initiated conversation with staff rarely and when she did speak at any length, it would be to blame herself for causing the family so much trouble, and claimed she deserved to die and everybody would be better off if she was dead. She stated frequently that she knew she had an incurable physical illness and she would not be persuaded to the contrary. It seemed that despite the efforts of the nursing staff, there was little that could be done to either alter Mrs P. D.'s thinking regarding her health, or improve her mood.

Subjective assessment

The most obvious subjective experience of depression is sadness (or dysphoria), which may be stated quite plainly by the person. Such an expression may be followed by an account of an event or stressful circumstances that heralded the onset of feelings. Some individuals may indicate that they have been feeling this way for a long time and may be under treatment. The person may state he feels miserable and unhappy, and may express feelings of self-pity and worthlessness. Anxiety may also be a concomitant feature of depressive feelings, particularly in overt depressive illness. Complaints of irritability, a sense of urgency, feelings of impending doom or danger, and uncertainty are common, and reflect the stress to which the person is subject.

Lowered achievement, poor job performance, and poor concentration, as well as a feeling of disinterest about all aspects of life, are common expressions of depression. Some people may talk about suicidal thoughts they have had or simply state that, 'I'd be better off dead' or, 'The world would be better off without me'. In sharing such a comment the person may be asking for help and displaying confidence in the nurse. Lowered volition may also extend into personal relationships with a resultant loss of support and self-esteem for the person.

Altered sleeping patterns are common and may include difficulty in falling asleep (initial insomnia), waking in the middle of the night, or early-morning wakening during which the person ruminates about all his or her problems. This period is often considered a danger time when suicide is quite likely. Anorexia is also a common feature of depression accompanied by loss of weight, although, paradoxically, some people tend to over-eat when feeling low.

Many depressed individuals will express their feelings of hopelessness, lack of interest, despondency, and their sense of personal worthlessness. These sorts of comments are useful information that should be recorded in the nurses' notes, using the person's own descriptions.

There are a wide range of somatic symptoms associated with depression, including general aches and pains, weight loss, nausea, loss of sexual libido, fatigue, headache, impotence, amenorrhoea, chest pain, constipation, dizziness and palpitations.

Individuals suffering from what is termed 'psychotic depression' may also complain of hallucinations, which are usually auditory in nature. The quality of these experiences tend to mirror thought-content, with voices elaborating on topics such as worthlessness, guilt, suicide, and the hopelessness of life.

A note should be made here on substance abuse and depressive behaviour. An increase in alcohol consumption, cigarette smoking, or the use of other substances (including prescribed anxiolytics and hypnotics) may be noted by the depressed person or by significant others. This may often be a reaction to stress and in the context of depression may either be a means of escape from unpleasant feelings or may contribute to a sense of lost control, lowered self-esteem, and self-blame. This latter point is particularly true of those with a past history of alcoholism or substance abuse where succumbing to the habit is seen as failure.

Objective assessment

Sadness, dysphoria, and depression are emotions easily transmitted non-verbally; in fact, they are often more readily expressed non-verbally than by verbal communication. Facial expression, posture, and activity level may be the principal cue for action by the nurse. Agitation, anxiety, decreased volition, reduced spontaneity, withdrawal, and decreased interaction with others may also be indicators of depression.

Activity level

Speech content tends to reflect the thinking processes with expressions of lowered self-esteem and self-worth. Severely depressed individuals will often simply reply with monosyllabic answers to questions and rarely, if at all, spontaneously initiate interaction. Speech tends to be laboured and slow, with paucity of content as if it is a great effort to talk at all. The focus of conversation may continually turn to somatic symptoms, guilt, worries, hopelessness, and their suffering in more mildly depressed and agitated individuals. Decision-making processes may be retarded, reflecting slowed thinking and self-doubt.

Diminished interpersonal behaviour also extends to general hygiene and dress, both of which may be neglected. Psychomotor retardation (slowed physical response and mental activity level) tends to be a function of the degree of depression. Severely depressed people may find it too difficult even to move; their responses are delayed and extremely slow. The overall picture then, is one of diminished activity and interest in themselves and others.

In contrast, some depressed individuals may be agitated, displaying extreme restlessness as a measure of their distress. Expressions of anger and irritability with a minor or no obvious precipitating event, are common signals of something being amiss. Very demanding behaviour and abruptness should similarly be regarded, in the first instance, as cues to the nurse.

Insomnia

Insomnia usually involves difficulty in getting off to sleep, or waking in an agitated state shortly after dropping off to sleep. Early morning wakening is also common and the nurse may find these people wandering about the ward or simply lying awake pondering their worries or worthlessness. Occasionally people may respond to depression with hypersomnia, sleeping for long periods as if escaping from their feelings.

Diurnal variation

A common feature of psychotic depression is that it tends to be worse in the morning, perhaps when the body's rhythm is at its lowest ebb, with improvement during the day. Acts of self-harm may be more likely to occur early in the day, particularly when the person has awoken at 3 or 4 a.m. in despair and alone. (Less severe depression is characteristically worse in the evening, the mood having deteriorated as the day progressed.).

Delusions

People with the rather more qualitatively severe psychotic depression may show evidence of delusions and hallucinatory behaviour. Delusions will consist of beliefs of worthlessness and sinful behaviour based on objectively unsubstantial evidence. Somatic delusions may also occur and, in the extreme, the person will believe he has cancer of the bowel or some other similarly dreadful condition despite evidence to the contrary. Psychotic individuals may become so withdrawn that they do not eat or drink, and hence run a grave risk of experiencing nutritional, electrolyte, and fluid balance problems. As Kiloh (1984) points out, many of these people would have died before effective treatment measures were developed. A more detailed description of the withdrawn person is given in Chapter 11 and is also relevant to depression.

Problem list

It should be quite clear that, given the type of information that can be gleaned from the person or his significant others, identifying 'depression' as the problem is quite inadequate as a basis for planning care. Listed below are a number of problems that may be identified in the sad, dysphoric, or depressed individual.

Feelings of guilt
Sadness
Anxiety
Low self-esteem
Feelings of unworthiness
Hopelessness/despair
Episodes of tearfulness
Agitation/restlessness
Difficulty in sleeping
Early-morning waking
Constipation
Suicidal thoughts
Irritability
Outbursts of anger
Withdrawal
Auditory hallucinations
Delusions
Diminished decison-making
Poor concentration
Hypochondriasis
Increased bodily complaints.

GOALS OF CARE

The goals of management fall loosely into two principal groups. In the first instance there are those aimed at providing symptomatic relief as short-term measures. Secondly, more long-term goals are intended to help the person change his outlook on life, behaviour, and decision-making processes. These latter goals depend to a great extent on the precipitating events leading up to depression or sorrow, and the individual's personality; in many cases, a precipitating event may not be readily apparent.

Some appropriate goals might be to

- improve self-concept and self-esteem
- reduce the impact of significant stressors
- provide a graduated programme of decision-making
- assist the person to regain interest in activities of daily living

- reduce preoccupation with somatic complaints
- establish a normal sleeping pattern
- maintain normal hydration and nutrition
- prevent acts of self-harm
- reduce agitation.

NURSING ACTION

Tearful people

People may cry for a number of reasons, such as frustration, anger, happiness, or sorrow, the latter being the most common reason. Crying is an important emotional expression, and in our society may be considered something of a catharsis due to the constraints we acquire about allowing our feelings to show in such a way. Most of us learn, for example, very early in life that it is better not to cry, to wipe away the tears and even 'put on a happy face'. People who do not express sorrow through tears are often said to be strong and it is probably still true that 'boys don't cry'; it is seen as being weak. As well as being a reason for believing that a person who is crying has reached a state of intense emotional arousal, this conditioning may also suggest that onlookers tend to be very poor at handling such situations. A person in tears often makes us feel uncomfortable, perhaps reminding us of our own vulnerability or making us fear that things may be beyond our control or ability to help.

This discomfort is reflected by comments such as 'don't cry' and suggestions that the person should get a grip on himself in an attempt to bring emotion back to a controllable level. Sometimes touching the person is a signal that he should try to stop crying. In fact there is no need to say or do anything, other than to stay close and provide some tissues. This shows respect for the person's feelings and allows the emotion to be expressed and the catharsis to run its course; emotions which are not experienced get blocked. Facilitating the expression of the emotion is an important therapeutic tool. Once the tears have finished the person may give a cue that he wishes to talk about his feelings, with the possible conclusion of resolving some important issue. At the very least, crying is an indication that something is wrong and may be the initial expression of stress. An empathic (rather than sympathetic) response from the nurse may help the formation of a valuable therapeutic relationship. In other cases a problem may be solved quite easily once the cause of distress is known. For some people the act of crying along with some gentle support is all the relief that is required.

Stressors

There are two groups of stressors that the nurse needs to consider in caring for someone who is exhibiting depressive behaviour. In the first place, there are those that can be identified as having precipitated the behaviour. The nurse may be able to assist the person to make decisions that will alleviate their impact, or use appropriate stress-reduction methods, such as relaxation, as an interim measure. Stressors such as hospitalization or the effects of some illness may be managed by providing support, the opportunity to express thoughts, or perhaps through education. For many, illness can be confronting, making a person aware of vulnerability and mortality, to which he responds with depression. The process of self-exploration provides an opportunity to resolve feelings and come to terms with what is happening. More concrete stressors such as pain should be managed appropriately.

The second group of stressors are those which may add to the already high level of stress that the person is experiencing. In a sense we are looking here at iatrogenic, or treatment-caused, stress. One of the most common stressors is the individual's lack of understanding about what is happening to him, which is frightening, and engenders a sense of being out of control of one's life. Providing information to the person regarding his illness, treatment, procedures, and hospital routine, for example, is vital. For

instance, performing a dressing procedure every four hours, might be routine for a nurse, but may be a dreadful experience for the hospitalized person, who is each time reminded of his mutilated body (colostomies, grafts, sinuses, amputations). Added to this may be some degree of physical discomfort during the procedure for which pain relief may not have been given. The depressed person needs to be protected from these additional stressors as much as possible, remembering that he may find it difficult to complain, object, or voice his feelings.

Helping behaviour

It can be very difficult to relate to depressed individuals because of their negative view of themselves and the world, as well as their general unresponsiveness. Not only is it difficult to form a relationship with such a person but the nurse may find it difficult to understand completely how the person is actually feeling. Rejection by the nurse would contribute to the person's feelings of unworthiness, despair, and helplessness. The answer lies in a quiet, warm, empathic approach which demonstrates that the nurse cares and the individual is important. A relationship can be built slowly, by listening and talking with the person, engendering a sense of trust. When important cues are given by the person, the nurse can respond appropriately by exploring feelings. To be avoided is an over-cheerful approach and suggestions that the individual should 'cheer up' or 'pull up his socks'.

A great deal of patience is needed on the part of the nurse in carrying out activities and in talking with the person. Both need to be paced, allowing time for physical and verbal responses, both of which may be considerably slowed. The proposed plan of care should be shared with the person, acting to involve him in treatment and reassuring him that recovery is highly probable. This involvement and reassurance should be continually reinforced despite the fact that the person may not be able to see past the present to better days.

Symptomatic relief[*]

Effects of depression such as constipation, poor sleep, anorexia, and weight loss contribute to the sufferer's poor sense of well-being. Good sleep and nutrition will contribute to the person's strength and ability to withstand stressors. A great deal of encouragement may be required regarding diet. Meals should be small, nutritious, frequent, and should consist of foods that the person will like and can easily digest. Those with severe depression and withdrawal should also have their fluid balance monitored. Roughage in the diet can also assist in alleviating constipation and mobilizing an otherwise reluctant gastrointestinal tract.

Encouragement and assistance should be given with hygiene, with the individual accepting as much responsibility as possible. Simple activities such as applying make-up or shaving, and washing and combing hair are important and contribute to a sense of well-being. The appearance of the individual can be appropriately reinforced. Where possible these people should not be allowed to languish in bed but should ambulate as much as possible. Success provides motivation for the possibility of future achievement and is intrinsically positively reinforcing. Expectations that are too high are stressful, and increase the probability of a sense of failure.

See the relevant chapters of Part Two for nursing action relating to sleep disturbance, withdrawal, activities of daily living and anxiety.

Dealing with feelings

We have already suggested that the approach displayed by the nurse should be sensitive and unrushed, aiming to develop a meaningful therapeutic relationship with which the depressed person can cope. The function of this relationship, as well as to assist the person in living from day to day, is to help him grow as a person through self-exploration and decision-making.

The three principal feelings that depressed people need to understand are sadness, anxiety, and a mixture of guilt, anger, and helplessness. The person can be brought to a position of acknowledging the existence of these feelings and then attempting to identify their origin. They can be seen as a reaction to stress which, for the moment, is overwhelming or threatening to overwhelm the person. Once this is achieved there are two avenues open for exploration. First, the stress can be reduced by decision-making and changes to lifestyle such as relaxation, exercise, and diet. Even though anxiety may not be evident in some depressed people, these stress-reduction methods are nonetheless important changes in behaviour. Exercise is stimulating, engenders a sense of well-being, and builds strength. Relaxation aids sleep and enables the body's immune system to function effectively. Diet is essential to body maintenance and well-being. The problem with more severely depressed people, of course, will be that changes in lifestyle require self-motivation, which is incompatible with depression. However, one would expect that even moderately depressed individuals would be referred for more intensive and long-term management. Changes in lifestyle help the person develop behaviours which are positively reinforcing.

The second avenue worth exploring with the depressed person, concerns the mental mechanisms and behaviours used which result in depression in the face of stress. Avenues can be explored, for example, which increase the likelihood of obtaining positive reinforcements from other people, rather than the person engaging in negative and self-defeating behaviour, which results in feeling bad about himself. Feeling negative about ourselves is a learned condition and as such can be unlearned. People can rationally evaluate the benefits of changing their attitude to one of being positive about self, by casting off previously acquired conditioning.

Some people may appear to lack the social skills required to relate well to others and hence obtain positive reinforcement. Although social skills training is a complex treatment, the nurse can help the individual explore changes in behaviour that could be of benefit. The object here is to improve sociability, and thereby increase the possibility of positive reinforcement from others. It is important that the person identifies areas requiring improvement rather than simply having them pointed out, which could be excessively confronting.

Helplessness can be unlearned by assisting the individual to learn that control is possible and more rewarding than behaving dependently; assertiveness training can facilitate this process. Personally beneficial decision-making can be learned by a gradual process starting with simple decisions and moving to the more complex. Helplessness and lack of control are often expressed in term of how outside influences are preventing the individual from functioning, being happy, or achieving. The person can become aware that helplessness is an internal state which he has the power to change.

Similarly, exploring alternative ways of viewing life and the world can help in preventing self-defeating behaviour that tends to reinforce a negative view of self. In the later stages of the helping relationship more confronting topics can be discussed, such as unrealistic ideals, self-expectations, and dependent behaviour. Some people have such unrealistic expectations of themselves and their behaviour that failure is nearly always seen as the outcome of any undertaking. Some people are conditioned to believe that whatever they do is just not good enough.

These latter therapeutic interventions should be approached with care. Changes takes time, and in the context of the general hospital setting there is the risk that the nurse may attempt to do too much too quickly. In many cases, self-exploration and self-evaluation at this level may not be attempted and indeed should be left to experienced counsellors after discharge. However, occasionally the opportunity may present for analysis of these problems. Essentially the therapeutic relationship is one of support and providing an environment in which the person feels safe in expressing feelings such as anger, helplessness, sorrow, and guilt; these are all complex emotions not normally expressed without sanction in our society. The nurse provides this environment by being aware of the cues given by the individual for the need to deal with behaviour and feelings.

Somatic therapies, antidepressant medications, and/or electroconvulsive treatment are frequently used in conjunction with these approaches, and are described in Chapter 3.

Referral

Some individuals with moderate to severe depression may require more specialized treatment involving perhaps chemotherapy and more intense psychotherapy. The person may choose to commence treatment while in hospital and be prepared to see a psychiatrist or psychologist. Alternatives may be explored, however, and the decision made to begin a treatment programme after discharge; an appropriate agency could be discussed.

Significant others

The depressed person's significant others can play an important role in his management. Regular visiting can be a vital tonic to the hospitalized person, serving to reduce feelings of isolation and prevent a sense of rejection. The ward routine should be designed to allow visiting at any time to accommodate those who cannot visit at normal times due to work or family commitments. Hospital visiting can, for some, range from being an uncomfortable experience to frank unpleasantness. Every effort should be made to make visitors welcome and to provide full explanations of what is happening to the person under care. Equipment and treatment which nursing staff tend to take for granted, such as drains, catheter drainage bags, traction, nasogastric tubes and intravenous infusions, can be quite horrifying to the uninitiated.

The nurse working with the depressed person could spend a little time with the individual and significant others, discussing progress and the more positive aspects of the visit. For those very close to the person, the feelings of that person can be discussed openly, with the benefits of visiting highlighted in terms of the possible good. Some individuals may also agree to discuss the actual problems confronting them, seeking help with their resolution.

It is also important to note that the person's interactions with significant others may be a stressor, a source of his feelings. In these cases the nurse can observe the interaction and at a later date use this information as a means to discussing the problem with the person; it might be noted that he or she is only ever upset after a visit — a valuable insight to both himself and the nurse.

In the case of people hospitalized for long periods, an avenue worth exploring is the possibility of going out for a few hours with the family. This idea may need to be proposed by nursing staff, as the person and significant others may find it difficult to make such a proposal tending rather to wait on decisions by the hospital staff, thinking that it is not an acceptable interruption to ward routine.

Risk of self-harm

Thoughts about wanting to die or otherwise obtain relief from the distress are commonly contemplated by people suffering a severe depressive illness or feeling depressed because they have a chronic illness that has a progressively deteriorating course. Nurses need to be aware of the risk of self-harm in such people, and have an assessment made of the potential for this behaviour. As well, nurses should be prepared for depressed people to state their desire to die and be able to respond appropriately when these statements are made. The subject of self-harm is considered in Chapter 10, and readers should refer there for details of nursing interventions.

EVALUATION

Evaluation of the interventions undertaken to assist the depressed person through a period of distress is based not only on how the individual feels and by changes in behaviour, but also on the person's own evaluation of his care and progress. Factors assisting in evaluation include

- documentation of therapeutic interactions with the person, so that progress in self-exploration can be evaluated effectively
- noting extent and content of verbal interactions with other people, particularly visitors and relatives
- observing level and frequently of self-initiated social contact with other people
- effects of medically prescribed care
- effects of paramedical interventions
- changes in observed and expressed mood
- expressions of ideas or beliefs indicating a continuing or diminishing degree of depressive feelings.

Good evaluation will maximize communication between all staff, who should be aware of how far the depressed person has progressed in achieving the predetermined goals.

REFERENCES

Beck A T 1967 Depression: clinical, experimental and theoretical aspects. Harper & Row, New York
Davison G C, Neale J M 1978 Abnormal psychology: an experimental-clinical approach. John Wiley, New York
Kiloh H 1984 Depressive illness. International Medicine, February
Kubler-Ross E 1969 On death and dying. Macmillan, New York
Lewinsohn P H 1974 A behavioural approach to depression. In: Friedman R J, Katz M M (eds) The psychology of depression: contemporary theory and research. Winston-Wiley, Washington

Miller W R, Seligman M E P 1973 Depression and the perception of reinforcement. Journal of Abnormal Psychology 82

Mitchell R E, Cronkite R C, Moos R M 1983 Stress, coping and depression among married couples. Journal of Abnormal Psychology 92

Raphael B 1975 (a) Grief. Modern Medicine of Australia, September

Raphael B 1975 (b) The presentation and management of bereavement. Medical Journal of Australia 2

Rehm L P 1977 A self control model of depression. Behaviour Therapy 8

Robinson L 1977 Psychological aspects of hospitalized patients. Davis, Philadelphia

Seligman M E P 1975 Helplessness. Freeman, San Francisco

Anger is but a short madness.

Perecles 490 BC

9

The person who is angry or aggressive

UNDERSTANDING ANGER

Anger is a fundamental human emotion commonly experienced by each and every individual throughout his life.

As both an objective and subjective disturbance of mental health, this state of arousal is manifested in a variety of ways best considered as a continuum ranging from complete non-communicative withdrawal to acts of violence perpetrated against other individuals. A nurse can expect to experience, and to be subjected to, displays of anger occurring anywhere along the continuum in everyday interactions with other staff, and people in hospital. Although this chapter concentrates on displays of anger occurring towards the extreme of outward aggression, it should be noted that this latter stage of emotional arousal is intrinsic in many of the manifestations of emotional or behavioural disturbance dealt with in other chapters, namely, anxiety, depression, withdrawal, self-harm, hyperactivity, sleep disturbance, alcohol and substance abuse.

Nurses are frequently exposed to angry outbursts and acts of aggression from people in hospital and/or their significant others, and often find their ideals as members of their profession at odds with their own feelings as individuals in handling such situations; there is conflict between their perceptions of the caring role and the response that anger or aggression inevitably engenders. An awareness

123

of the origins of anger and aggression and the causal factors that may precipitate such feelings, as well as competence in effective intervention, can do much to lessen the intensity of these outbursts or prevent them occurring at all.

Although anger is a universal, commonly felt emotion there has been little systematic research into the phenomenon, and the quantity of literature apportioned to this subject is apparently disproportionate to its occurrence in interpersonal relations and communication. As Rothenberg (1971) states:

'It is enormously strange that so little attention has been paid in psychiatric and psychological literature to the phenomenon of anger. Problems of violence, destructiveness and hate are so much with us in the current scene, and there seems to be a crying need for clarification and understanding of such processes and any processes related to them.

'. . . as clinicians we devote a considerable portion of our thinking and practice to unearthing, clarifying, and tracing the permutations of anger in our patients . . . We interpret the presence of anger, we confront anger, and we help the working through of anger. Yet not a single modern psychiatric or psychological volume deals with this topic, and an extensive search of periodical literature reveals only a sprinkling of experimental articles and fewer theoretical ones.'

As nurses needed primarily to be able to identify angry feelings and intervene when they are expressed, this chapter will deal simultaneously with anger and aggression.

DEFINITION

The derivations of the word 'anger', and of terms denoting behaviours associated with angry feelings, reveal the underlying unpleasantness of the emotion of anger and the potential destructiveness of the overt display, and covert suppression, of this emotion (see Table 9.1).

The following definitions of anger and aggression, although each from a different source and differing in their descriptive terms, convey a similar suggestion of intensity of feeling and subjective unpleasantness.

Rothenberg (1971) defines the expression of anger as 'an assertive, alerted, communicative

Table 9.1 Derivation and meaning of terms associated with anger

Term	Latin derivative	Meaning
Anger	'angere'	To strangle or a strong feeling of displeasure about one's throat
Hostility	'hostilitas'	To act as an enemy or to be unfriendly and antagonistic
Aggression	'aggresio'	To move toward another for the purpose attacking, or to behave in a destructive manner
Violence	'violentus'	The tearing of flesh or the act of violating

state that arises as an alternative to and a defence against anxiety.'

One American dictionary expands the simpler English dictionary meaning of 'anger' ('hot displeasure'), describing anger as 'a feeling of extreme displeasure, indignation, or exasperation toward someone or something; synonymous words include hostility, rage, wrath, and ire.' (American Heritage Dictionary of the English Language 1970)

Other sources define aggression, a manifestation of anger, as follows.

'. . . an instinctive force, probably deriving from muscle physiology, which, being influenced by the experiencing of frustrations, lends itself to destructive aims.'

(Keyes & Hofling 1980)

'Response to frustration by attacking either the frustration source or a substitute.'

(Kaluger & Unkovic 1969)

'Destrudu; ideas and/or behaviour which are angry, hateful or destructive; activity or action, especially when carried out in a forceful way.'

(Campbell 1981)

('Destrudu' is an antonym of 'libido', describing an instinctual death drive, as originally postulated by Freud.)

ORIGINS OF AGGRESSION

Although it is the manifestation of aggression through behaviour that is particularly important to nursing, an understanding of the origins of aggression is necessary to comprehend how and why this behaviour is expressed.

There are several theories about the origins of aggression, however there is still no generally accepted theory which conclusively determines its exact origin. Following are versions of these theories indicating the diverse range of ideas.

Instinctual drive

The earliest writings on the subject were by Sigmund Freud in 1920 (Freud 1932), postulating aggression as a basic, instinctual drive manifesting itself as destructive wishes and in conflict with the life or sexual instinct (the libido). Similar psychoanalytic views of instinct, or an innate drive, were maintained by others through to the middle of this century, including Alfred Adler (1930), Karl Menninger (1942), Franz Alexander (1941), and Heinz Hartman & Rudolph Lowenstein (1949). Man shares basic, instinctual drives of a self-preservative and sexual-social nature with other mammalian species, but his hostility and aggressive behaviour have no correlation in any other biologically similar species. No other species fights and injures its own so persistently as man; there is very little evidence of intraspecies destructive behaviour and interspecies destruction, apart from the need to obtain food, in species other than man.

Aggressive behaviour is not therefore purely a response to a basic, instinctual drive. This is further supported biochemically by the fact that there is an absence of any common chemical or physiological source comparable to that present with other instinctual drives such as self-preservation (hunger) or libido.

Biological

Biological studies by Malliani et al (1968) have examined the relationship between rage and electrical stimulation of the hypothalamus, and Valzelli (1981) indicated a correlation between aggressive behaviour and changes in serotonin levels.

Psychosociological

Other fields of study include the concept of aggression occurring when an individual's personal space or body buffer zone is entered, the influence of lunar cycle on the incidence of aggressive behaviour, and learning theory and man's interaction with his environment.

Learning theory

The basis of the learning theory hypothesis is the idea that man is born with the potential to act aggressively, but whether he learns to do so depends upon contingencies in his environment. Dollard & Miller (1939) suggested the existence of an aggressive drive which is engendered by frustration. This drive may be innate and unconscious, or learned and either conscious or unconscious. According to Hayes et al (1980), modelling others' behaviour is responsible for the acquisition of aggressive acts, and sensory reinforcement from the environment determines their maintenance. This idea becomes more explicit when one considers the learning-developmental aspect of human behaviour.

The most common emotional behaviour in infancy is anger, characterized by the approach/attack behaviour of motor or verbal aggression. This anger-expressing behaviour changes with age: initial crying changes to diffuse unco-ordinated movement, such as thrashing of arms and legs, as the infant gains muscle control; this expression changes as the power of speech is developed, allowing anger to be expressed by verbal abuse. The child's incomplete maturation and restraints of the environment continually provoke anger, while conflict with authority and social problems are prominent anger-provoking stimuli throughout childhood. With maturation this angry behaviour modifies, as socially accepted behaviour responses are substituted for infantile responses and restraint is learned; the individual utilizes the unconscious mechanism of sublimation. Sublimation is described by Gillis (1980) as 'a mechanism that we all use a great deal in daily life in order to circumvent the frustration of wanting things we cannot have or of being unable to act according to what we feel . . . a means of 'shunting off' the energy of an impulse or urge arising in the unconscious mind, by changing its direction or aiming it at something more accessible and more acceptable.'

The varying incidence of aggressive behaviour amongst individuals can be explained by the inability of some individuals to learn this adaptive process, resulting in the maintenance of infantile-like control over their angry feelings when confronted with frustration.

Frustration

Frustration, whether it arises unconsciously through conflict of instinctual drives (Menninger 1942, Durbin & Bowlby 1939), or consciously from the environment was considered by these early theorists to be inherent in aggression: 'Aggression is aroused when desires are frustrated' (Durbin & Bowlby 1939). The study of the nature of this frustration has rendered as many theories as the origins of aggression.

Maslow & Mittelman (1951) — frustration involves a danger to the integrity of the personality, damage to the feeling of security, or lowering of one's self-esteem.

Symonds (1949) — frustration arises through a blocking of motivation, even when adequate means of resolution are present.

Maier (1949) frustration occurs when learning is inhibited and some other form of response is adopted.

Shaffer (1936) — frustration is a situation in which accustomed reactions fail to yield satisfactory results.

Aggressive behaviour in adults can arise out of the frustrations of basic needs in early childhood, such as the need to be loved, the need for food, the need to explore, the need for expression of one's individuality; it may be more tangible, resulting from environmental or external impositions (traffic jams, inclement weather); or aggressive behaviour may be personal in origin, stemming from obesity, height, a physical handicap, social status,

educational deficiencies, or the behaviour of others.

It can be seen that the emotion of anger and its expression through aggression can be explained utilizing several different fields of study including the psychoanalytical, biological, environmental and developmental, and has conscious and unconscious components.

The situation where a previously passive, well-integrated individual becomes subject to violent outbursts of uncontrolled anger following brain trauma, demonstrates the credibility of all the varying theories on the origins of aggression.

A theoretical model showing the interelationship of the origins and manifestations of aggression is depicted in Figure 9.1

NURSING CARE

ASSESSMENT

All individuals have the potential for aggression and may express it in various ways other than the most obvious — verbal or physical attack. Some may experience anger but be unable to express it at all.

When an individual is hospitalized and placed in a 'patient role' there appears to be an associated increase in the potential for experiencing anger. Nurses therefore need to be able to identify and understand the various forms of aggressive behaviour demonstrated by people who are in hospital. Some of the more commonly occurring forms are

1. Withdrawal or anxiety — these displays of emotion are considered in detail in Chapters 12 and 7 respectively, but as a form of aggression they may result from a fear of the individual's own aggressive or destructive impulses when placed in a situation where these impulses may be discharged, i.e. the person is unconsciously fearful of the consequences of outwardly displaying his inner feelings.
2. Guilt and depression can be the result of anger towards oneself, experienced, for example, when one has held aggressive

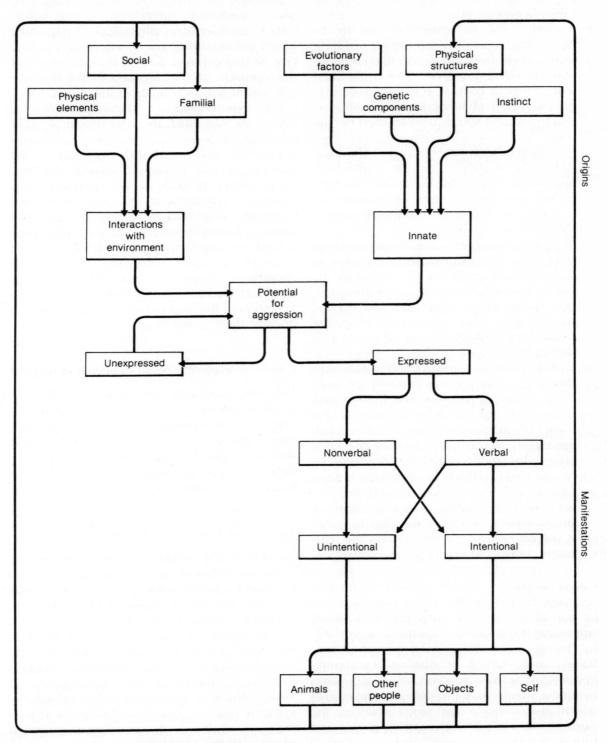

Fig. 9.1 A theoretical model aggression.(After Lanza 1983.)

feelings towards another who dies or is/has been injured.

3. Passivity and an inordinate desire to please are behaviours sometimes resulting from a slight from any action that could be considered aggressive. The individual fears a loss of control, possibly previously experienced in childhood temper tantrums; adulthood and subsequent learned behaviour, and social constraints, prevent repetition of such infantile angry behaviour.

4. Antisocial activities can be displays of aggression where the individual has little or no superego control or conscience, and has failed to learn the mechanism of sublimation.

5. Suppressed anger is not always obvious but occurs when an individual consciously withholds the expression of anger in any form. This unexpressed anger increases the potential for aggression and occurs, for example, when aggressive feelings are held towards someone on whom one is dependent.

6. Displacement of aggressive feelings involves directing these feelings towards an innocent object or person not in any way responsible for the original feelings. This form of aggression can often explain apparently unprovoked and unreasonable anger directed towards nursing staff by hospitalized individuals and their significant others. Some acts of self-harm or sabotage of treatment are a form of displacement, in which the person 'takes it out on himself, rather than on the frustrating person or object or on a substitute.

Aggression is a means of relieving tension resulting from frustration and can therefore be considered a stress response. Individuals communicate a stress response non-verbally by being unusually silent, wringing their hands, and staring or making threatening gestures. As a stress reaction, anger/aggression results in involuntary physiological responses which also indicate the angry state to the nurse; these include increased pulse rate and blood pressure, vasodilation, increased production of saliva, possible perspiration, and characteristic alterations in the voice. Other, unobservable, physiological responses which are occurring are an increased production of hydrochloric acid in the secretions of the stomach, and an increase in the lymphocyte count and fatty acids in the blood.

The maintenance of these physiological responses can lead to a pathological state resulting in some of the more commonly occurring 'stress-related disorders', for example, nervous dyspepsia, nervous vomiting, cardiospasm, irritable colon, nervous diarrhoea, hyperventilation, amenorrhoea, migraine, essential hypertension, anorexia nervosa, neurodermatoses, asthma, ulcerative colitis, and peptic ulcer. The identification of anger as a possible underlying cause of such conditions should be considered by the nurse, as interventions can be taken whilst a person is in hospital to reduce symptoms and prevent their recurrence.

Causes of anger/aggression in people in hospital

The concept of patienthood and the increase in stress associated with illness and hospitalization receive attention in most nursing literature. Several factors associated with illness and hospitalization may predispose or precipitate feelings of anger and displays of aggressive behaviour.

Feelings of helplessness and loss of control

Apart from the actual symptoms and discomforts of physical illness, being sick has profound psychological effects. The person may be unaware of the depth of this disturbance but does have feelings of being helpless, at the mercy of his illness, and unable to maintain control over what is happening to him. Control over his own destiny becomes the responsibility of others, engendering anxiety and fear. This threat to the individual's integrity causes frustration manifested in feelings of anger, a disturbance of emotion obvious to the observer.

Feelings of dislocation

Hospitalization isolates the person from his established way of life and family. The familiar reference points in an individual's life, the places he knows, routine habits, the expected reactions of familiar people, and relationships with loved ones are disorganized upon entering hospital.

Threats to individuality

The hospital system by virtue of its organization and function presents a threat to the person's individuality. Although a fundamental objective of all nursing care is to preserve individuality, a person is unaware of this when first hospitalized. He may perceive himself as one of hundreds of other sick people in bed, no longer belonging to himself or able to take care of his own bodily needs and functions; he is now a property to be cared for, fed, washed, and treated. A reaction to this perceived loss of individuality can be aggressive behaviour, aimed at exerting some control over the environment and asserting independence.

Hospital mistakes and failures

These do not necessarily solely refer to mistakes and failures in treatment or surgical procedures, although they would be justifiable causes of anger. Many mistakes perceived by people in hospital are in fact miscommunications between their care-givers and themselves, misunderstanding of information, or misinterpretation of instructionns. Failure to successfully treat illness does occur, but the failures perceived by a person are often of their expectations of treatment, which may have been initially unreasonable. The angry feelings and resultant aggressive behaviour often appear to the nurse to be disproportionate in their intensity, and can be examples of the phenomenon of displacement of feelings onto substitute objects or persons.

Not unreasonably, the hospitalized, helpless-feeling individual often has the constant fear that he may suffer further harm as a result of carelessness or lack of skill on the part of those caring for him.

Perceived assault

Performing procedures on or touching people without first asking their permission has been claimed by them to be a direct cause of evoked angry responses. Apart from being an inconsiderate insult to an individual's dignity, this action also serves to increase the person's fear of loss of individuality. Moreover, it is an example of an aggressive response to intrusion of personal space or body buffer zone. Hospitalization tends to heighten territorial perception.

Inadequate privacy

People in hospital have also described experiencing anger at the lack of privacy available when staff perform procedures or inspect wounds, incisions, or drains. Resultant feelings of fear and discomfort arise.

Staff attitude and approach

Naturally the attitude of staff towards their responsibilities and their approach to people can potentiate increased anxiety and anger if staff are unaware or forgetful of the effect of non-verbal communication.

Mental illness

Anger and aggression are sometimes associated with more comprehensive disorders of mental health, when the threshold of self-control is decreased. The incidence of violence becomes more common when there is involvement of drugs, including alcohol, and especially where there is an addiction or a feeling of desperation or frustration associated with the addiction. When thought disorder is present and the person is detached from reality, violence can result as a consequence of the content of the disordered thinking or from an increase in perceived

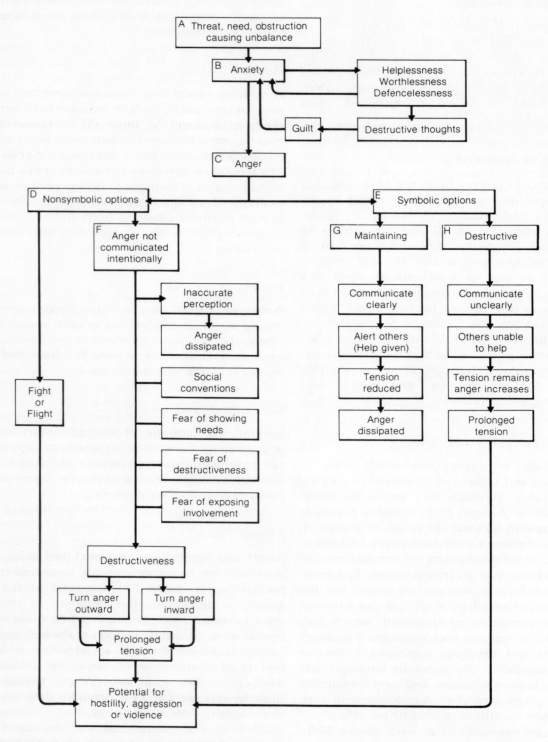

Fig. 9.2 The process of anger.(After Duldt 1981.)

threat to the individual. Non-directive aggression occurs in some states of delirium, and, in manic disorders, more directive acts result from a decreased tolerance to frustration.

In summation, the basic underlying psychological mechanism involved in the causation of anger/aggression in hospitalized individuals is the presence of factors which increase fear and anxiety, producing an increase in the potential for anger, and ultimately resulting in displays of aggressive behaviour.

Figure 9.2 presents a conceptual model of the process of anger, developed by Bonnie Duldt (1981). It depicts the theoretical relationships between causal factors of anger.

GOALS OF CARE

- Assist the person to recognize angry feelings and encourage their appropriate expression.
- Guide the person towards a constructive rather than a 'no-win' outcome to anger.
- Promote feelings of security and preservation of the person's individuality.
- Lessen the person's anxiety, thus facilitating and expediting recovery.
- Promote and maintain people's safety.

NURSING ACTION

Early management

When confronted with a person who is angry the nurse needs to communicate an acknowledgement of that person's situation. Let the person know you realize he is angry by saying, 'I see you are upset' or, 'I can tell you are irritated', accompanied by non-verbal communication indicating you do understand and empathize with him, and have a genuine concern for his feelings (see Ch. 4).

Actively listen to the person, showing you are attentive and interested, and attempt to identify with him the precipitating cause of the anger.

Remain rational, calm and dependable, making constructive remarks rather than

commanding or retaliating with argument; assist the person to regain self-control, and defuse the situation.

If the person's aggressive behaviour is of a violent nature and the nurse or other people are in danger of physical harm, do not hesitate to remove them from danger. Immediate assessment must be made by the nurse of her ability to manage the situation; if assistance from other staff may be required then this should be sought before attempts are made to intervene in the violent situation. It can be comforting for a frightened, violent person to see he is capable of being restrained effortlessly if need be.

General management

Knowledge of an individual person's frustrations can assist the nurse to perceive the cause of the person's anger and predict potential sources of aggressive behaviour.

Always seek permission from people before touching them in order to perform any procedure, and attempt to provide as much privacy as the ward structure allows.

When it is known that a person has a low tolerance for frustration, reducing stimulation (e.g. the level of activity in the vicinity of the person) lessens the potential for confusion; this will alleviate anxiety and reduce the possible occurrence of angry feelings.

Avoid delaying attendance to the hospitalized person's needs, thus reducing causes of frustration, and never knowingly give false information to placate 'petulent' individuals; constant attention-seeking or demanding behaviour is indicative of anxiety and is often a form of aggressive behaviour.

Caution should be shown when humouring a person's expression of anger, as this strategy of 'laughing it off' is not always appreciated by an individual who is in distress. If a mistake has been made, or an anomaly exists which has precipitated anger, then admit it, discussing the situation with the person.

When it is considered that aggression is likely to be repeated as a pattern of behaviour or that further expressions may cause others distress, it will be necessary for the nurse to set limits on the person's behaviour. This is achieved by

1. Informing the person what constitutes acceptable behaviour and the consequences of unacceptable behaviour (e.g. summoning security officer, separation from other sick people, restricting visitors, discharge from hospital).
2. Allowing the person to assume responsibility for his own behaviour.
3. Making it clear to the person that he has the choice of behaviour.
4. Clarifying limits to behaviour before negative consequences are enforced.
5. All staff being aware of the plan and actually carrying it out.

These limits are not intended to be applied in a punitive way but rather as a means of allowing the person to express himself in socially acceptable, non-distressing ways. At all times the person is seen as the decision-maker regarding his own behaviour.

Dissipating stress responses and diverting anxiety can be achieved by encouraging the person's physical activity. A programme can be designed, with the assistance of paramedical staff, appropriate to the individual's particular physical capacity, even if this only allows a timed pattern of breathing exercises to reduce accumulated tension and frustration. Moreover, alternative aggressive physical activities should be avoided, as according to Green & Quanty (1977), participating in aggressive activity either increases the original aggressive behaviour or maintains it at the same level.

In all interventions by staff in displays of anger and aggression by people in hospital, it is important that there is a consistency of approach by all nurses. This not only provides a sense of security for the person but allows him to establish conformity in his expression of feelings, and learn responses of others to these feelings.

EVALUATION

Identifying anger in people and intervening appropriately to alleviate these feelings is essential to promote mental health. The success of interventions undertaken can be evaluated by the observation of people, their ability to discuss their feelings rationally with nurses, and by an overall lessening of anxiety and inappropriate expressions of anger. Where continuous aggressive behaviour is displayed this may well be subject to more control by the person, and there should be indications of the person learning responses to his feelings which ultimately lessen the intensity and incidence of aggressive behaviour.

FEELINGS OF THE NURSE

When considering the effects of anger on people and assessing the management of this emotion, it is useful to consider the feelings and responses of nurses. Foremost, nurses must consider their own reaction to anger. How do they react to someone else's open expression of anger? Do not take a hospitalized person's verbal or physical attack personally. Rarely is it directed at a particular nurse for reasons of personal aggravation. If upset by the individual's behaviour, the nurse should have the opportunity to discuss what has happened and her reaction to the behaviour; normal composure should be regained before contact with any other ill person. Anger is an accepted emotional response to appropriate provocation, and is a relatively automatic response when we are threatened in any way. Nurses should not feel guilty for harbouring angry feelings towards a sick person, but should identify that they are angry and the object of their anger.

When anger is consciously identified, we are much more capable of dealing effectively with the emotion. If it is rational to have the angry feelings, then adopt a problem-solving approach to determine what can be done to change the situation. Remaining angry and refusing to recognize or deal with the person's feelings is a non-therapeutic response.

Ward meetings, at which angry behaviour is discussed, are useful in providing staff with the opportunity to share their responses and feelings with one another and to formulate plans to manage any further predicted behaviour.

Never be reticent about telling a person that his behaviour or attitude is making you angry. Remembering that aggression has a compo-nent of learned behaviour derived from environmental responses, the nurse has a role as a behavioural model; if people are not made aware of the effect of their behaviour they will maintain it until they can observe a response. Moreover, by the nurse stating his or her feelings to the person and at the same time maintaining a warm, positive approach, he or she is demonstrating to people that they can feel and express anger directly and appropriately without damaging interpersonal relationships.

REFERENCES

Adler A 1964 Superiority and social interest. North Western University Press, Illinois

Alexander F 1941 The psychological aspects of war and peace. The American Journal of Sociology 46: 504–520

American heritage dictionary of the English language 1970. Bowmar/Noble, Los Angeles

Boettcher E 1983 Preventing violent behaviour. Perspectives in Psychiatric Care XXI (2): 54–58

Burrows R 1984 Nurses and violence. Nursing Times, January 25th: 56–58

Campbell R 1981 Psychiatric dictionary, 5th edn. Oxford University Press, New York

Dollard J, Miller N 1939 Frustration and aggression. Yale University Press, Newhaven

Duldt B 1981 Anger: an occupational hazard for nurses. Nursing Outlook (9): 510–518

Durbin E J M, Bowlby J 1939 Personal aggressiveness and war. Columbia University Press, New York

Freud S 1932 The complete psychological works of Sigmund Freud. Hogarth Press, London

Gillis L 1980 Human behaviour in illness, 3rd edn. Faber & Faber, London

Green R G, Quirty M B 1977 The catharsis of aggression. In: Berkowitz L (ed) Advances in experimental social psychology 10: 1–37

Hartman H, Dris E, Lowenstein R 1949 Notes on the theory of aggression psychoanalytic study of the child. International University Press, New York

Hayes S, Rincover A, Volosin E 1980 Variables influencing the acquisition and maintenance of aggressive behaviour, modelling theory versus sensory re-inforcement. Journal of Abnormal Psychology 89: 254–262

Kaluger G, Unkovic C 1969 Psychology and sociology. Mosby, St Louis

King M 1982 Look back in anger. Nursing Mirror 155(16): 52–54

Knowles R 1981 Handling anger: responding versus reacting. American Journal of Nursing (12):2196

Keyes J, Hofling C 1980 Basic psychiatric concepts in nursing, 4th Edn. Lippincott, Philadelphia

Lanza M 1983 Origins of aggression. Journal of Psychiatric Nursing and Mental Health Services 21(6): 11–16

Maagdenberg A 1983 The 'violent' patient. American Journal of Nursing, March: 402–403

Maier N R F 1949 Frustration: the study of behaviour with a goal. McGraw-Hill, New York

Malliani A, Carli G, Marcia G, Zanchetti A 1968 Behavioural effects of electrical stimulation of group 1 muscle afferents in acute thalamic cats. Journal of Neurophysiology 31: 210–220

Maslow A H, Mittelman B 1951 Principles of abnormal psychology 2nd edn. Harper and Row, New York

Menninger K 1942 Love against hate. Harcourt, Brace & World, New York

Richardson J, Beline-Nauman D 1984 In the face of anger. Nursing, February: 8–11

Rothenberg A 1971 On anger. American Journal of Psychiatry 128: 454–460

Shaffer L F 1936 The psychology of adjustment. Houghton Mifflin Co, Boston

Symonds P M 1949 Dynamic psychology. Appleton-Century-Crofts, New York

Valzelli L 1981 Physiological bases for aggression. Raven Press, New York

Sitting alone in the half light of the electric fire and staring into the middle distance his sense of hopelessness was becoming more intense by the minute. There were no possible answers to any of the insurmountable problems which filled his mind. No-one could help; there was no-one to ask. Tomorrow! The thought came with horrifying awareness. Another day, just like today, hopeless, painful, to be followed by another and yet another.

Sleep, that was the answer. Oblivion through the dark night. Why not tomorrow too, and the day after. After taking the whole bottle of oxazepam and all the amitriptyline he felt much better, as if making a decision lightened the load in some way.

10

The person who commits acts of self-harm

SELF-HARM: A MENTAL HEALTH PROBLEM

DEFINITION

'Self-harm' describes behaviour that is directed towards deliberately causing physical damage or death to self. Other terms which are more commonly used to describe this behaviour are 'suicide' and 'parasuicide.' 'Suicide' refers to an act of deliberate self-injury as a result of which the person dies. 'Parasuicide' is a term that has been proposed to replace what was previously labelled as 'attempted suicide' (Henderson & Williams 1974). This care in the use of words is not without good cause. As well as being an emotive word, 'suicide' is too broad a term to differentiate between the behaviours involved in actually killing oneself, and deliberate self-injury not intended to culminate in death (Hoff & Resing 1982).

We have used the term 'self-harm' because it is unambiguous, more accurately describes behaviour rather than its outcome, avoids the emotion involved in the word 'suicide', and leaves open the question of cause, which may be highly complex. It not only includes unsuccessful attempts at killing oneself in which there is an intention to die, and self-destructive behaviour in which there is an ambivalence about actually wanting to die that may decrease the intensity of the suicidal action, but also deliberate self-injury not intended as a suicide attempt. It is a fallacy to assume that every act of self-injury has death as its goal. One other important point supporting this argument is the suggestion that only a minority of those who commit deliberate acts of self-injury have an identifiable mental illness (Henderson & Williams 1974). What is likely is that an act of self-harm will usually involve considerable distress on the part of the individual.

PRECIPITANTS OF ACTS OF SELF-HARM

The scenario outlined at the beginning of this chapter describes the type of circumstances most people would associate with deliberate self-injury. Although the act might be predictable in the circumstances described, the outcome is not. If the outcome is death, it is often easier to understand how the person must have been feeling and the justification for his action. However, if death does not occur, the whole situation becomes less comprehensible. A possible outcome, one familiar to many nurses, is that the person presents to casualty having demonstrated a change of mind. In our case-history, this may come about due to the sense of relief felt by making a decision. Many other individuals who have slashed their wrists or taken an overdose are even less easy to understand due to the lack of a tangible motive. This inability to understand why some people would wish to cause themselves injury sometimes affects the way in which nurses and doctors treat these people.

A significant contribution to the understanding of self-destructive behaviour was Emil Durkheim's (1897) classic work *Le Suicide* (translated into English in 1951). According to Durkheim's sociological viewpoint, which is still frequently used as a theoretical basis for study of self-harm, suicide is related to the degree to which an individual is integrated into and regulated by society. On the basis of this idea Durkheim described four types of suicide.

Egoistic suicide occurs when society is poorly integrated; individuals have too few ties with the community and are deprived of reasons for living.

Anomic suicide occurs when society is poorly regulated; the acknowledged relationships between an individual and society are broken, for example in the loss of a relative, close friend, job or money, and the individual believes he can no longer continue his expected lifestyle.

Less common types are *fatalistic* and *altruistic*. The former occurs under excessive societal regulation such as in prison, the latter under excessive integration, when societal customs or rules demand a self-sacrificial suicide, for instance hara-kiri and suttee.

Karl Menninger (1938) also provided a major contribution to the understanding of self-destructive behaviour by developing the Freudian psychoanalytical theory of an inherent hostile drive. He identified the basic causes of suicide as the wish to kill, the wish to be killed, and the wish to die; he is responsible for the 'anger turned inwards' hypothesis of suicide. Menninger also described chronic suicide (e.g. alcoholism), focal suicide (e.g. impotence) and organic suicide (e.g. psychophysiological illnesses).

Loss, aggression and depression have been identified as predictors (Hirsch 1960). Frederick (1971), suggests that stress, loss, behaviour changes, the lack of supporting people, and rejection are causative factors of deliberate self-harm. In a review of work investigating the causes of parasuicide, Henderson & Williams (1974) have identified a number of factors which may describe the circumstances of the act. They suggest that these factors are not likely to be independent but may interact with other factors such as demographic characteristics and situational circumstances. These factors are

1. A depression factor. Here there are the typical features of depressive illness such as guilt, worthlessness, self-blame and hostility towards self, and helpless/hopeless feelings.
2. An extrapunitive factor which involves feelings of hostility towards others, usually family members. An example here might be an adolescent cutting her wrists

as a result of intense feelings of anger towards her parents.

Deliberate self-harm is particularly prevalent among females aged 15–30 years (Holding et al 1977).

3. An alienation factor. As we have discussed previously, successful interaction with and acceptance by a social network is important in the maintenance of mental health and psychological functioning. The alienation factor refers to a sense of non-acceptance, or perceived separation from others.

4. An operant factor. The act of self-harm is a communication to others that the person wishes their behaviour towards him to change. He uses the act to achieve a positive result. It is an attempt to condition the behaviour of others.

5. A modelling factor. This suggests that, like other behaviour, acts of self-harm may be learned from others as the way to deal with certain situations such as excessive stress. Inappropriate ways of dealing with life's circumstances may be learned from poor parental coping mechanisms and attitudes.

6. An avoidance factor. Here the person experiences a personally overwhelming state of anxiety that culminates in deliberate self-injury. It is thought that this may explain the sense of relief felt by the person on committing the act. This is described in the scenario at the start of this chapter.

Another motive for self-harm might be described as 'existential'. Having thought clearly through all the alternatives, such an act may be a logical conclusion to circumstances. A person with a terminal illness would be an example of someone who may make this type of choice. The right to take one's own life in this existential sense is an emotive issue, with ethical and legal implications giving rise to a debate important to nurses and other health professionals.

Self-mutilating behaviour may also occur in persons who are hallucinating, as a response to the demands of voices or out of despair and frustration. These acts are usually impulsive and violent.

Hoff & Resing (1982) suggest a number of signs that assist in the assessment of high suicide risk. These include a suicide plan, history of suicide attempts, lack of personal and social resources, recent loss (separation, death, job, financial), physical illness, alcohol addiction, and social isolation.

Studies in adolescent suicide suggest that poor family characteristics such as conflict, poor communication, strict and punitive parenting, and parental attitudes of helplessness may be found (Newnes 1982).

What this data suggests is that acts of self-harm result from complex psychological processes and cannot be seen as simply 'silly', attention-seeking devices, or as the result of intractable depression. There are probably very good reasons behind these acts, and nursing care should be directed towards understanding the individual and providing effective care based on that understanding.

SOCIETAL ATTITUDES

One of the most important influences on the treatment of people who deliberately injure or poison themselves are negative societal attitudes. As members of the greater society, health workers and health systems have internalized these attitudes and this is reflected in the care provided. It seems strange, for example, that previously suicidal people are often discharged on medication such as amitriptyline that is potentially lethal if taken in large doses. When the person is received into casualty having taken an overdose, for whatever reason, the staff are surprised if not furious at such behaviour. In a very well portrayed scenario, Ryland & King (1982) describe the anger and negative judgement that is frequently displayed towards these people. It is an indictment of the health-care system that organizations need to exist which provide an emergency telephone service to those in distress. Casualty services, in our experience, are inadequately equipped to handle those who deliberately self-harm.

Current attitudes towards these people have their roots in history. Frederick (1971) claims that, 'Prior to the 1950s, except for the effects of a few courageous practitioners, suicide went untreated as a mental health problem and was hardly ever discussed.' The same author showed that suicide was strongly taboo among both professional and non-professional groups as late as 1971.

The churches since the 5th century, and many philosophers, have interpreted suicidal acts as sinful, wicked, futile, and foolish (Newnes 1982). In many respects suicide ranks with euthanasia and abortion in the extent of controversy that the subject creates for society and the health professions alike.

With these antecedents it is understandable that we tend to find acts of self-harm difficult to comprehend. In addition these acts do tend to contradict what is, for most of us, a strong instinct for survival, and the fact that we are organisms designed for maintenance of homeostasis. Nurses should explore how they feel about people who commit acts of self-harm and attempt to resolve negative feelings. It is not uncommon, for example, for nurses to feel very angry towards people who repeatedly present themselves to hospital having deliberately poisoned or damaged themselves. The probability of nurses having contact with this group is reasonably high, as some 40% of those who indulge in self-destructive behaviour have done so previously, and approximately 20% will repeat the behaviour within a year (Kessell & McCulloch 1966). Ryland & King (1982) suggest that these people are frequently the victims of projected anger and frustration that nurses and doctors feel about other issues. This projection of anger towards self, the institution, employers, hard work, low pay, circumstances, and other facts of life onto the individual can be perceived as prejudice. The result is highly judgemental and negative attitudes.

NURSING CARE

Nurses in general hospitals are most likely to have contact with people who are *recovering* from the effects of acts of self-harm. However, individuals do commit self-destructive acts on general wards, and on occasions commit suicide. The following case illustrates the reality of that possibility.

CASE ILLUSTRATION

Mrs S. H., a 48-year-old recently widowed woman, had been in hospital for 10 days for investigation of a number of problems relating to her bowels. On recovery from exploratory surgery, she had been told that she had cancer of the colon. Mrs S. H. had suspected for some time that something was seriously wrong, and was anticipating bad news. Apart from declining her meals and requesting to be alone, Mrs S. H. appeared to the nurses to have reacted to the unfavourable prognosis very well. She remained responsive and pleasant to the staff throughout the day and into the evening, although stating she was tired and would like some undisturbed time to rest.

During the night Mrs S. H. hanged herself in the shower cubicle of her room.

ASSESSMENT

The assessment and resultant management of those who have committed acts of self-harm may be considered within three broad areas. These are risk factors, immediate personal crisis, and prevention of future overwhelming distress.

Risk factors

Easly assessment of immediate risk of further acts of self-harm is of vital importance in determining future care. For the nurse in the hospital setting this will involve preventing further acts during hospitalization or after discharge, or after physical treatment is completed. In particular, discharge from casualty is critical due to the short-term contact involved. Risk does not just involve the person who has already injured or poisoned himself, and may be evidenced in any person due to the reasons we have already discussed. The community nurse may identify features of risk during home visits, casualty nurses frequently receive phone calls from those on the brink of harming themselves, and any hospitalized person could be said to be at greater risk than the general population simply by virtue of being ill. This is particularly true in terminal and very debilitating disorders, and following disfiguring surgery.

One of the most popular myths about people who deliberately harm themselves is that when a person says they will, or may, attempt such an act, then he or she will not. Any statement or inuendo that alludes to self-harm should be taken seriously. Those who say they will, often will, particularly if this covert plea for help has been ignored. Robins et al (1959) found that 69% of those who committed suicide had communicated their intention, 41% by a direct explicit statement, usually to more than one person.

Behaviour that indicates the need for help is often labelled as 'attention-seeking' and this is indeed an apt description. Most people believe that the standard treatment for attention-seeking behaviour is to ignore it. Unfortunately, this is an ill-conceived belief not based on fact; it is probably an avoidance behaviour on the part of health workers who cannot understand quite how to handle these people. If a person is seeking attention, there is usually a good reason for it, and the treatment is to identify that reason. If attention-seeking involves a threat to life, there is even more reason to take note.

It should not be assumed that one act of self-harm will not be followed by another. A person who actually wished to die may plan better the next time, even in hospital. Others may be in as much distress as prior to the first act of self-harm, and may do something else to themselves. Many individuals assume that if they outwardly show their intent then they will be prevented and closely observed, and so will attempt to harm themselves to ensure this attention. More subtle indications of intent may be observed. For instance, those who intend to kill themselves often spend a great deal of time putting their affairs in order in much the same way as do terminal patients. Similarly, if a person has demonstrated the ability to construct well-developed plans for

suicide, the risk that another attempt may occur should be considered as high (Hoff & Resing 1982). It is important for the assessor to attempt to evaluate the circumstances and planning involved in the act. A history of acts of self-harm is also important in assessing risk and may be obtained from the person or from significant others.

A significant degree of depression, anxiety, anger, or agitation should be noted and evaluated carefully in the context of the person's feelings prior to an attempt on his or her life. Expressions of life being a waste of time, futile, and hopeless, or about how significant others would be better off if the person were dead, are important and worth exploring further. An empathic understanding of the existence of overwhelming stressors and their impact on that individual is vital in assessing risk.

For some people self-harm is the best available means of communicating distress. If healthy forms of communication are not quickly established, further unhealthy expressions are likely. This is particularly true when stressors, such as family conflicts, are not examined and alleviated.

The illness model and suicide

Although committing an act of self-harm is not necessarily the behaviour of someone who is seriously disturbed, it has been associated with what are termed 'psychiatric illnesses'. Psychotic depression, for instance, is noted as a significant precipitant, with a mortality through suicide of approximately 15% (Bhanji 1979); alcoholism is present in about 15% of suicides (Barraclough et al 1974); schizophrenia in 3% (Bhanji 1979); and a personality disorder in 33–50% of those who commit suicide (Overstone & Kreitman 1974).

Other problems of significance are the presence of hallucinations and persecutory delusions. Hallucinatory voices are frequently very persistent and the person's likely response can be evaluated by determining their content and how he or she feels about them. Self-harm may result not only from the insistent

Table 10.1 Risk factors for future acts of self-harm

Previous acts of self-harm
Verbal threat of self-harm
Non-verbal clues of intent
Drug or alcohol abuse
Loss — real, perceived, symbolic
Depressive symptoms and other psychiatric predisposing
  factors
Impulsivity
Low frustration tolerance
Family conflict
Self-destructive hallucinations
Alienation and isolation
Physical illness and disability
Poor ability to communicate and interact with people
Poor personal resources and support systems
Extreme stress
Poor coping mechanisms
Existence of suicide plan
Readily available means

demands of voices but also from having insight into the unremitting nature of the symptoms. Impulsivity in those with psychotic symptoms is particularly important, since these people have a high risk of self-mutilation.

A summary of risk factors is provided in Table 10.1.

Immediate personal crisis

The assessment of the psychological state of these people involves two areas of potential personal crisis. On the one hand there are the causal factors that have brought about the wish to commit an act of self-harm; on the other is the effect of hospitalization and, in the case of those who have already harmed themselves, the treatment itself.

Establishing the events and personal feelings that preceded the act are an important part of evaluating risk and identifying the particular problems facing the person. This is no easy task and requires the nurse to communicate effectively to develop a trusting relationship and a forum for open discussion.

It is quite common for these individuals to feel quite guilty, after treatment for self-poisoning or self-mutilation, as a reflection of societal attitudes towards these acts. In some cases the response of overworked and

stressed casualty staff may have accentuated these feelings. (See Ryland & King 1982, pp. 40–41, for an interesting case history involving this phenomenon.) Distress may actually increase in the knowledge of what the person has done to himself, or in the anticipation of what other people are going to think. These feelings may be expressed openly, or covertly as anger, ambivalence, depression, or withdrawal.

Prevention of further overwhelming distress

The assessment here involves finding psychological, sociological, and physical factors that are in the long-term contributing to distress and the inability to resolve stressors effectively. Many of the precipitating factors of self-harm have already been discussed in this chapter and involve many possible causes. A comprehensive survey of stressors and coping mechanisms is important, and in most cases this will be carried out by members of the psychiatric team. However, the nurse may develop a sufficiently close relationship with the person to identify clues and features of his life which are important in the overall assessment. It is from the person's day-to-day interactions with others that the most vital information can be gained, and the nurse at the bedside is the one most likely to see the natural behaviour of an individual in hospital. In particular, observation of interaction between the individual and significant others may assist in future management.

Referral

The assessment of these people is often very difficult and requires skills not always available to the nurse. Most hospitals have psychiatric liaison staff or other similar personnel who can carry out this vital task. Nursing staff should utilize this service either directly or through the medical officer as soon as possible after admission. Similarly, individuals who are to be discharged from casualty should have the opportunity to be assessed, particularly for risk, prior to leaving. All casualty nursing staff should be taught or should learn basic psychological assessment skills to precipitate immediate nursing management if there is any possible delay in obtaining skilled help.

GOALS OF CARE

Although many of the goals that the nurse and the person in distress set are highly specific to the particular problems of the individual, some general goals may be identified. As in all care planning, the nurse and the individual should co-operate together in determining the direction of care. People who self-harm are likely to feel much more secure in the knowledge that goals can be achieved, and that staff are cognizant of the problems facing them. These general goals are to

- prevent further acts of self-harm
- determine the stressors responsible for the person committing or wishing to commit an act of self-harm
- develop more constructive means of communication
- eliminate or resolve stressors
- examine problem-solving alternatives with the individual.

NURSING ACTION

The most important factor in achieving these goals is the development by the nurse of a warm and trusting relationship that will facilitate co-operation and enable the person to freely express his feelings. This is not always easy, particularly if the nurse experiences negative feelings towards the person as a result of his behaviour. Awareness of these feelings in the nurse is the first step in being able to form a therapeutic relationship, and the nurse should not be discouraged by his or her own reactions, which are (after all) only a reflection of those attitudes of society at large. Self-harm is a serious and common problem that ranks with disorders such as

myocardial infarction in terms of hospital admissions (Mills et al 1974) and requires particular attention. Remember that we are much less judgmental of those people who have had a myocardial infarction due to considerable self-harm through smoking, obesity, lack of exercise, or poor dietary habits.

The element of risk of further acts of self-harm is an important feature of nursing care and the following is essential.

- All people recovering consciousness following acts of self-poisoning or self-mutilation *must* be continuously observed until an assessment of further suicidal intent has been made by a medical officer or member of the psychiatric team. Semiconscious people have been known to start removing sutures and other paraphernalia of surgical repair. Further attempts are always possible when consciousness has been reached.
- Staff should ensure that an individual is not in possession of articles or drugs that could be used for a further attempt. This may require searching the person's belongings and should be done in his or her presence with a full explanation of why it is necessary.
- There are many articles available in the immediate hospital environment, such as knives, mirrors, surgical implements, or any object with a sharp edge, that can be used to cut wrists or throat. The authors have found that a thermometer when broken will cut fairly hard plastic, and would thus be ideal for sawing at skin. The insertion of metallic objects into electric power points in the vicinity of their bed is another strategy that has been employed by people in hospital in an attempt at self-harm.
- In order to facilitate observation, the person should be nursed in the company of others rather than in isolation. This does not warrant warning room-mates of the person's problem. However, if the

individual is actively suicidal and desperately intent on harming himself, one-to-one specialized nursing may well be the chosen care approach.

- Never allow the person to be alone. People in hospital have been known to drown themselves in baths, jump out of windows, and hang themselves, given the opportunity. The quiet, early hours of the morning after a sleepless night and when nurses are giving 'hand-over' reports are common times for these events.

- Ensure that the person swallows prescribed oral medication. Hoarding of tablets is not uncommon and is easy for the determined person, even in the psychiatric setting under close observation. Liquid forms of medication should be given where possible. Although drug trolleys should never be left unattended nor medications left on bedside lockers in any circumstances, this is vital in the presence of an at-risk individual.

- All appropriate personnel should be alerted to the person's self-destructive behaviour and to the level of risk.

Observations that are especially pertinent for these individuals involve mood, what the person says, expressions of emotion, and interactions with others. Although it seems contradictory, sudden elevations in mood may precede an act of self-harm. This is particularly true if the person has been severely withdrawn and is gradually recovering: in the withdrawn state, motivation (even to commit suicide) may be dulled, but as the person feels better motivation returns. An elevation of mood may signify that the person has finally devised a fool-proof plan or made the decision to act. Increasing withdrawal and depressive symptomotology is also important. Changes in mood, of course, may also indicate improved mental health and should be reflected back to the individual as a means of reinforcing positive behaviour.

Despite the close observation often required in caring for these people, an appropriate and increasing level of independence should be fostered. This is aimed at relieving feelings of guilt and worthlessness in the initial stages. A more lasting objective is to encourage the sense of responsibility for behaviour that is the cornerstone of growth. Reinforcement for positive decision-making should be given by the nurse when applicable, and when certain goals have been achieved. Independence should be thought of as accepting responsibility for decision-making and organization of the routine tasks of daily living.

Self-esteem can also be improved by identifying the individual's strengths and abilities and encouraging their utilization. In the psychiatric setting, activities and occupational therapy are utilized for this very reason. It is possible to use similar resources in the general hospital setting in much the same way.

Later on, exploration of the reasons for self-destructive behaviour is an important aspect of the management of these people. Nursing care plans should include encouraging discussion with staff members of the specific problems that have contributed to distress. Healthy coping mechanisms should also be discussed for obvious future benefit. Since anger and frustration are commonly a feature of self-harm, alternative means of expressing these emotions must be explored with those individuals who have this problem. This process of growth may be rather prolonged and it is worthwhile discussing with the person support systems that are available should distress threaten to overwhelm. Where applicable, referral can be made directly by the nurse or through the psychiatric team.

In many respects the intense counselling often required to help these people in the long-term is beyond the resources of the general nurse in a general hospital setting. It is surprising, however, how much can be achieved in a relatively short time given the appropriate relationship and sufficient effort. What is important is that people are not dispeople are not discharged without referral or assessment by skilled personnel.

EVALUATION

The attainment of goals can be described in terms of how the person feels about himself or herself, and future risk of self-harm. Evaluation of risk should be made regularly and the care modified as necessary. In the long-term, effectiveness of care is not easy to determine, since we cannot be absolutely sure of the extent of growth.

NURSES' FEELINGS

The presence on general medical and surgical wards of people who are recovering from acts of self-harm frequently causes the nursing staff to complain of added stress. Societal attitudes, and consequent staff attitudes, towards these people, and the conflict of these attitudes with the basic ethics of

nursing, are partly responsible for this stress. However, the nurses' responsibility for preventing further self-destructive behaviour is also a significant stressor. Nurses assume that they can be and are responsible for the lives of those for whom they are caring. While it is reasonable to expect that a person in hospital can be prevented from attempting to harm himself, it is not reasonable to assume that any staff member is responsible for that person's life; that responsibility belongs ultimately to the individual. All staff should diligently try to prevent acts of self-harm by their approach and competent nursing practice. However, despite these actions, individuals will still occasionally succeed in harming themselves. Blythe & Pearlmutter (1983) state, 'There is no way one human being can prevent another human being who is determined to kill himself from doing so, at least not indefinitely.'

REFERENCES

Barraclough B, Bunch T, Nelson B, Sainsbury P 1974 A hundred cases of suicide: clinical aspects. British Journal of Psychiatry 125

Bhanji S 1979 Affective disorder. In: Hill P, Murray R, Thorley A (eds) Essentials of postgraduate psychiatry. Academic Press, London

Blythe M, Pearlmutter D 1983 The suicide watch: A re-examination of maximum observation. Perspectives in Psychiatric Care XXI 3: 90–93

Durkheim E 1951 Suicide. A study in sociology. The Free Press, New York

Frederick C J 1971 The present suicide taboo in the United States. Mental Hygiene 55:178

Henderson S, Williams C L 1974 On the prevention of suicide. Australia and New Zealand Journal of Psychiatry 8:237

Hirsch J 1960 Suicide, part IV: predictability and prevention. Mental Hygiene 44:382

Hoff L A, Resing M 1982 American Journal of Nursing, July: 1107–1110

Holding T A, Buglass D, Duffy T C, Kreitman N 1977 Parasuicide in Edinburgh — a seven year review

1968–74. British Journal of Psychiatry 127: 133–43

Kessel N, McCulloch M 1966 Repeated acts of self-poisoning and self-injury. Proceedings of the Royal Society of Medicine 59: 89–92

Macdonald N 1982 An unhappy ending. Nursing Mirror March 10

Menninger K 1938 Man against himself. Harcourt Brace & World, New York

Mills T, Williams C, Sale I, Perkins G, Henderson S 1974 The epidemiology of self-poisoning in Hobart 1968–72. Australia and New Zealand Journal of Psychiatry 8:167

Newnes C 1982 A cry for help. Nursing Mirror, February 10

Overstone I M K, Kreitman N 1974 Two syndromes of suicide. British Journal of Psychiatry 124: 336–45

Robins E, Gassner S, Kayes T, Wilkinson R, Murphy G 1959 The communication of suicidal intent: a study of 134 consecutive cases of suicide. American Journal of Psychiatry 115: 724–733

Ryland R, King M 1982 An overdose of attitudes. Nursing Mirror, June 9: 40–41

Home they brought her warrior dead;
She nor swoon'd nor utter'd cry.
All her maidens, watching, said,
'She must weep or she will die.'

Then they praised him, soft and low,
Call'd him worthy to be loved,
Truest friend and noblest foe;
Yet she neither spoke nor moved.

Stole a maiden from her place,
Lightly to the warrior stept,
Took the face-cloth from the face;
Yet she neither moved nor wept.

Rose a nurse of ninety years,
Set his child upon her knee —
Like summer tempest came her tears — 'Sweet my
child, I live for thee.'

The Princess, Tennyson

11
The grieving person

UNDERSTANDING GRIEF

Grief is the emotional experience that occurs due to loss; this loss may be either real or fantasized, depending on the individual's perception of what constitutes a loss. Raphael (1975) describes the reaction to this loss, the emotional experience, as '. . . a complex amalgam of sadness, anger, guilt, despair.' As such it is experienced in varying intensities by everyone perhaps many times in a lifetime; its desired resolution may be a period of growth and understanding. In addition to knowing grief personally, there are very few of us who have not been confronted with someone who is bereaved, grieving or in mourning. This of course is particularly true of nurses: it is a part of our daily experience — an integral aspect of nursing practice.

Although loss is usually taken to mean death in the literal sense, it does in fact cover myriad circumstances. These include loss of a relationship, job, health, body part or organ, financial status, independence, self-image, sexuality and so on. Loss may be considered as a stressor: the individual is forced to adjust or adapt to changed circumstances because of the impact of the loss on his life and values.

It is interesting to note that on the Holmes & Rahe social readjustment scale (see Ch. 4), quantitatively at least, death of spouse is perceived as the most stressful life event. Certainly, in western societies, death is an event not easily confronted: '. . . a dreaded

143

and unspeakable issue to be avoided by every means possible in our modern society' (Kubler-Ross 1975). As Robinson (1977) points out, our society places a high value on youth, and death, until recently, was a taboo subject, not for discussion. This social attitude has meant that we are generally poorly equipped to handle experience of death — both our own and other people's. Start discussing death among a group of people, even nurses, and the conversation will be labelled very quickly as 'morbid'.

NORMAL GRIEF VERSUS PATHOLOGICAL DEPRESSION

Grief and the process of mourning should be considered a normal reaction to perceived loss rather than as a pathological or abnormal condition. Lindemann (1944) compares 'normal' grief in terms of its symptomatology with 'morbid' grief reactions where loss is unresolved. While grief is normal, there is a certain morbidity associated with the process of bereavement where there is poor resolution (Raphael 1977, 1978, Stedeford 1984).

Unresolved grief may lead to a whole host of physical and psychological problems in much the same way as does exposure to intense stress over a long period of time. These problems seem to fit generally into the categories of anxiety states, depression, and physical illness. The difference between intense grief and agitated depression is not all that obvious as regards symptomatology, at least in the early stages of grief. In addition, the use of the word 'depression' tends to be rather loose, and often denotes sadness rather than a diagnosable illness (see Ch. 8). Attempting to differentiate between the two is complex, and perhaps not a part of the nurse's role. However there are a number of general points worthy of mention here. Depressive symptoms tend to worsen over time, whereas one might expect the grieving person to demonstrate a pattern of decreasing intensity of symptoms. In a normal grief response feelings tend to be associated with

and directed towards the object of loss. The depressed individual may be less 'feeling-specific', turning anger and despair inward rather than expressing them appropriately. In psychoanalytic terms depression involves a greater degree of regression and resultant self-preoccupation. Stuart & Sundeen (1979) make the comment that, 'Depression is, in a sense, abortive grieving', where the person avoids grieving or mourning, presumably because the feelings are too uncomfortable. In denying feelings expressed towards the object of loss, the individual instead internalizes them and the focus of attention becomes the person's own guilt and feelings of unworthiness. Behavioural and cognitive explanations of depression (see Ch. 8) would suggest that some people would be more likely to develop depression due to loss because they have learned maladaptive thinking and responses, and/or possess personality traits which predispose them to this reaction.

With this in mind, there are two major implications for intervention. First, grieving may be regarded as a painful experience, albeit normal, during which the person may require support in the expression of feelings. This support involves not only reassuring and comforting, but also allowing and encouraging the uninhibited ventilation of feelings and fears, and the eventual movement toward insight and reality-based perception of the loss and its meaning. Secondly, there is evidence to suggest (Raphael 1978, 1981) that assistance in the resolution of the bereavement crisis may assist in the prevention of more damaging pathological conditions.

THE HELPER

A third, and most important, area of consideration in intervention involves the feelings of the helper. Being in contact with the dying is in itself a personal confrontation, a time at which we become aware of our own vulnerability and the reality of death. For some, a person who is dying or who dies may be a painful reminder of some previous loss, bringing feelings of grief back into our conscious awareness. The death of young people and children is a particularly difficult experience and it is not unusual to hear nurses expressing anger at the 'system', 'medicine', God, and themselves for what is seen as a tragedy. When the nurse is experiencing strong feelings, perhaps even grieving, he or she is in a poor position to actually help the dying and the bereaved. When intervention does occur it is an added stress on the nurse that can be difficult to manage.

The nurses' feelings

A useful strategy for nurses is to take time to consider their own feelings about death and to imagine how these will affect them. Bereavement and death awareness seminars should be an integral part of all nurse education programmes at a very early stage, prior to their being confronted with dying people and grieving relatives/friends. If the nurse feels he or she may have difficulties with helping the dying or bereaved, then it is important to talk to someone who can help in an attempt to resolve feelings. Nurses are very often the key people to whom the grieving and their relatives turn for support, and the nurse should be well equipped to offer sustenance and help. Another important avenue for the nurse to take is to be aware of feelings and the stress that may have occurred as a result of a person's death. In helping people in hospital and their relatives to grieve, we aim to allow expression of feelings. In this respect the nurse is no different, and needs to express, rather than suppress, anger, guilt, and anxiety when they occur. Unfortunately, nurses are still expected to keep on smiling, maintain a stiff upper lip, and cope in the face of violent or miserable death.

It is worthwhile remembering that it is acceptable to show emotion; in fact it is healthy.

THE ENVIRONMENT

Other factors that operate to make dying an unsatisfactory or poorly managed event are the nature of the hospital's physical and social environment, and the structure of nursing. Hospitals may be considered to be alien places with rigid schedules, deadlines, rules, roles, uniforms, and plenty of hustle and bustle. Dying is the antithesis to the aim of this structure and its function — to make sick people well at all cost. Despite the importance of counselling the bereaved or the dying, this is a difficult proposition under the conditions of staff shortages, poor preparation, and rigid role expectations experienced by many nurses and health-care workers. This is not the case, however, in hospitals and clinics specializing in the care of people with cancer, and particularly those who are terminally ill. These agencies provide resources and facilities to manipulate the milieu on behalf of the terminally ill, diminishing the cold, clinical hospital atmosphere.

Hospice care

Fortunately, 'hospice care', an enlightened approach that attempts to treat the dying more sensitively, has been developed. A good summary of the goals of hospice care may be found in Shaw (1984). These are

- To facilitate and sensitize community support for home care for a person who chooses to die at home, with particular consideration of cultural and religious needs.
- To facilitate appropriate institutional support as necessary, and sensitize caregivers to ensure that the needs of the dying person and family are met.
- To provide appropriate assistance to caring families, to encourage mutual support amongst those who are grieving, and when necessary to facilitate counselling of the bereaved.

The accent is on living until death, and prevention of premature separation from family, friends, and home. In addition, there is preparation for death and bereavement, aiding the resolution of grief.

LOSS

Most of the significant work on loss seems to involve the dying person. However, much of the thinking in this area can be extrapolated to loss in general. Kubler-Ross (1969, 1975) has been responsible for much of our understanding of dying people and the process of dying, and much of what follows stems from her work.

Confrontation with the knowledge that one is dying raises a whole host of anxieties, not least of all about death itself. What will happen to the family, the children? How will they feel? What about money? Will it be painful? Will I be burden? And so on. Death is also a separation, and there is the problem of regret and thoughts about things not yet done. Regret can also conjure up anger, particularly in younger age-groups where there is a sense of being cheated. Death may also lead to feelings of sadness and even despair, depending on the context and the person.

DEFENCE MECHANISMS

Rational feelings about death (and loss) seem to manifest themselves in a number of ways. One way of dealing with anxiety is by utilizing a mental defence mechanism: in this case, when an individual becomes aware of impending death, the fact is promptly denied. Denial is effective and manifests itself by the person simply not acknowledging that death will occurr and ignoring all the evidence. Denial is more likely to occur in the initial stage of awareness and may last right up to the time of death. Anger is a very commonly experienced emotion and may be directed at relatives, friends, self, doctors, nurses, and God, or just the world in general. It is important to note that the grieving person is not actually angry with other people but with his circumstances; there is a tendency for some people to personalize another's anger and become resentful or angry themselves, which is stressful and unhelpful. People with burns,

paraplegics, and quadriplegics often direct extreme anger about their loss at others or internalize it towards self.

Dying people may also attempt to bargain regarding their death, often with God, as a means to putting if off and asking for more time. Sadness or despair (loosely called 'depression') is also likely to occur as the individual mourns or grieves in preparation for death. Separation from family is particularly sad, but there may come a time when the person actually completes the separation before death. This can be very difficult for those close to the individual: they may feel rejected, and perhaps guilty, if the person has completed his business with everyone. Some people reach the stage of calm acceptance, not resignation, about death, and feel comfortable about letting go of life.

An understanding of the feelings involved in grieving helps us make some sense of what the individual is saying and enables us to listen and respond more intelligently. By allowing the person to express feelings, the stage of acceptance may be reached.

There is not always time to prepare for loss, of course. Death may be sudden, leaving significant others shocked and numb with disbelief. Violent death and suicide often result in anger on the part of those left behind and may be a cause for more prolonged and specialized counselling (Stedeford 1984). The outlook for the bereaved in these cases tends to be rather worse (Raphael 1975), with a much greater perception of trauma and disaster (Raphael 1981).

HELPING THE GRIEVING PERSON

An important starting point in caring for those who have experienced loss is to accept the person's feelings as quite normal and needing expression; otherwise, there is a tendency to attempt to protect the person from the sadness, the anger, guilt and the general pain of grief. As with other emotional expressions, crisis immediacy is important because it is at this point, when sadness or anger is evident, that the individual is most capable of being open. By demonstrating a warm, safe, and supportive attitude, the nurse can gently encourage discussion about the loss and the feelings associated with it. On no account should feelings of fault, sadness, anger or regret be negated, rather they should be respected and allowed expression. Sometimes the person may simply require support, by having someone quietly close and listening, particularly when shocked and numbed by unexpected, sudden loss.

Relationships with those who are close to us are often very complex and rarely perfect. Imagine, if you will, the feelings of a woman who has had a violent argument with her husband over his drinking and the poor general state of their marriage. He leaves in tears and promptly gets killed in a car accident. She would be likely to feel tremendous guilt and self-blame. In another situation, a young couple bring home their new baby and, as is usual in the early days, the child becomes central to the ministrations of the mother. The father feels a mixture of hurt, resentment, and love. One night the child is discovered dead in its cot. The father's anger at such a catastrophe becomes turned inwards because he secretly wished the child not to be there.

Children may be affected in a similar way by the death of a parent, somehow feeling they were responsible. In addition there is a sense of intense rejection, that they were not loved by the person who has left them. This may also occur in broken marriages where children find it difficult to ascribe causality to events not involving themselves.

The message from the nurse is that it is alright to talk about loss, to have feelings and to acknowledge them. In encouraging discussion about the circumstances of loss, the relationship with the person, their life together, and how they feel are useful starting points. When guilt, anger, hostility, or resentment appear they can be explored in terms of the reasons for the person's feelings. Telling the person not to feel guilty is not helpful; working through it is.

When death finally occurs after a very long illness, relatives may feel a sense of relief, quite naturally, but then decide that this is unacceptable, with resultant feelings of guilt. It is not uncommon for the grieving person to have unfinished business with the person who has died. This becomes complicated when a relationship has been ambivalent, perhaps between father and son. The son fails to tell his father how much he really loves him, perhaps after years of suppressing the feeling amid anger or distrust. The son may experience profound sadness, guilt, or resentment, which becomes turned inwards. Sometimes a loved-one may harbour a secret that was never shared — again the result is intense guilt.

Loss then, often involves complex emotions that need to be listened for by the nurse. This also applies to other forms of loss, perhaps involving changes to body function, body-image, sexuality, and lifestyle. The nurse should encourage the person to discuss how he feels about the lost organ, changed image, the past, and the future (which may appear extremely frightening). Specialized counselling has become an area of particular attention for people with paraplegia, quadriplegia, and burns. One innovation has been to provide counsellors who are 'ex-patients' and are able to offer advice, answer questions, and work through feelings from first-hand knowledge.

In recent years the preparation for loss has become a part of the preoperative management for mutilating surgical procedures such as mastectomy, amputation, bowel resection and stoma formation. Supportive counselling is also provided after the operation has been performed. In the case of the dying, the relatives and dying person can prepare for the separation, bereavement, and the period of mourning. During this time unfinished business — both practical and psychological —can be taken care of. Nurses should ensure that adequate preparation has indeed been made and feel free to fill any gaps in knowledge and emotional preparedness. Where necessary referral should be initiated.

Denial presents a difficult problem, since it

is effective in guarding against intense anxiety — the psychological pain of awareness. The nurse should not attempt to break down this barrier but should patiently wait for cues that the person is ready to discuss the evidence and what is happening to him. Anger is usually displaced onto the world, immediately involving relatives and staff. The nurse should not personalize the individual's anger but should accept it for what it really is. Rather than distancing himself or herself from the person by avoidance and/or rejection, the nurse should maintain the relationship, engendering trust, providing support, and helping the person not to feel alone. A useful strategy is to ask the person to redirect the anger, and confront it as an expression of his situation, but care must be taken not to berate the individual.

Like the bereaved person, the dying person needs to be able to mourn, to grieve, expressing his regrets, memories, failures, and feelings. Even today some people are not told they are dying and so never have the time or opportunity to grieve for what they are losing or to take care of unfinished business. At the very last minute there may be panic and despair with the awareness that things have not quite been squared away. This sometimes poses a problem for nurses who are left to look after a person who is obviously dying but has not been told. Nurses frequently ask what they should say if the person asks them if he is dying. A good reply makes the person consider why he asked the question and what his feelings are. 'Why do you think that?', 'Do you think you are?', 'Have you been thinking about death lately?' are all good responses. People may indicate their awareness in other ways: referring to being 'a hopeless case', stating that 'I'm not getting better', commenting on their length of stay, or mentioning that most people who have cancer die. The nurse should attend to these cues from the person, because they indicate a willingness to talk that has required some degree of courage. People may also choose the individual member of staff in whom they have confidence and with whom they feel safe; an opportunity may be lost if the nurse fails to respond.

Night can be a particularly lonely time for the dying, accompanied perhaps by the fear of losing all possible control by going to sleep. Regular visits by the nurse can reassure the individual that he is not alone. This may also be a time when people may feel more like talking, when things are quiet and there is no hustle and bustle. Pain-relief and the individual's comfort are of course vital if mental growth is to take place. Some people like to take control of this aspect of their care, giving directions and making sure everyting is just right. The nurse should attempt to feel comfortable about this, allowing the person to lead and not fighting to maintain an upper hand. This is also a common feature of the behaviour of people who are in hospital for a long term or have permanent disabilities (burns or paralysis, for example).

A great deal of confusion and anxiety can be prevented by ensuring that the person is aware of treatment and of the actual disease processes that are taking place. Stedeford (1984) notes, for example, that the individual may believe cancer is contagious and hence refrain from touching others. Protective isolation contributes to the person's sense of fear, loneliness, and psychological isolation. The masks, gowns, gloves, and rituals inhibit communication. Although these barriers exist, it is advantageous to spend time with the person rather than rushing in and out, using hands and eyes more to express verbal content since these are all the individual can see. Regular visits to these people are imperative.

A CONCLUDING NOTE

Perhaps the most important single factor that interferes with nurses caring effectively for the grieving is their own personal fear. Transcending that fear is not easy, and the ability to confront loss requires a degree of self-awareness and self-growth. Nurses can do much to help themselves, and ultimately the grieving person, by thinking about the problem and talking about it with others. Death is inevitable and will happen to everyone, even nurses; struggling with the problem now is far better than leaving it until it is too late.

REFERENCES

Kubler-Ross E 1969 On death and dying. Macmillan, New York

Kubler-Ross E 1975 Death, the final stage of growth, Prentice Hall, Englewood Cliffs

Lindemann E 1944 Symptomatology and management of acute grief. American Journal of Psychiatry 101:141

Raphael B 1975a Grief. Modern Medicine of Australia, September: 55–57

Raphael B 1975b The management of pathological grief. Australian and New Zealand Journal of Psychiatry 9: 173–180

Raphael B 1977 Preventive intervention with the recently bereaved. Archives of General Psychiatry 34

Raphael B 1978 Mourning and the prevention of melancholia. British Journal of Medical Psychology 51: 303–310

Raphael B 1981a Postdisaster morbidity of the bereaved. A possible role for preventative psychiatry, Journal of Nervous and Mental Disorders 169:4

Raphael B 1981b Personal disaster. Australian and New Zealand Journal of Psychiatry 15: 183–198

Robinson L 1977 Psychological aspects of the care of hospitalized patients. Davis, Philadelphia

Shaw M W 1984 The challenge of ageing, Churchill Livingstone, Melbourne

Stedeford A 1984 The dying patient and his family. International Medicine, February

Stuart G W, Sundeen J 1979 Principles and practice of psychiatric nursing. Mosby, St Louis

Solitude is dangerous to reason, without being favourable to virtue . . . Remember that the solitary mortal is certainly luxurious, probably superstitious and possibly mad.

Miscellanies, Samuel Johnson

12

The person who is withdrawn

DEFINITION

Withdrawal, as a form of behaviour, is the act of retreating from interpersonal contact and social involvement.

Mild and transitory withdrawn behaviour is a defence mechanism used by an individual to cope with potentially overwhelming stress, for instance in response to psychological shock or trauma. The behaviour ceases as the initial reaction subsides and the individual develops other mechanisms of coping with the situation. On occasions, this reaction is not transitory, the withdrawal becoming increasingly more severe and prolonged to the extent of interference with healthy functioning.

CAUSES

Illness and hospitalization are significant stressors to most people. Consequently, withdrawal in varying degrees of severity will be seen by nurses in a considerable number of people. These people may display aspects of withdrawn behaviour as a mechanism to cope with their reaction to the anticipated or perceived psychological effects of being hospitalized, e.g. anxiety, decreased self-esteem, loss of individuality, independence, and control of their well-being; as a reaction to bad news regarding their illness or prognosis; as a response to potentially overwhelming fear; or as a natural response of the very young or very old who may be lacking the ability to understand what is happening to them and who may not possess as large a range of available coping skills as other age-groups.

Apart from a direct response to the excessive psychological stress inherent in illness and hospitalization, withdrawal can also be a symptom of a number of mental illnesses, being most commonly observed in what are defined as depressive and schizophrenic disorders. Some individuals admitted to hospital for investigation of physical discomfort or dysfunction suffer from depression, which is an underlying causative agent in aggravating physical disease. In these people, withdrawn behaviour in the form of conscious isolation from, or avoidance of, interpersonal interaction, may be an expression of distrust of others or may arise from feelings of failure and low self-esteem. More profound depression, in which there is significant retardation of both mental and physical activity is frequently characterized by severe withdrawal arising from anergy, and loss of drive and volition; the ability to initiate contact, move about and interact is lost. Similarly, a person subsequently found to be suffering from a schizophrenic disorder may initially be hospitalized for investigation of possible physical causes for his withdrawal, loss of motivation, and reluctance to interact. These behaviours often result from the disturbances in thinking and feeling and the deterioration in social functioning characteristic of some schizophrenic disorders. Preoccupation with delusions and an internal fantasy world is another cause of withdrawal patterns.

NURSING CARE

CASE ILLUSTRATION

Mr W. D. is in hospital for stabilization of his physical condition prior to major surgery. In the days prior to the date booked for his operation, Mr W. D. becomes progressively less communicative with nursing staff, refusing to eat or drink and passively resisting all nursing care. He neglects personal hygiene and lies inactive in bed, seeming disinterested in his surroundings. He does not respond actively to visitors, although he does recognise their presence. Although refusing food and fluids, practically mute, occasionally incontinent, and unresponsive to environmental stimuli, Mr W. D.'s conscious state is not impaired. However, continuation in this state will seriously compromise his physical health.

Mr W. D. is demonstrating withdrawn behaviour in response to the significant psychological stress associated with his imminent surgery.

ASSESSMENT

A person may be withdrawn when initially presenting to nursing staff or may become withdrawn at some stage when under nursing care. The withdrawn or withdrawing individual initially appears aloof, detached, removed, and apart. These people lack spontaneity in initiating contact with others and generally avoid interaction. There is an apparent apathetic attitude which extends to an inattention to appearance, grooming, and personal hygiene. With an increase in the extent of the withdrawal, there is a progressive decrease in, or absence of, verbal communication and an increase in attempts to isolate self from others. The person may appear unaware of surroundings, and a decrease in general motor activity can result in inadequate food and fluid intake, constipation, and urinary retention. When the state of withdrawal is extreme, as may be the case when an individual is severely depressed or experiencing an acute psychotic reaction to severe psychological stress, physical health can deteriorate rapidly. There may be total non-compliance with the basic activities of daily living, problems of nursing care being compounded by the person being incontinent, mute, and totally refusing to eat or drink. The person could also be hallucinating and perhaps experiencing delusional ideas, further complicating attempts to provide basic care.

GOALS OF CARE

The goals of care are

- to maintain adequate nutrition and fluid balance

- to provide a safe environment
- to maintain continuity of care despite non-compliance
- to increase the individual's feeling of security
- to increase the person's responses to environmental stimuli and interaction with other people
- to increase levels of physical activity
- to prevent the complications that may result from continued withdrawal.

A further long-term goal is, upon recovery, to ascertain the reasons for the individual's behaviour, and if appropriate, explore with him alternative methods of coping with the precipitating factors.

NURSING ACTION

Early management

Despite the withdrawn person's apparent reluctance to communicate and recognize the presence of others, it is still essential for the nurse to establish contact and build rapport. This reluctance, or inability, to speak on the part of the withdrawn person is not indicative of an altered state of consciousness; the failure to respond to verbal stimuli in that case would be due to a lowered conscious state. The person is totally receptive to stimuli received through all his senses and thus the extra communication skills required in nursing become important in enabling the nurse to identify and respond to the non-verbal communications of the individual. These skills will also enable the nurse to convey trust, warmth, and respect, and thus establish rapport in the absence of verbal communication.

To be able to establish this contact and rapport, nurses need to assess the degree of withdrawal in terms of the level of functioning and communication of the individual, and to commence working at that level themselves. When meeting the withdrawn person for the first time, state your name and explain that you are going to be involved in providing care and will be there to assist as needed. Avoid talking too much as this can add to stress; respect silence, but remain attentive and provide feedback to any response. Appropriate physical touch becomes a very meaningful communication at these times.

Since the individual remains receptive to environmental stimuli, but consciously or unconsciously ignores them, the nurse should provide sensory stimulation, thus helping the person maintain contact with the environment and preventing further withdrawal. To achieve this, do not allow the individual to be alone for long periods of time; ensure that he has the opportunity to be in the company of others, and that a nurse is present for short periods of time. These times can be gradually increased in frequency and length as rapport is established.

During periods of contact, always expect the individual to respond and allow sufficient time for this, but do not necessarily always seek a verbal response. Tolerate silence. Provision of a radio or television, and reference to people, objects, and happenings relevant to the person will maintain and enhance contact with the environment. At all times let these people know that they are noticed and important by using their name whenever approaching them, checking that they are eating adequately and are comfortable, and by reinforcing healthy behaviour.

Ensuring the maintenance of adequate nutritional and fluid intake, and elimination is essential, as these activities can be neglected by the withdrawn person. Details of facilitating interventions in these areas of care are dealt with in greater detail in Chapter 18. Aspects of care particularly relevant and beneficial in these situations are: remaining with the person during meals; feeding if necessary; and monitoring bowel and bladder habits to facilitate early recognition of indications of constipation and urinary retention.

General management

The preceding guidelines, apart from being necessary at the commencement of nursing care, should also be followed and modified appropriately until the person's problem is resolved. However, there are certain other points related to the behaviour pattern of withdrawal which nurses should attend to throughout their care.

Withdrawn behaviour, of the type most commonly seen by the nurse, is an expression of the individual's emotional distress. In order for people to be able to recognize the specific nature of their distress, they have to be able to explore and talk about their feelings. The nurse therefore must provide and promote a supportive and secure environment in which the individual can feel safe to discuss these feelings. The nurse should appropriately encourage the person to express emotions and should also be available and receptive when the person chooses to do so. At first, when verbal expression is too difficult a task, the nurse could suggest that the person gives vent to emotions through the less threatening medium of writing down thoughts and feelings. Later, as the extent of the withdrawn behaviour diminishes, the person should be encouraged to openly verbalize emotions as much as possible.

Physical health should be attended to as well as emotional state. Physical activity is just as important as interaction and verbal communication in fostering an alteration in the pattern of withdrawn behaviour.

Involvement of the individual in extensive physical activity is often limited by constraints of the general ward situation and the willingness of the person to participate. However, passive exercises can be undertaken with the assistance of a physiotherapist or occupational therapist, with the aims of maintaining physiological function and involving the individual in his or her care. If non-compliance is extreme, then routine attention to skin and general pressure care provides a basic but essential form of physical activity.

When an individual withdraws from reality, one of the first changes in behaviour may be a significant loss of interest in personal hygiene and attractiveness, associated with a loss of, or lowered, self-esteem. By paying close attention to grooming and general personal hygiene and encouraging the person to carry out these activities, the nurse can assist in increasing self-esteem and allaying any

feelings of uselessness and worthlessness. It is important for the nurse to help the withdrawn to take responsibility for his own personal hygiene and grooming.

Planning effective interventions that will help each individual depends primarily on an accurate initial assessment of the aforementioned problems. The nurse must be alert to the need to differentiate between a behaviour pattern of withdrawal and the display of behaviour characteristic of a pre-morbid personality type. Such a personality type may manifest as a quiet, aloof, uninvolved person, these traits being formed early in life, possibly as a result of a childhood inability to establish relationships (Kahana & Bibring 1964). These traits bear a close resemblance to the initial presenting characteristics of a withdrawn behaviour pattern. The difference between the two lies mainly in the attitude of the person to his environment, compliance with maintaining health care and general functioning, and differing levels and extents of response. If the individual is not demonstrating an uncharacteristic withdrawal but merely maintaining a usual and long-term personality trait, then many of the interventions suggested for the withdrawn individual may in fact be the antithesis of what is required. The naturally quiet, aloof person may, for instance, feel more comfortable in a single room, spending as much time as is practical alone, whenever privacy is possible. This being the case, the nurse should respect the individual's desire to remain emotionally and physically distant, as this will not compound an emotional state or complicate illness or recuperation. Physical touch by the nurse should be avoided unless it is necessary in providing direct care. The nurse should not pressure the person with continual verbal probing into thoughts and feelings, nor reciprocate quiet uninvolvement, but remain available and receptive.

EVALUATION

The effectiveness of interventions in the care of the withdrawn person should be evaluated by continually assessing levels of functioning and the response to nurses, other people, and general environmental stimuli. Expecting or forcing too much too quickly from these people will retard recovery and can precipitate further withdrawal.

Ongoing care can also be achieved by monitoring the person's performance, on a daily basis, in a programme of low-level goal-setting. Each daily goal must be easily and quickly achievable by the individual.

If during the process of care it becomes apparent that the nursing management is not being effective, then reassessment should be undertaken, bearing in mind that withdrawn behaviour may be symptomatic of a depressive illness. In such a state, the individual could be experiencing a loss of ability to relate to other people, associated with feelings of sadness, apathy, and a general loss of energy. Depression is a common reaction to illness, especially in those who are responding to some form of loss (Donnelly 1979). This loss can be directly related to aspects of their illness, or may involve a real or perceived change in their role within the family or work situation, or a loss of actual function. The loss can either be obvious and tangible such as that which results from an amputation or radical surgery, or more subjective, as in spinal cord injuries, cerebrovascular accidents, chronic debilitating disorders, and terminal illness.

A further point to be considered in caring for those displaying withdrawn behaviour, is whether the person was depressed or withdrawn prior to admission to hospital. The behaviour in hospital may be due to pre-existing stress and not to illness or hospitalization: there may be no correlation at all between the withdrawn behaviour seen by the nurse and illness or hospitalization. In this case, many of the interventions undertaken by nurses may prove to be ineffectual.

FEELINGS OF THE NURSE

It is important to be aware that there is a vital difference between non-compliance in withdrawal and non-compliance due to rational decision-making. A person who is making a rational decision regarding treatment has every right to refuse any care. In the case of withdrawn people, where the disturbed behaviour pattern is interfering with the health and nursing care, it is more therapeutic to gently insist that care be given rather than to avoid the problem. More than one nurse may be required at one time to facilitate delivery of care when non-compliance is evident. Do not hesitate to seek assistance as required.

Providing nursing care to a withdrawn person is demanding and emotionally tiring. It is not always easy to give and sustain emotional warmth and personal care to an unresponsive person who may appear deliberately non-compliant and negative. To provide this care, endeavouring to establish rapport and maintain a close relationship with the individual, requires a great deal of patience, and may be interspersed with feelings of frustration and anger. These unpleasant emotions can be distressing to nurses who feel such emotions are incongruent with their professional ethics and incompatible with good nursing care. At times the nurse may consider that a person is failing to respond quickly enough or is becoming increasingly withdrawn despite intense efforts to alter the situation. This state of affairs is disheartening to the nurse, who may experience a sense of failure, particularly if the person continues to reject approaches. At these times it can be easier to consider that any efforts are going to fail, or that the person is not going to ever allow formation of a relationship; however, the nurse must be able to maintain a consistent, accepting approach at all times.

REFERENCES

Donnelly T 1979 The neuroses. In: Visdin G, Lewis T (eds) Psychiatry in general medical practice. McGraw Hill, New York
Kahana R, Bibring G L 1964 Personality types in medical management. In Zinberg N (ed) Psychiatry and medical practice in a general hospital. International Universities Press, New York

The forest appears more dense now, the track you have been following for miles very much resembles one you traversed earlier, in another direction; you no longer know how far or in which direction you must go. It is getting dark and you seem to have been walking for hours, unaware of the progress of time. You are hopelessly lost — not knowing exactly where you are relative to the environment, and how long you have been there; but are you disorientated? The apprehension, the inability to think clearly and find a solution to your problem cause a feeling of anxiety and uncertainty. In the fading light, things around you momentarily appear to be something they are not, and your heightened alertness causes you to hear sounds you cannot immediately recognize. You are anxious, muddled, perplexed; but are you confused?

13

The confused and disoriented person

DISORIENTATION

Many people state that they are 'disorientated' when they find themselves lost in unfamiliar surroundings or wake up after an unusually prolonged sleep not knowing the time of day. This phenomenon can be experienced by anybody and is generally not considered to be symptomatic of any pathology, since the person can regain knowledge of his whereabouts or the time when in receipt of the necessary information. A state of true disorientation is more profound and can be an indicator of an individual's lack of clarity of thinking and cognitive dysfunction.

Orientation may be defined as the ability to recognize one's surroundings and their temporal and spatial relationships to oneself, or to appreciate one's relations to the social environment (Freedman et al 1976).

A mentally healthy person is orientated in three spheres: to time, place, and person. To be orientated to time, one would be expected to know the approximate time of day, the day of the week, and the month or season and the year. Orientation to place involves knowing, or being able to work out where one is in terms of the surrounding environment. Correctly identifying people in your environment and knowing who you are in relation to them, constitute being orientated to person. A person deficient in any one, or all three, of these areas is considered to be disorientated.

CONFUSION

'Confusion' is a word often used in everyday language to describe an inability to distinguish one thing from another, or to readily understand or process information. This feeling, state or emotion can be experienced by an individual and not be apparent to an observer, in which case it is described as 'subjective confusion'. Objective confusion is obvious to others, being manifest in a person's speech and behaviour. As a clinical sign, objective confusion is a more complex syndrome than the feelings of bewilderment often experienced by the healthy individual.

Confusion in a clinical sense refers to an impairment of cognitive functioning characterized by a state of perplexity, muddled thought processes associated with delays or an inability to perform routine acts, and disorientation resulting in a disturbed awareness of the immediate environment. Confusion is a clouding of consciousness that is a state between, at one extreme, maximal alertness, and at the other, stupor and coma. In those with neurological trauma, for example, confusion (and disorientation) is an important sign of deterioration. Associated with, and compounding the state of confusion, are impairment in memory and judgement (Sainsbury 1980).

CAUSES OF DISORIENTATION AND CONFUSION

Disorientation and confusion are commonly coexistent symptoms of, and sequelae to, a number of disturbances of physical and mental health, and will be encountered frequently by nurses in any ward of a general hospital. Many nursing hours on a busy ward can be spent on the disturbances of behaviour that are associated with these symptoms. The states of confusion and disorientation can be either acute, lasting hours or days, or chronic and unremitting, depending on their causation.

ACUTE CAUSES

There are several causal factors responsible for acute disturbances in which confusion and disorientation are prominent features. The underlying pathophysiology in these states is a reversible disruption occurring in the metabolic processes of the neurons of the brain. It is this transient interference in brain function that produces the confusion often displayed in the following commonly occurring states of ill-health.

- post-anaesthetic recovery
- severe infectious diseases, e.g. meningitis, encephalitis, pneumonia
- conditions in which there is a fluid or electrolyte imbalance
- hypoglycaemic states
- head injury causing brain trauma
- cerebrovascular accidents
- transient ischaemic attacks
- post-ictal confusion following epileptic seizures
- vitamin deficiencies, especially of the B group.

A typical case of confusion and disorientation occurring in a general hospital is depicted in the following case illustration.

CASE ILLUSTRATION

Mrs D. L., a 55-year-old widow, is admitted to a medical ward, undernourished, and generally in a poor state of health. She is moderately dehydrated, and hyperpyrexic, with an increase in pulse rate, and respirations. Physical and radiological examination indicate lobar pneumonia and routine treatment is commenced immediately.

Although lethargic and drowsy following admission, during her first evening in hospital Mrs D. L. becomes restless and agitated, insisting she must get up and prepare breakfast for the children. She begins to misinterpret aspects of her immediate environment and misidentifies the nurses as her children, expressing her anger at their apparent disobediance of her instructions to get ready for school.

As the night progresses and the ward lighting is dimmed, Mrs D. L.'s agitation increases, her speech becomes accelerated and incoherent, and her initial aggression changes to apparent fear and increased motor (physical) activity. She does not appear to know where she is or the identities and intentions of the people around her; nor does she realise she is unwell.

Unable to settle Mrs D. L. and fearful of the lady causing herself some harm, the nurse in charge summons a doctor who prescribes sedating medication.

Over the next few days Mrs D. L. remains confused and disorientated although no longer as agitated. At first she is unable to perform properly the basic activities of daily living and remains totally disorientated to time, place and person. This state diminishes progressively over the ensuing days. By the end of one week in hospital Mrs D. L. is completely settled and fully aware of her surroundings; her pneumonia is responding to treatment and the electrolyte imbalance and nutritional state have been corrected.

CHRONIC CAUSES

Confusion can be a permanent state, in which the interference in brain function is continuous, rendering the individual permanently unable to re-orientate himself or to diminish his muddled thinking. Conditions in which this degree of chronicity exist include

- dementias (including permanent brain trauma)
- metastatic disease
- advanced stages of Parkinson's disease and Huntington's chorea.

The second case, illustrated below, depicts a more chronic manifestation of confusion and disorientation.

CASE ILLUSTRATION

Mr D. M., an 80-year-old retired salesperson, has for the past 2 years been living in a retirement home. Over the previous months his social functioning and ability to care for himself have deteriorated progressively to the stage where he has been referred to hospital for assessment of his general health.

Prior to admission, Mr D. M.'s behaviour had become a concern to the staff of the home. He was wandering away from his surroundings, leaving taps running in the bathroom, and continually allowing food he was cooking to burn; he had also left electric radiators switched on unnecessarily in his absence.

In hospital, Mr D. M. was noted to have poor concentration, and was unable to remember which was his bed or the names of any of the nurses or doctors. He would, however, tell repeatedly and in great detail stories of his younger days. On occasions he would become angry and insulting, claiming that other people were taking his belongings. This mood quickly changed to one of mischievousness, making lecherous comments to individual female nurses. Mr D. M. appeared unable to make decisions for himself, and became bewildered and anxious when attempting to do anything that necessitated

some thought. He required assistance with washing, dressing and ambulating, and was occasionally incontinent of urine.

Apart from hypertension and evidence of cardiovascular disease, Mr D. M. had no other apparent acute physical illness.

NURSING CARE

ASSESSMENT

People who are hospitalized for reasons other than organic brain disease often lose track of the date, the day of the week, and even the month if their stay extends to a lengthy period. In such cases simple questioning to test orientation to time may evoke incorrect replies; these are not necessarily diagnostic of impaired brain function. However, if on questioning, an error in the year is made repeatedly, then this is of diagnostic significance, as is an error in the time of day if this involves mistaking meal-times (Freedman et al 1976). Continually becoming lost within the ward environs, and an inability to find the way back to bed or to the toilet, may be indications of disorientation to place. This disorientation will of course be complicated by any impairment in memory.

Misidentifications of nursing staff will commonly occur when confusion and disorientation are present; individuals often think they are in a different situation and that the people around them are not who they claim to be. On other occasions a person may correctly state the name of the hospital, but incorrectly claim it is a restaurant or hotel, or misplace it geographically.

The perplexity and muddled thought processes characteristic of confusion may be evidenced, in those who are hospitalized, by an apparent inability to perform what are considered routine activities of daily living. The acts of putting on clothing, washing, or eating may not be able to be performed, or may take an extraordinary amount of time to be completed. This is not due to any dysfunction of motor activity, but arises from muddled thinking that results in a basic inability to work out the sequential steps necessary to perform the action.

Often associated with a confusional state are feelings of anxiety. Disorientation, the tendency to misinterpret environmental stimuli and misidentify people, can cause the individual to be suspicious of, and hostile towards, those around him. This uncharacteristic aggression appears unreasonable to other people, who see the behaviour as unprovoked and having no apparent precipitant. If the confusion is arising from a serious delirium, the person may also be experiencing illusionary and hallucinatory phenomena, further aggravating the state and complicating nursing management.

The nurse must, therefore, be alert to the potential complexity of interrelated emotions and behaviours experienced and demonstrated by an individual suffering from an illness in which confusion and disorientation are primary signs. Each display of emotional distress requires separate interventions, necessitating an understanding of the psychopathological process in its entirety. Intervention and management of the various interrelated disturbances (e.g. anxiety, thought disorder, aggression) associated with states of confusion are examined in separate chapters (see Chs 7, 9, 14).

GOALS OF CARE

When planning nursing care the goals to be considered are

- to identify, where possible, the cause of confusion and disorientation
- to prevent further physical and psychological deterioration
- to alleviate and/or prevent anxiety and reduce stress
- to provide safety and protection
- to obtain and maintain compliance with the activities of daily living, nursing, and paranursing treatment
- to preserve rewarding qualities of life
- to regain contact with reality.

NURSING ACTION

The first problem to be confronted by the nurse is actually initiating contact with the confused person and establishing communication. Bearing in mind that the individual may be misidentifying staff, and unaware of his situation, the nurse's approach should be in a calm, non-threatening manner. Unrealistic expectations by the nurse of responses to attempts at meaningful communication will result in frustration for both nurse and individual. In particular, compliance — which is an important initial goal in establishing a relationship — may be threatened.

The muddled thinking experienced by the confused dramatically alters and slows down the ability to process information, and to understand what is being said. To diminish the effect of this problem, the nurse's speech should be clear and unhurried, with uncomplicated, straightforward vocabulary which avoids terminology or phraseology that could be open to misinterpretation. Providing ample explanation prior to performing any procedure or activity also facilitates the prevention of unnecessary anxiety. Do not assume that because these people do not appear to comprehend what is being said they will not care to be concerned about what is happening around them.

These explanations may also play a part in the process of establishing a contact with reality through reorientation and focusing attention. The nurse becomes associated with the role of helper, a person to be trusted and who is non-threatening.

As the ability to process information is impaired, the amount of information available to the brain in the form of sensory stimuli should be limited. This can be achieved by ensuring a quiet restful environment, a feature often lacking in institutions such as hospitals.

A common feature of those being treated in intensive care units is delirium which includes confusion and disorientation as central symptoms. This state is due not only to toxicity in many serious illnesses but also to the environment (Baxter 1975), which is overloaded with monotonous sensory input such as monitors beeping and respirators 'whooshing'. Because of this problem very special attention needs to be paid to rest, reorientation, and personal contact in acute care areas where the environment is not as beneficial as needed. In contrast, it should not be assumed that these people should be isolated from others; too much peace and quiet may constitute sensory deprivation.

Since cognitive functioning is impaired, the need for the individual to use problem-solving thinking should be maintained at a minimum, and this can be achieved by avoiding excessive or complex decision-making on his part. In many cases basic decisions involved in daily living may have to be made by the nurse; these may include the choice of clothing or food. The nurse may even have to assist in the performance of basic tasks such as dressing, washing, and eating, as the degree of confusion may preclude the person from being able to perform these activities of his own volition.

Making frequent, brief contacts is reassuring, lessens agitation, and assists in reorientation. Moreover, this facilitates the building of rapport with the person, who will begin to trust staff and feel safe and secure. This may produce a subsequent diminution of hostility and increase compliance with the endeavours of the nurse, particularly in regard to essential daily functioning. By reducing the level of anxiety and establishing a sense of security, the frequent use of the call buzzer can be diminished.

Confusion typically becomes worse with the onset of darkness. This phenomenon is often a problem in the care of the elderly, and is frequently witnessed in wards of hospitals where people may be recovering from recent surgery or suffering from any of the causes of confusion previously mentioned. This problem can be alleviated by anticipating this exaggeration of distress and leaving a dim light in the vicinity of the individual during the night. Explanation of such things as the changing reflections and shadows occurring at night will prevent misperceptions of objects and move-

ment (illusionary misperceptions), with a subsequent decrease in anxiety.

Before examining the problems and interventions involved in helping the disoriented, it is of interest to consider the involvement of impaired short-term memory. Although it is ultimately the display of disorientation (rather than its cause) that is of concern to the nurse, it is worth considering whether the problem is arising solely as the result of an inability to remember where one is, what date it is, or various personal relationships. If this is the case, and the impairment in memory is of sufficient severity, the individual may not regain the ability to remember specific data for long enough to remain orientated. It is difficult to ascertain the extent to which impairment of memory and concentration are involved in any state of disorientation, and it is possibly unnecessary to make the differentiation. When planning care, the principles of management will be the same regardless of the cause; only the on-going management and ultimate success of any intervention will differ, and will become evident during continual evaluation of the care plan.

Identifying problems and planning appropriate care is facilitated by examining separately the three spheres of orientation: time, place, and person.

Time

Individuals disorientated to time are unaware of their disorientation and unable to orientate themselves without assistance. The most obvious resultant problem is the individual's inability to order daily activities chronologically. Providing a clock, daily newspapers, and a radio or television set enables access to information from which the person can extract the data necessary to locate self in relation to the date and time of day.

On all contacts with someone who is disoriented reference should be made repeatedly to the date or time in association with daily events: e.g. 'Good morning. It's 9.00 a.m., breakfast is over and it's time to have your morning shower'; or, 'It's 12 midday and lunchtime. The meal for today, Tuesday, is . . .'

Establishing and maintaining a daily schedule of events provides both a feeling of security for the individual and stable reference points in relation to the time of day.

Place

Spatial disorientation causes a person to become continually lost, even in a familiar environment. Constant supervision is therefore necessary to ensure protection and safety. At every opportunity, orientate the person to his present whereabouts; this increases awareness of surroundings and facilitates orientation. Conversation on these occasions should include frequent reference to the ward name, the name of the hospital, and its location. Even explaining the location of the hospital in relation to the person's own home may provide extra information through which spatial relationships can be understood.

Physical evidence, such as hospital brochures, hospital charts, photographs, pictures, and addresses, which may assist in confirming the individual's present situation should be provided. Draw attention to and explain any everyday background hospital noise such as moving trolleys, paging system, and equipment in operation; this will tend to further familiarize the person with his environment and lessen suspicion and anxiety.

If the person is independently ambulant, clearly mark the bed or room with his name in large letters, thus providing a constant reminder of place, and an aid to self-relocation.

Always identify yourself and others by title or designation when initiating contact, e.g. 'I am Nurse White, and this is your doctor, Dr Black. We will be helping you in your recovery during your stay in this hospital.'

The strategy of leaving a dim light at night has already been mentioned. Not only does this help diminish typical nocturnal confusion, but it also serves to lessen the disorientation that may occur on waking during the night in unfamiliar surroundings. By being able to see

clearly, the person can quickly recognize markers which serve as reminders to present location.

All the previously mentioned interventions aid the process of searching for and recognizing environmental stimuli or data, which every person utilizes to orientate themselves in relation to their surroundings.

Person

Disorientation to person renders individuals unable to correctly identify people and their relationship to them. There may also be difficulty in establishing a sense of personal identity.

This can be alleviated by always addressing the person by name in conversation; providing personal belongings, familiar possessions, mementos, and writing the individual's name on visible personal possessions are other strategies that facilitate the resolution of this problem.

Talking with the person about himself and his family, continually reinforcing reality, will assist him in regaining identity relationships. Visits from relatives and friends should also be encouraged; the recurring presence of those people with whom the person was most familiar will further enhance the regaining of personal orientation.

A full explanation of the goals of care and nursing strategies to significant others may have two important benefits. In the first place, full involvement will help in reducing anxiety and future alienation from the person who is ill. It is not difficult to understand how distressing it must be for those close to someone who is confused and disoriented. No longer is the person in control; he may be emotionally labile, perhaps acting in what appears to be silly ways, and generally unlike his former self. Secondly, teaching appropriate ways for relatives and others to respond provides them with a basis for confidence and is therapeutic for all involved. The effect of regaining contact with familiar people and loved ones is likely to be a far more powerful reorientation for someone who is confused than the relatively new relationships in an institutional setting.

PLANS FOR ON-GOING MANAGEMENT

The guidelines for nursing care mentioned so far concentrate mainly on aspects of psychological management; aspects of physical care will also need attention. The duration of the state of confusion will necessitate plans for on-going management, many of which will revolve around the need to promote and maintain physical health.

Of paramount importance is the need to provide a safe environment and to prevent injury to the person and others; this may necessitate the use of bed-rails. A quiet, but not isolated, environment should be provided, the objectives being to reduce stimulation and thus lessen agitation, and the prevention of misperception of environmental stimuli. Constant observation is necessary, with particular attention being paid to vital signs, conscious state, fluid balance, degree of orientation, restlessness, and general physical condition. Record overall improvement in all levels of functioning and behaviour, as well as signs of further mental and physical deterioration. The intake of adequate nutrition can be ensured by providing a nutritional, easily digestible diet supplemented with nutritional fluids. In the long-term, an environment conducive to eating, a varied diet consisting of preferred foods, and attractively presented servings will encourage appropriate nutritional intake.

Incontinence will often occur during a state of confusion, and interventions should be initiated to prevent the person experiencing this unpleasant and degrading situation. At all times the nurse must attempt to maintain the personal dignity of the individual, since much of the conversation as well as the actions and behaviour of the confused person could create embarrassment on recovery.

Disruption to sleep and disturbance of the sleep-wakefulness cycle have been described as being associated with states of delirium. Adequate rest is important in preventing physical exhaustion and complications, and in promoting recovery. The various strategies available to the nurse to intervene in problems of sleep disorder will be examined in Chapter 18.

FEELINGS OF THE NURSE

Providing nursing care to those experiencing confusion and disorientation can be tiring and frustrating. Difficulties will be encountered in performing routine, essential nursing procedures and initially in establishing communication. Tolerance, acceptance, and patience is required in relating, especially as the confused may be non-compliant and suspicious, to the point of being overtly hostile. The nurse should not succumb to the feeling that the person is being deliberately unco-operative, beligerant, or irrational, as may well seem to be the situation to the ill-informed member of staff. Remain supportive, consistent, and accepting, and encourage consistency in approach and management by nursing colleagues by ensuring that the care plan clearly identifies the particular problems and is continually evaluated and revised as changes in the condition warrant. Some of the nurse's primary functions are to play a central role in enabling the individual to regain contact with the environment, and to facilitate the resumption of lucid thinking.

While supporting people through a period of confusion, the nurse will realize the extent to which relatives and close friends of the person can be distressed by the objective display of confusion and disorientation. Significant others will be disturbed by the uncharacteristic content of speech, and by behaviour, especially if there is a failure to recognize, and misidentification of, close family members or friends. The nurse can provide much support and explanation to relatives and friends at such times, and act as an important link between them.

When muddled thinking, agitation, and disorientation give way to a clear sensorium, relaxation, and full contact with reality, the nurse can share with the person and his family the relief from pressure, frustration, and concern.

REFERENCES

Baxter S 1975 Psychological problems of intensive care. Nursing Times 71: 22–3, 71: 63–5
Freedman A M, Kaplan H I, Sadock B J 1976 Comprehensive textbook of psychiatry, 2nd edn, Vol 1. Williams & Wilkins, Baltimore
Kreigh H Z, Perks T E 1979 Psychiatric and mental health nursing. Reston, Virginia
Sainsbury M T 1980 Key to psychiatry, 3rd edn. Australian and New Zealand Book Company, Sydney

Is this a vision? Is this a dream? Do I sleep?
Merry Wives of Windsor, Shakespeare

14

The person who is hallucinating

THE NATURE OF HALLUCINATIONS

SENSORY PERCEPTION

The experience we know as sensation is the result of a complex physiological and psychological process. In very general terms, physical stimuli are selectively received by sensory organs and translated into electrical messages which are then carried by sensory nerves to the brain where coding and/or interpretation takes place. It is through this process that we form a concept of reality and then use this concept to respond to events as they occur. Even the absence of only one major sensory system, such as vision or hearing, results in enormous problems of adaptation for those affected. Does, for example, the concept 'tree' have the same meaning for a sightless person as for someone with normal vision? As one writer succinctly puts it, 'All our meaningful behaviour, all our awareness of physical reality, all our ideas about the universe ultimately spring from impressions our sense organs alone can provide' (Coon 1982).

One of the most interesting physiological features of the sensory nervous system is the fact that only a certain range and type of physical stimuli can be received. This prevents us from being overwhelmed by the enormous amount of physical activity that occurs in the environment. The result of this phenomenon would seem to be that only potentially useful material is made available for future interpretation and coding by the brain. We are also able to supplement this process by selective attention. In a crowded room where there are many conversations going on, we are able to listen to just one, and everything else becomes background. However, the mention of certain key words, such as our name, may serve to bring to awareness a conversation nearby and we become distracted from the previous focus of attention.

The interpretation of sensory messages involves more than physiological processes. Experience, our memory of information already coded, affects our perception to a significant degree. We know for example that a car is much smaller than a house, yet at a distance the disparity in size diminishes. This occurs despite the fact that the retinal images must retain their proportionality, i.e. an object 10 metres long will have half the retinal image of an object 20 metres long. Many of the common illusions are explained by the effect of experience, or our knowledge of how the world actually functions.

An illusion is a misperception involving a false interpretation of signals actually received by a sensory organ. Figure 14.1 shows two common line illusions.

In the Ponzo illusion, the top horizontal line appears longer to most people, yet both are the same length. This may be explained by our experience in the three-dimensional world in which true perspective exists. We know that the top line is further away than the bottom one, as in railway tracks. Since the retinal images are the same the brain assumes that the top line must be longer. In the Müller-Lyer illusion, both lines are the same length, yet the left figure appears longer. In our world of

corners this figure represents the internal corner of a room and the right figure the outside corner of a building. Since insides of rooms are smaller than the outsides of the building we assume that the left figure must be longer to account for the same retinal images. It is interesting and supportive of this explanation that Zulus, who live in a world virtually devoid of corners, do not experience this illusion (Gregory 1973).

This very brief discussion is intended to highlight perception as not simply the result of a physiological process (although that is a significant part of the process), but complicated by higher cognitive functioning.

DEFINITION AND TYPES OF HALLUCINATIONS

An hallucination is a sensory perception that occurs in the absence of any external signal (Field & Ruelke 1973). What this amounts to is that whatever is perceived does not objectively exist in the real world, but the person subjectively experiences it. Any of the senses may be affected, giving rise to gustatory, olfactory, auditory, visual, and tactile hallucination. The most commonly experienced type are auditory; it is suggested that these are more primitive and result when thought processes regress to a perceptual level (Field & Ruelke 1973).

One type of fleeting hallucination worth mentioning here are hypnogogic phenomena, because they occur in otherwise normal individuals and are not thought to be indicative of any underlying psychopathology. These experiences take place in that brief period between being awake and asleep and are usually auditory in nature. The person will suddenly become aware of hearing their name called, for example, and awake to find no-one there.

The most important feature of hallucinations, particularly from the point of view of those who have not experienced them, is that to the sufferer the sensation is very real. It is so real that this internally created perception

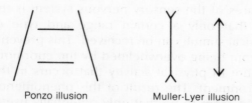

Ponzo illusion   Muller-Lyer illusion

Fig. 14.1 Line illusions. (a) Ponzo illusion. (b) Muller-Lyer illusion.

is projected onto the real world as if it actually exists. For all intents and purposes the perception *does* exist for the person, but not for an observer, and the problem is one of interpreting reality.

There are some people who experience hallucinations yet display few, if any, other psychotic signs or symptoms. When contact with reality is good these individuals may learn to live with their voices (Alchin & Weatherhead 1976) and will simply complain of them as being bothersome (especially when there is no other competing sensory input) (Stuart & Sundeen 1979). This type of situation should be contrasted with that of the acutely psychotic person who is totally withdrawn from reality with disordered thought processes and disorganized personality, who will readily respond to hallucinations as manifestations of reality.

CONDITIONS IN WHICH HALLUCINATIONS ARE A FEATURE

Hallucinations are most commonly a feature of overt psychiatric illness, and in particular of psychotic conditions called 'schizophrenia' and 'delirium'. The type of hallucination experienced can often give a clue as to the actual illness, since they very often reflect the individual's thought processes and underlying personality. In the illness known as 'paranoid schizophrenia', for example, threatening and persecutory voices reflect the paranoid thought processes specifically diagnostic of the condition. Olfactory hallucinations, in which poison gases may be smelled, are also seen in this disorder. Severely depressed (affective psychosis) people can experience voices which tell them of their worthlessness and guilt, as well as sometimes proposing suicide as a solution to their problem.

In the general hospital setting hallucinations are often encountered in those suffering from delirium or toxic confusional states. The classic example here is that of delirium tremens (alcohol withdrawal) in which the person experiences horrifying visual and tactile hallucinations involving snakes, spiders, beetles, and other similar creatures. Imagine yourself lying on a bed in a room, quite helpless, as snakes slither out of the walls, huge spiders spin their webs and drop onto the bedclothes, insects crawl over your skin, bats circle the room, and rats nibble at your toes and fingers. Terror and panic are common emotional consequences of such experiences, as might be expected.

Alcohol withdrawal is not the only cause of delirium and we should consider also fluid and electrolyte inbalance, hypoxia, medication, extreme fatigue, sensory deprivation, and sensory overload. People in intensive care units, who are undergoing extreme physiological stress as well as the psychological trauma of treatment, are a particularly vulnerable group for hallucinations. Hallucinations may also occur in people under intense stress and in those with sleep deprivation.

Hallucinations may also be induced by certain drugs such as LSD (lysergic acid diethylamide), psylocybin (mushrooms), amphetamines, mescaline, DMT (dimenthyltriptamine), and, in high doses, marijuana. People who use these substances state that the nature of the hallucinations is often influenced by the mood prior to intoxication. These people on occasion may present to casualty out of fear (their own or their friends'), from overdose, or after an accident. LSD has been known to cause hallucinations hours, days, or years after use, and a most disturbing feature of some of these drugs is that they may precipitate chronic psychosis in susceptible individuals.

EXPLANATIONS FOR HALLUCINATIONS

There are a number of theories that attempt to account for hallucinatory experiences but, as in many areas of psychopathology, the evidence is as yet inconclusive. Biochemical theories suggest that stress may result in the release of certain neurochemicals which cause hallucinations (Stuart & Sundeen 1979). For schizophrenia in general there is evidence that dopamine, a neurotransmitter, plays a part in the production of symptoms, since phenothiazines used for its treatment affect dopamine levels in the brain (Cooper 1984).

Other explanations see anxiety as the central issue in the development of hallucinations. Psychoanalytic theorists suggest that the defence mechanism of projection as a means of alleviating anxiety from repressed impulses is exagerrated to the extent of assigning internal thoughts to an external source.

Field & Ruelke (1973) indicate that in the early stages of the development of hallucinations they are a means of relieving anxiety and are so effective that they become a useful mechanism. Others feel that they occur due to a weak ego in which the person's sense of self is diminished, and hence internal thoughts and feelings may become confused with external events.

NURSING CARE

ASSESSMENT

Hallucinations rarely occur as an isolated problem, being usually symptomatic of an acute or chronic psychotic condition. The assessment of the person is likely to be rather broad, consisting of many aspects of personality and behaviour, out of which hallucinations may be one of many problems. Nevertheless, the assessment of the type, extent, content, and the reactions of the individual to hallucinations is important in overall treatment and on-going assessment.

Subjective experiences

Getting someone to admit to or talk about their hallucinations is often very difficult. Acutely psychotic people with severe thought disorder and fragmented personality find it almost impossible to join in a discussion involving insight. Many are reluctant to discuss their hallucinations for fear of being considered mad. Others simply have difficulty in distinguishing between hallucination and reality, and if the hallucinations are being used as a means of alleviating anxiety, there may be good reason to avoid treatment. For these reasons the nurse needs to be warm, non-judgmental, and empathic to develop the trusting relationship required to elicit valuable information.

Some people are able to describe their hallucinatory experiences with great clarity, as well as how they feel about them. Others are able to outline only ideas expressed by voices, or simply complain of vague mumblings or fleeting visual experiences. Where possible the actual content of hallucinations should be recorded in the person's own words to avoid misinterpretation and to facilitate ongoing evaluation of symptoms. An attempt should be made to identify possible situational influences that appear to affect their occurrence, such as the relative quiet at bed-time or the presence of certain people. Emotional experiences are also important; anxiety, anger, or depression may occur before or after an hallucinatory experience. A history of epilepsy is significant since, a hallucination may precede a grand mal or temporal lobe episode. In the case of voices, suggestions of suicide, self-mutilation, strange acts, and violence require particular attention, since these people may act quite spontaneously on what they hear.

It is worthwhile asking the person directly whether they understand their experiences as being hallucinations and to what extent they are confused with reality. This information aids in judging the severity of the mental state as well as the extent to which behaviour may be affected by hallucinations.

CASE ILLUSTRATION

The following extracts quoted from a true account of an episode of delirium tremens serve to illustrate graphically one person's experiences of hallucinations and thought disturbances.

' . . . then there were voices. Not too loud, not persistent, but whispers in passing, subtle giggles or a firm intonation from just outside the window. . . . I tried to talk back once or twice, I remember, but no one replied. . . . Suddenly a mass of green spiders materialised in the well of the toilet and swarmed up towards me. . . . Then the insects arrived, but insects of a nature I had never seen before. Large, multi-coloured masses moved and crawled over the walls; vicious heads and tentacles lashed from them. . . . Visions came and went, my perception of distance altered and then the strangers came. They started to talk outside the sitting room window, in loud voices. Male voices of a coarse nature. 'Get him, the bastard,' I heard them say quite plainly. They were hatching some vile plot to get me and I could not understand why. . . . I can remember people chucking themselves out of windows and crashing onto the pavement, their brains running red patterns of blood into the gutter. . . . I can remember pillows and jackets growing faces, taking on life-forms like dogs and puppies and then fading and dying. Everything started to die. . . .' (McQueenie 1984).

Objective assessment

In many cases it is not what the individual says but his overt behaviour that provides the information suggestive of hallucinations. Withdrawal, in which the person is preoccupied and almost totally excludes others and events around him or her, may indicate the presence of hallucinations. Similarly, the person may talk to himself and even argue with the voices to the extent of displaying outbursts of anger or violence. Inappropriate gestures and facial expressions frequently occur in response to the content of hallucinations, as well as a preoccupation with a point in space. In response to voices the person may tilt the head as if listening, or become absorbed in a radio or television which is turned off.

Sometimes someone who is hallucinating may appear surprised for no apparent reason, look around furtively, or seek clarification from others that what they saw or heard was really there. Attempting to avoid hallucinating experiences may result in a fondness for noise and activity, covering the head with pillows, or otherwise trying to shut them out. Hallucinations may be so bothersome that the person becomes very restless, hardly stopping to sit down, or may result in a considerable degree of anxiety bordering on panic. This is particularly true of persecutory, obscene, or threatening voices.

Impulsive behaviour may sometimes occur in response to a visual or auditory hallucination, and acts may be violent, suicidal, or self-mutilating in their most dangerous forms. It is always important to attempt to ascertain from these people what tempted them into an impulsive act, particularly if psychosis is suspected.

Clarification regarding any of these behaviours is vital, because other quite benign causes may exist. Relatives or others who know the individual well may also provide valuable information about recent behaviour. It is also likely that admission of the existence of hallucinations may have been made to a trusted family member.

It is often neither easy nor appropriate to attempt to assess hallucinatory behaviour in isolation. Other psychotic behaviour should be taken into consideration in developing an overall picture. When behaviour indicative of hallucinatory experiences does not appear to fit into the general assessment, other explanations should be sought. One of the pitfalls with objective assessment of other people's behaviour is misinterpretation, particularly if evidence is less than conclusive. The labelling of a person as hallucinating may be readily accepted by other staff, who will then respond quite inappropriately without further clarification. Written data, such as reports, should describe the evidence seen by the nurse rather than give a simple statement that hallucinations are occurring.

Problem list

When hallucinations are known to exist, the information obtained from the person and nursing observations form the basis for care and serve as a means for identifying specific problems. The content of the assessment that is required for developing a problem list has been summarized by Alchin & Weatherhead (1976) and is modified here:

1. Behavioural problems associated with the hallucinations, such as self-mutilation, suicide, violence, or strange practices.

2. The extent to which the person understands his hallucinations for what they are.
3. Overall contact with reality.
4. The emotional impact on the individual (anxiety, depression).
5. The effects on the activities of daily living such as nutrition, hygiene, sleeping habits and relationships.
6. The individual's understanding of the causes of his hallucinations.

The sorts of problems that might be elicited from the assessment could include the following:

- severe anxiety due to content of voices heard
- sudden impulsive acts of self-mutilation when alone
- sleep disturbance due to hallucinations
- poor nutrition due to preoccupations with hallucinations and withdrawal
- lack of understanding of nature of hallucinations — poor contact with reality
- poor/no insight into hallucinations and cause
- bizarre, inappropriate, and purposeless behaviour resulting from hallucinations
- 'voices' as companionship that is preferred to reality.

GOALS OF CARE

The general goals of nursing care of people who are hallucinating are to:

1. Reduce the effects of the hallucinations, i.e. anxiety, loss of sleep, poor nutrition.
2. Identify the possible cause of the hallucinations, e.g. anxiety, drugs, or stress.
3. Eliminate dangerous or self-destructive behaviour that is resulting from hallucinations.
4. Help the person to understand the true nature of his hallucinations and assist in establishing contact with reality.
5. Reduce or eliminate the occurrence of hallucinations.

The individually stated goals and their priority will depend on the severity of the hallucinations, their effect, and the mental state of the individual. In the case of self-mutilating behaviour, its elimination in the short-term is vital. Similarly, the reduction of anxiety may be most important.

In less severe cases or when initially disturbed people have been stabilized, long-term goals such as developing insight may be set and a meaningful treatment programme implemented. When hallucinations are symptomatic of a severe psychotic illness, more general goals aimed at developing insight or reducing symptomatology may be more appropriate — for example, to idenfity the possible causes of the overall psychotic reaction that incorporates hallucinations. In contrast, hallucinations may be the most disturbing symptom for a person and perhaps the principal expression of psychosis, in which case specific goal-setting is appropriate.

It should not be assumed that the goals of care and treatment cannot be discussed with these people. The advantages are much the same as for discussing goals and treatment with any individual. In severe psychotic illnesses this may of course be potentially threatening, if not impossible, and may have to be postponed until the acute stage has subsided and contact with reality has improved.

NURSING ACTION

Emergency care

Being confronted by a person experiencing vivid hallucinations can be both a frightening and difficult situation for anyone, especially when behaviour constitutes a threat to self or others. On these rare occasions safety is of primary importance and the nurse should not hesitate in calling for help. Physical restraint within the usual ethical and legal boundaries may be required to prevent self-mutilation or acts of violence. When this sort of behaviour is predicted the medical officer may have ordered a neuroleptic agent as treatment, and this may be given. However, the administration of regular medication as a palliative measure is preferable and is the outcome of a thorough and adequate individual assessment. On the behavioural aspect of care it is vital for the nurse to remain calm and reassuring. The basic approach should be to restore contact with what is happening around the person and the consequences of behaviour. Direct statements about behaviour should be made firmly but without threat. Similarly, actually asking the person what he is doing may cause the cessation of behaviour or the redirection of thinking.

In cases of delirium due to drug intoxication or alcohol withdrawal, any sort of reasoning or redirection of behaviour may be fruitless, and the use of medication may be the treatment of choice. The value in this course of action is that the person can rest and does not become exhausted, impulsive acts are diminished, and general care is facilitated. The prevention of the many potential complications of delirium may be facilitated by keeping psychotic behaviour under control.

Patients who are hallucinating vividly may strike out, or grab hair, uniform, or flesh, as a result of fear. This is particularly true for those with delirium tremens who see horrifying snakes and spiders coming at them. Nurses should remember that this is not an affront to them personally. In remembering this, a negative attitude towards the person may be prevented and better care facilitated; so much depends on the attitude and behaviour of the nurse if successful care is to be given.

General management

Fortunately, most people who are hallucinating present less of an acute problem and more attention can be directed towards general care.

Much of the care of people suffering from what may be called 'psychotic illnesses' or 'psychotic symptomatology' depends on initial control and maintenance with psychotropic medication. The administration of these medications and the evaluation of their effectiveness is an important initial stage of treatment. This early intervention will facilitate sleep and other aspects of care such as maintaining hygiene and nutritional status. In addition, psychological treatments may be more readily implemented with greater potential for success.

The evaluation of the effectiveness of medication aids in determining the optimum dosage required. Excessive neuroleptics result in drowsiness and other unwanted side-effects, whereas insufficient amounts may not control hallucinations and their effects at all. Accurate documentation of behaviour and subjective experiences enables an accurate evaluation over a period of time.

Psychological care

The foundation of caring for the hallucinating person lies in the trusting relationship that is developed by the nurse. In order to facilitate this relationship the nurse must attempt to understand hallucinating experiences and how the individual must feel. A block to effective nursing care sometimes occurs due to the inability of nurses to acknowledge the problem that exists and virtually negating it, since it is too difficult to conceptualize. Those who are hallucinating are sometimes reluctant to discuss their experiences and need to feel safe to divulge information because of the risk of rejection. The treatment regime requires a degree of co-operation on the part of these people, and trust engenders compliance.

This relationship provides the opportunity for the discussion of other matters as well as the hallucinating experiences. The effect of this is to devalue (Field & Ruelke 1973) the hallucinations and concentrate thoughts on people and the environment; in other words, on reality. It is a question of replacing the hallucination with something else that is of more use to the person in terms of relating to others and day-to-day functioning.

Hallucinations may be sufficiently severe to impair normal communication and decision-making processes. In these cases instructions may need to be precise, clear, and given step-by-step for procedures such as eating, bathing, or dressing. Even simple decision-making may be threatening for these people, and attention should be given to developing a well-ordered plan of care that is systematic and as uncomplicated as possible. Contacts with the person should be brief but frequent: they are a means of observing behaviour, maintaining contact with reality and preventing preoccupation with hallucinations, and diminishing anxiety.

With improvement the individual can accept a graduated increase in responsibility for self and complexity of decision-making. This will result in increased self-esteem as experiences become more rewarding.

Familiar objects around the person and regular visits by significant others may also reduce anxiety. In the case of relations and friends, valuable information can be obtained regarding individual's normal eating, drinking and hygiene habits.

An attempt should be made to help the person understand the true nature of hallucinations. At suitable times this may be overtly explained, although the subject should not be debated. A related technique is to make reference to hallucinations as the person's own subjective experiences, rather than as actually existing, by describing them as being 'like voices' or 'as if someone were talking'.

It is important for the nurse not to humour these people because, rather than being an expedient way of reducing anxiety, it only serves to reinforce the individual's view of reality. The result is a perpetuation of the mechanism as a coping behaviour. It should be remembered that one of the principal goals of care is to diminish or alleviate the experience altogether.

Stuart & Sundeen (1979) suggest that explaining to the person that his or her experience is not real for the nurse is preferable to negating the reality of the experience. To someone who is hallucinating it *is* real, the object is to reinforce the idea that it is a subjective experience rather than an objective reality. As indicated, this reinforcement may be either covert (subtle) by talking of other things and redirecting attention, or overt through explanation of the hallucinatory experience.

Observation and anticipation of behaviour is important to prevent impulsive acts when the individual's attention to voices is intense. Documentation of the content of hallucinations should be ongoing to assess the need for formal observation and to evaluate the effectiveness of care.

In the psychiatric unit the management of these people is facilitated by a team approach in which all health workers are involved. The responsibility for implementing and maintaining treatment in the general ward falls very much on the shoulders of the nurse. Effective plans of management and good communication among nursing staff can make care-giving much more efficient and can be of enormous benefit to the person.

THE FEELINGS OF THE NURSE

Severely hallucinating people can create tremendous disturbance in a ward, creating a significant degree of stress for staff. Nurses should be encouraged to talk about their feelings towards these disturbed people and discuss the effects on them personally. It is understandable to have negative feelings towards psychotic people, since they are frequently non-compliant, do not fit the usual sick role, and are difficult to understand. What is destructive to good care is to leave these feelings unresolved and allow negative attitudes to develop.

REFERENCES

Alchin S C, Weatherhead R 1976 Psychiatric nursing a practical approach McGraw Hill, Sydney

Coon D 1982 Essentials of psychology. West Publishing Co, St Paul

Cooper J E 1984 Schizophrenia and allied conditions. International Medicine, Australian Edn

Field W E, Ruelke W 1973 Hallucinations and how to deal with them. American Journal of Nursing 73:4

Gregory R L 1973 Eye and brain: psychology of seeing, 2nd Edn. McGraw Hill, New York

McQueenie K J 1984 The day the strangers came. Nursing Times 80(26): 51–4

Sainsbury J 1980 Key to psychiatry. Australia and New Zealand Book Company, Sydney

Stuart G W, Sundeen T S 1979 Principles and practice of psychiatric nursing. Mosby, St Louis

15

The hyperactive person

DEFINING HYPERACTIVITY

The disturbance of concern here is not the excessive, uncontrolled energy of the hyperactive child, nor the over-exuberant enthusiasm of an adult, but the behaviour symptomatic of a pathological disturbance, of a type of severe mood disorder.

Disorders of mood, or the more technically correct term 'affect', are detailed in Chapter 2, mention being made of 'normal' variations in mood; just as some individuals seem to have an almost permanent melancholic personality, many appear to live their lives from day to day on a 'high', ever active, cheerful, and gregarious. When these characteristics reach a level at which they become detrimental to the individual's personal, occupational, and interpersonal functioning, intervention by others, including nurses, becomes necessary. Manifestations of hyperactive behaviour will be seen to be occurring in association with other displays of emotional and behavioural disturbance, including extreme anxiety, anger and aggression, confusion and disorientation, hallucinatory experiences, thought disorder, sleep disturbances, and as the result of substance abusing behaviour. Hyperactivity is increased motor activity to the point of almost ceaseless motion, with the inability to rest or relax. The individual may demonstrate continuous agitation ranging to the extreme where activity is accelerated, ceaseless, and wild. A proportional increase in the rate of mental activity may accompany the motor activity. In this state, described as 'psychomotor activity', the individual puts into physical execution all the ideas that occur to him, resulting in a level of physical activity paralleling that of the mental activity.

Excluding cases where the cause is related to organic factors, hyperactivity is considered to be an unconscious defence against depression. In such cases, manifested in episodes of mania, the underlying content of the mania does not differ from that of a major depressive illness (see Ch. 2); the difference is in the expression of conscious and unconscious thoughts and feelings arising from the loss of the inhibitive superego. Freud (1924) explained this phenomenon in psychoanalytic terms by suggesting that the underlying dynamics involved in both depression and mania are the same: in the former the ego succumbs to the overwhelming thoughts and feelings, whereas in mania the ego, no longer under the control of the superego, overcomes the threatening feelings and attempts to dismiss them by allowing previously suppressed impulses to be expressed, and manifested by hyperactive behaviour.

NURSING CARE

ASSESSMENT

Hyperactivity is a manifestation of a serious disturbance of mental health. Unlike some displays of emotion or behaviour (such as anger, aggression, tearfulness, and anxiety), excessive hyperactive behaviours are always associated with a pathological condition. The two most commonly encountered states in which hyperactivity will be witnessed are mania, and states where the precipitating factor is of an organic nature. The latter include specific organic brain damage, delirium, drug intoxication, and behaviours associated with intellectual handicap without evident brain damage. In hyperactivity arising from organic factors, whether they are the result of damage to brain tissue or an acute alteration in the metabolic processes occurring in the brain, the resultant behaviour is usually purposeless and outside the conscious control of the individual. The behaviour associated with mania is generally purposeful, contrived, and under conscious control; however, the degree of control is seriously diminished.

Hyperactivity in mania can therefore present in a different manner to hyperactivity resulting from other causes, and consequently the nursing management will be in accordance with the nature and cause of the hyperactive behaviour.

The type of disturbance in feeling and behaviour described in this chapter usually necessitates management in a psychiatric unit. However, individuals may become manic while in wards of the general hospital or require admission to such wards while suffering an episode of mania, necessitating management of this disturbed state by ward nursing staff. Many individuals who become hyperactive while in hospital are suffering from a chronic mood disorder characterized by recurring episodes of mania interspersed with longer periods of healthy functioning. The occurrence of physical ill-health, trauma and/or hospitalization in such individuals can act as both physiological and psychological stressors of sufficient severity to precipitate a relapse and subsequent emergence of manic symptomatology. There are, however, a number of people who become hyperactive and manic while in hospital, who have no previous history of any serious disorder of mood. These individuals may have a predisposition to developing problems associated with a severe mood disorder, and it is not until they are subjected to the stress associated with a change in their physical state that manifestations of the disorder occur; psychoses occurring in post-partum women are examples. Hyperactivity and other signs of mania may already be evident when an individual is admitted to hospital, and are often the reason for the admission, the individual being frequently drug toxic, dehydrated, or suffering from exhaustion or exposure, or having sustained a fractured limb or cardiac distress as a result of the effects of activities performed while manic.

Nurses should thus be aware of the problems of the person who is manic in order to be able to understand the needs of the person, plan nursing care, and assist him effectively in retaining optimal physical and mental health.

The following case illustrates an example of manic behaviour occurring in a person in a general hospital.

CASE ILLUSTRATION

Mr H. A. had been brought into hospital by ambulance after he had collapsed at home. He appeared to be in a state of exhaustion, moderately dehydrated, and had a markedly increased heart rate. Clinical evidence of hyper-thyroidism was later confirmed by abnormal thyroid function tests. Due to his poor physical health he was admitted to a medical ward. On the ward Mr H. A. declined to stay in bed, preferring to move continuously, involving himself with the other ill people and being generally disruptive. He would enter the nursing station continually, attempting to assist staff in performing their duties and advising them on alternative ways to manage situations. His speech was rapid and continuous, often jumping from one topic to another with such abruptness that other people were unable to follow his conversation. The ward's public telephone was monopolized by Mr H. A., who would make numerous calls arranging appointments with various professionals and organising the many schemes that he had devised. His activity level appeared to be increasing; he talked more and more rapidly, slept very little, and could not take time out for meals. Aggressive outbursts towards staff were common, Mr H. A. becoming irritated easily when thwarted in his activities. However, his mood would change rapidly, aggression being replaced by over-friendliness and elation, at which times he would make suggestive remarks to the female staff, often alluding to his sexual prowess. Although generally resisting nurses' requests and delivery of nursing care, Mr H. A. was markedly distractible and attention to his physical health needs could be provided with his co-operation.

All aspects of the manic, hyperactive person's behaviour are exaggerated, irrational responses to internal and external stimuli. He is pressured in his thoughts and actions, producing an increase in the rate and extent of physical activity and speech. Talk is rapid, incessant, and jumps from one idea to another without pause — characteristics indicative of the rate of mental activity which are described as 'pressure of speech' and 'flight of ideas'. This accelerated mental activity produces an increase in self-confidence resulting in the continual formulation of new schemes, none of which is carried through to completion. The increase in self-confidence and loss of impulse control give rise to disinhibited behaviour in which the individual may speak and act in a way which is socially unacceptable and potentially damaging to his occupational and social activities. A diminished ability to concentrate is evidenced by a short attention span, distractibility, and intolerance of obstacles which threaten to thwart any plans and actions. Rapid swings in mood, irritability and aggressive outbursts are witnessed by those who attempt to apply any restraint to his activities. Effective communication with the individual is difficult as his pressure of thought and shortened attention span render him unable and unwilling to listen.

If manic prior to admission to hospital, the loss of impulse control and judgement may have caused a previously cautious and prudent individual to have indulged in wild spending sprees, purchasing and ordering expensive items without consideration of financial implications. He may, for instance, have bought an exotic sports car, made bookings for an overseas holiday, and signed contracts for the purchase of real estate, none of which could be afforded. Inappropriate and impulsive decisions at work could have placed his means of livelihood in jeopardy; and expansive, often profane, language may have damaged his relationships with family and acquaintances.

Although the hyperactive person may seem to be elated and 'on a high', subjectively he is usually angry, fearful, and feels constantly threatened. He is suspicious and hostile, particularly if experiencing delusional ideas. When delusions are part of the syndrome, the content is grandiose in nature (delusions of grandeur); the person believes he is a celebrity or someone important, typically a media personality, member of a Royal family, or a religious figure.

Continuous hyperactivity over a period of

days subjects the body to excessive levels of physiological stress, the person being constantly active, sleeping very little, and failing to maintain adequate nutritional intake and fluid balance. Sleep, if occurring at all, may average only one or two hours a night; the individual is unable to concentrate sufficiently to eat proper meals, and may neglect to drink and maintain regular bowel and bladder habits. Fatigue and the potential for serious physical distress may therefore become the paramount reason for others intervening and insisting on the person's admission to a hospital. Such intervention often entails enforced hospitalization and necessitates invoking relevant provisions of Mental Health Acts. The manic, hyperactive person, by virtue of his lack of insight, judgement, and impaired mental state, will often dispute the need for treatment; he resents the interference by others and resists hospitalization. If this situation exists, the nursing management of the hospitalized individual is complicated by active non-compliance with care planning, and by the prevailing antagonism towards nursing staff and others instrumental in arranging his admission to hospital.

GOALS OF CARE

- To provide an environment in which the person can feel secure.
- To decrease hyperactivity and promote self-control in behaviour.
- To establish and maintain adequate nutrition, fluid balance, and other activities of daily living.
- To preserve the person's self-esteem and personal dignity.

NURSING ACTION

Early management

Hyperactive behaviour is an exaggerated response to environmental stimuli. To diminish the degree of hyperactivity it is therefore necessary to lessen the amount of stimulation to which the individual is subjected. This entails providing the person with a single room, devoid of as much extraneous 'hospital noise' as possible; however it does not mean advocacy of complete sensory deprivation. A quiet room, away from other people, furnished only with essentials and without brightly coloured or harsh decorations, will provide a subdued, sedative environment.

Simplified surroundings limit the amount of sensory input and interpersonal stimulation, thus helping to diminish the pressure of thought and activity which otherwise would be perpetuated. To maintain this state of diminished stimulation, the number of people with whom the individual has contact should be kept to a minimum. In the early stages of management, friends and relatives should be discouraged from visiting and care should be provided by as few different staff as possible. The approach of these staff to the person should be in a firm, calm, relaxed manner, speaking only when necessary and then in a kind, low-pitched, undemanding voice. Nurses designated to be with the person must be able to control their feelings towards his behaviour and not show alarm or be provoked by his verbal hostility, profane language, or possible sexually suggestive or obscene behaviour. Simultaneously, the nurse must be able to exert non-antagonistic control over the person's more extreme behaviour.

General management

Promotion of rest, sleep, and adequate nutrition are important in maintaining the individual's physical and mental health. Continuous observation should therefore be made for signs of fatigue, and times provided during the day when rest is encouraged; monitoring of sleep patterns will indicate whether enough sleep is being obtained to ensure physiological rest. As the person's continued activity will preclude him from eating regular meals, foods that can be eaten at any time should be available; these may include snacks such as sandwiches and fruit. High protein food supplements will be necessary to sustain the high energy output. Fluid intake must also be encouraged to maintain adequate hydration. As with sleep, food and fluid intake should be monitored closely to ensure that levels are sufficient to cater for the increased need. Associated with intake is attention to elimination. Nurses must ensure regularity in the person's bowel and bladder habits, as there is a risk of constipation, faecal impaction, bladder distention, and urinary retention due to neglect of these functions. The overactive individual will feel the discomfort of these difficulties, but, as with other physical trauma, may disregard the symptoms. This apparent unawareness of physical discomfort also presents as an area of concern to the nurse in ensuring the person does not become too hot or too cold and is not suffering any trauma which he may have neglected to mention. An injury may be sustained during an episode of extreme excitement or agitation, and the nurse must always be alert to preventing the person from causing himself harm, either accidentally or deliberately.

As well as providing the person with a single room and a subdued atmosphere, other interventions can be incorporated in the management plan to facilitate the diminution of hyperactivity. Organizing a consistent, structured daily programme will assist the person in establishing a routine, and allow him to concentrate his energy in predetermined activities. The planning of these activities must take into consideration the limited concentration span of the individual and should aim at achieving tasks within his capabilities, i.e. those able to be completed in a short time. The hyperactive person is very competitive in all aspects of interpersonal and inter-group functioning and therefore involved discussions with others on the ward should be avoided until he is able to exert some self-control. However, graduated socialization will become a necessary component of the management plan at a later stage when the need to regain confidence arises. When organizing the structure of daily events, always involve the person in setting the goals of the activities, as this encourages understanding of what is expected

and places constraints on otherwise uncontrolled behaviour.

Writing has been found to be a beneficial activity for the hyperactive individual, allowing him to express the many and varied ideas continuously present in his mind. Apart from writing, nurses should provide the person with the opportunity to vocalize feelings of anger and frustration and encourage him to give vent to these, and other, feelings in a controlled and reasonable manner.

Physical activity is necessary as an outlet for the excess energy the person will have. Such activity can be in the form of single or one-to-one non-competitive games, or non-aggressive physical activity. Physiotherapists and occupational therapists should be utilized to provide activity for the person within the confines of the ward situation. Limited attention span and distractibility can be utilized by the nurse to shift the person's attention away from undesirable activities towards more acceptable behaviour. It will be found to be far more satisfactory to suggest an alternative activity than to prohibit the undesirable behaviour in which the person may be indulging. When talking to the individual about activities or acceptable behaviour, use uncomplicated, direct explanations and requests; do not give commands, or become involved in arguments. This will only serve to stimulate and antagonize the person, taking him close to his diminished threshold for frustration. Consistency of approach by nurses at all times is essential in assisting the person to regain control and in building a trusting relationship. The establishment of rapport and mutual trust is of paramount importance in the effective management of the hyperactive person. The nurse must not allow herself to be provoked by the person, remaining relaxed, and supportive but firm. Do not condone the individual's behaviour, or encourage him by playing along with him, or evoke his irritation by laughing at or deriding him. Listen to him, showing concern for his feelings, but quietly interrupt him if his conversation becomes pressured and illogical. The person will respond more favourably and feel secure if he realizes he can trust the nurse. Maintenance of this trust is essential, and should not be betrayed by misleading or attempting to manipulate the person, or by making statements or promises that cannot be verified or kept.

It will be necessary to set limits on the person's behaviour. This should be achieved by involving him in discussion of the proposed limits and clearly establishing what is inappropriate and what is acceptable behaviour. Limit-setting is not a punitive measure but a means by which staff can facilitate the process of providing the individual with constraints within which he can establish direction and control over his day-to-day living.

When the hyperactive crisis has passed and the person is able to tolerate interpersonal and intergroup activities, the nurse should be aware that the person's pressured, often disinhibited, behaviour may be irritating and unbearable to others. These individuals may not understand the nature of the hyperactive person's problems; the nurse must therefore anticipate the potential for friction between the person and others, and the likelihood of aggressive interactions. Preservation of the individual's dignity should be a constant consideration of the nurse, protecting him from that might be sources of embarrassment to him when he is functioning better and able to resume his relationships with friends, colleagues, and the general public. Such sources of embarrassment might include anti-social disinhibited behaviour or promiscuous sexual activities.

The person's relatives will find this behaviour very disturbing and distressing, their relationships possibly having been placed under a great deal of strain. They may require support, reassurance and information on aspects of the person's problems and their management. The nurse should be alert to this need and be prepared to ensure that the relatives and the person who has been ill are provided with the appropriate details and understand what is explained to them. Appreciation and understanding of the problems associated with the person's behaviour will promote compliance with management and facilitate in regaining a stable level of functioning.

EVALUATION

Accurate monitoring of all aspects of the person's daily activities will ensure that his physical health is not dangerously compromized by his hyperactive behaviour. The effects of interventions aimed at decreasing the degree of activity will be noticeable in the individual's interactions with staff and in his mood and general behaviour during the day and night. The desired effects of any psychotropic medication prescribed to sedate the person (see Ch. 3) must be noted, as it is possible that compliance by the person with such treatment will be poor. Hyperactive individuals frequently refuse to take prescribed medications and engage in various ploys to secrete or avoid swallowing oral preparations.

As the person shows signs of responding favourably to the management plan, provide him with appropriate positive feedback. His compliance, trust and reliance upon the nurse for support and direction will be evidence of the effectiveness of the interventions undertaken.

REFERENCES

Burr T, Andrews T 1981 Nursing the psychiatric patient, 4th Edn. Bailliere Tindall, London.
Campbell R 1981 Psychiatric dictionary, 5th edn. Oxford University Press, New York
Freud S 1924 Collected papers, Vol 4. Translated by Riviere T, Leonard and Virginia Woolf and the Institute of Psychoanalysis, London

Kreigh H Z, Perko T E 1979 Psychiatric and mental health nursing: commitment to care and concern. Reston, Virginia
Mereness D A, Taylor C M 1974 Essentials of psychiatric nursing, 9th edn. Mosby, St Louis

In Xanadu did Kubla Khan a stately pleasure dome decree . . .
(The opening line of the famous poem by Samuel Taylor Coleridge, composed while in an opium-induced dream.)

16

Substance use and abuse

This chapter and the next, on the alcohol user, differ somewhat from the other problem-specific chapters in this section. These two chapters are much broader in their treatment of what are actually descriptive mental disorders, diagnosable by certain criteria. Many of the problems discussed elsewhere in this section, such as anxiety, anger, withdrawal and hallucinations, may be exhibited by the drug abuser. The decision to single out the problem of substance use and abuse stems from its social prevalence and the high incidence among the population in hospital and community. Although alcohol comes under the medical classification of a substance, it has been selected for special treatment in this book because of its place as a significant physical and psychological health problem.

THE PROBLEM OF SUBSTANCE USE AND ABUSE

DEFINITIONS

The *Diagnostic and Statistical Manual of Mental Disorders III* 1980 (DSM III) uses the term 'substance use disorders' to describe the diagnostic class which 'deals with behavioural changes associated with more or less regular use of substances that affect the central nervous system'. Pathological use is divided into two sub-categories of substance abuse and substance dependence. For each substance certain criteria are given for diagnosis.

Substance abuse is differentiated from non-pathological use in DSM III on the basis of

- 'A pattern of pathological use' which may involve intoxication, inability to stop, continued use in the presence of a serious physical disorder which the person knows is exacerbated by the use of the substance, and need for daily use of the substance for adequate functioning.
- 'Impairment in social or occupational functioning caused by the pattern of pathological use.'
- 'Duration, lasting at least one month, of a pattern of pathological use.'

Dependence is diagnosed in the presence of

- Tolerance, which means that a desired effect is achieved only by using increased amounts of the substance.
- Withdrawal, a 'substance-specific syndrome' which 'follows cessation of or reduction in intake of a substance that was previously regularly used by the individual to induce a physiological state of intoxication' (DSM III).

This diagnostic classification specifically refers to the notion of a substance as affecting mood and behaviour. A somewhat broader view of the problem may be obtained, however, by redefining 'substance' slightly and giving it the same definition as the term 'drug'. A drug is 'any substance which when taken into the body may alter one or more of its functions' (Gaerlan 1980).

Thus a consideration of substance use and abuse may take into consideration effects on all body systems and not just the nervous system.

Our avoidance of the use of the phrase 'drug use and abuse' is justified by the following discussion regarding social attitudes, norms, and mores.

A SOCIETY AT RISK

One of the ways in which we make initial judgements of other people is by the process of stereotyping. More often than not this process involves becoming aware of a particular attribute of a group or individual and then formulating impressions of that group or individual on the basis of preconceived ideas associated with previous knowledge of the attribute. Moreover, we assign a whole lot of other characteristics to the individual or group because the characteristics are also associated with the original attribute.

Present a group of people, including nurses, with the terms 'drug addict', 'dependency', or even 'drug' and an example of stereotyping can be seen. The images conjured up involve typically, narcotics, LSD, 'shooting up', prostitution, crime, dirty needles and syringes, hepatitis, youth, pop music, cheating, death, and dole bludgers.

This stereotype reflects the social attitudes towards drug use which originated during the adolescent years of those born in the period of the post-war baby boom. The cultural revolution of sorts which occurred in the 1960s and 1970s and involved this group of young people, saw an increased awareness by society, and particularly among parenting groups, of drugs. A great deal of effort was expended by newspapers, magazines, the law, and even health agencies to publicize, and inadvertently popularize, the evils of drugs — particularly speed (amphetamines), heroin, LSD (lysergic acid diethylamide), and marijuana. The latter has certainly gained considerable notoriety and is still given a fair degree of coverage by the media.

The point is that the common stereotyping of the drug scene is only partially accurate; the problem is much more far-reaching. Ray (1978) makes the real issue very clear.

'If you weren't paying attention in the mid-sixties to early seventies, don't bother to look for the drug scene, it's gone. There are some occasional vignettes to be viewed, and some of us for a brief period may even be a part of a resurrected mini-drug scene. But the drug scene came and was conquered. It never went away, it became a part of us — part of our society — as earlier drug scenes have done before.'

The real drug users and abusers are Mr & Mrs Average Citizen, and the stereotype is, in numbers of the population, a minority group outside of the real problem. For this reason we shall refer to 'substance', rather than 'drug', use and abuse.

Mr & Mrs Average Citizen use and abuse daily a wide range of substances such as alcohol, tobacco, analgesics, tranquillizers, caffeine, and appetite suppressants. These substances are taken with the principal aim of altering mood, behaviour, or body function. These are the same basic reasons that some people use heroin, LSD, and marijuana. The difference is that these latter substances are illegal, and the former are not only legal but also considered socially acceptable. Alcohol and tobacco have been used for a long time, yet it is only in recent years that society has been prepared to consider their potentially damaging effects. As a part of a pharmacological revolution (Ray 1978) there has been an enormous increase in the number of prescription drugs marketed for use by the health consumer. Some of these drugs have been shown to have potentially harmful effects and may be abused by susceptible individuals; they include barbiturates, oral analgesics, substances containing amphetamine derivatives, and the benzodiazepines.

Many people use these socially acceptable substances to the extent of being unable to stop or being unable to function adequately without taking them. They are substance users and abusers.

In clarification of this latter criterion, taking prescribed substances is of course justified on the basis of a physical or mental health problem. What may happen though is that the substance becomes a crutch on which the person leans long after the time of maximum therapeutic benefit. After this time abuse or dependency may occur.

We have become a society of substance users and abusers in which it is considered acceptable to take substances to alter mental and physical functioning as long as they are not illegal. Not least of the reasons that the problem is largely ignored by society is the enormous amount of money derived from the sale of pharmaceuticals, alcohol, and tobacco.

A large portion of this money is earmarked as revenue to governments.

This discussion is not intended to minimize the problem of illegal substance abuse and the devastating effects of drugs such as the opiates, hallucinogens, amphetamines, and phencyclidine. It is intended to highlight the fact that substance use and abuse is an important health problem in the context of what can be considered normal social standards. The nurse in any health care setting is much more likely to meet an abuser of analgesics, tranquillizers, alcohol, solvents, or tobacco (or someone dependent on these substances), than a person using heroin.

CAUSES OF SUBSTANCE USE AND ABUSE

The predisposing factors which play a part in determining who will or will not be a victim of substance use and abuse are not readily identified.

Certainly one of the principal reasons that people use substances is that they obtain some sort of mental or physiological benefit. Overall the result is a sense of greater well-being and a sense of being able to function more effectively. This is true whether the specific reason for taking the substance is pain-relief, reduction of anxiety, or elevation of mood. Such a positive pay-off is potentially reinforcing, resulting in further likelihood of use.

The evidence of supporting specific psychological origins for substance abuse is generally inconclusive, suggesting at this stage that there is not a *type* of person who uses drugs. However, it has been suggested that users of hard drugs, for instance, commonly have a disrupted upbringing involving disturbed relationships with parents (Chein 1964, Gossop 1978). It is interesting to note the number of heroin addicts (47%) who have lost a parent either through death or some other cause during early childhood (Stimson 1973). Another factor might involve modelling in which the child learns substance-taking behaviour from parents. As mentioned previously, the social acceptability of substance use is really quite high; in fact it is highly valued. The difference in the degree of acceptability perhaps lies in the type of substance used.

It might be expected that individuals who have difficulty in managing the stresses and strains of life might be prone to relieving their problems through artificial means. The common use of legal anxiolytics/sedatives has certainly contributed to people seeking this way of managing their problems.

Other factors contributing to drug use are as follows (National Standing Control Committee on Drugs of Dependence 1971).

- medical introduction (i.e. originally prescribed for treatment of symptoms of an illness)
- experimentation or thrill-seeking
- boredom (housewives, unemployed)
- persuasion from others, not least of which is the media
- availability (e.g. doctors and nurses)

SPECIFIC SUBSTANCES AND THEIR EFFECTS

The types of substances most commonly abused are listed in Table 16.1. Several of the examples of substances appearing in this table are not discussed in the text due to the relative infrequency of use.

Table 16.1 Table of commonly abused substances other than alcohol

Group	Examples
A. Sedatives and hypnotics	Benzodiazepines — diazepam, oxazepam, nitrazepam Chloral hydrate Barbiturates — amylobarbitone, pentobarbitone
B. Opiates	Opium, heroin, methadone Narcotic analgesics — morphine, meperidine, pethidine, palfium, codeine
C. Non-narcotic analgesics	Pentazocine (Fortral) Dextrapropaxyphene (Digesic)

Table 16.1 (cont'd)

Group	Examples
D. Hallucinogens	Lysergic acid diethylamide (LSD) Hashish, marijuana and cannabis Tetrahydracannabinol (THC) Mescaline (extract of peyote cactus) Psilocybin (extract of magic mushroom) Phencyclidine (PCP, an animal tranquilliser) Less commonly available: MDA-34 (methylenedioxyamphetamine), DOM or STP (215 dimethoxy-4-methyl amphetamine), and two LSD-like substances — DMT (dimenthel treptamine) and DET (diethyltryptime)
E. Stimulants	Amphetamines (speed) — dextramphetamine, methidrine, benzamphetamine Caffeine — coffee, tea, cola drinks Cocaine Nicotine — cigarettes, cigars, pipe tobacco
F. Volatile substances	Petrol Aerosols and fire extinguishers Solvents — paint and lacquer, cleaners, degreasing agents, typing correction fluid, modelling glues Liquid gases — butane, propane
G. Non-prescription proprietary preparations	Analgesics — (Panadol, Panadeine, Aspirin) Cough mixtures — may contain codeine derivatives either alone or combined with antihistamines or ephedrine, in alcohol base Appetite suppressants — may contain amphetamines

NON-PRESCRIPTION PROPRIETARY SUBSTANCES

Substances in this group are freely available 'across the counter' to the general population and are widely abused by a considerable number of people of all age-groups. A major concern regarding the abuse of these substances centres around their potentially harmful effects on physical health. Many people believe that if a product can be bought from a corner store, supermarket or pharmacy without a prescription, it cannot be harmful. Unfortunately this is not the case and the most commonly abused proprietary preparations — analgesics, and 'cough and cold' preparations — can cause significant harm, and death. The Australian Kidney Foundation has placed non-narcotic analgesics fourth on the list of harmful, addictive drugs (after alcohol, nicotine, and sedatives).

Most non-prescription analgesic preparations contain, either separately or in combination, paracetamol, codeine phosphate, and aspirin, which function primarily to relieve pain. However, these preparations are also used by the population for reasons other than pain-relief. Consumers attribute analgesics with properties outside their recognized pharmacological action when giving reasons for their use, for examaple, 'to help calm me down', 'to get my strength back', or 'to help me sleep'. When persistent or recurring pain leads to the continued use of analgesics, the pain is frequently a psychosomatic concomitant of long-standing emotional conflicts.

Such substance abuse leads to psychological dependence and an increase in tolerance, but the most serious consequence of abuse is renal damage. Renal impairment can occur as a toxic effect of overdose or as a long-term effect of continued abuse over a prolonged period; gastric or duodenal ulceration and chronic gastritis also result.

The 'cough and cold' preparations include mainly cough suppressants, expectorants and nasal decongestants. These preparations may contain codeine derivatives, stimulants and antihistamines and, if in liquid form, have an alcohol base. They are abused for the mind-altering effects of these constituents, either directly by the user who is aware of their potential effect, or indirectly by the person who is unaware, yet develops a psychological dependence. The toxic effects of these proprietary preparations, particularly those containing phenylpropanolamine, has aroused considerable interest in members of the medical profession and pharmacists in recent years. Phenylpropanolamine (PPA) is a substance similar in structure and action to amphetamine, a powerful stimulant and well-known substance of abuse. Toxic effects and morbidity from drugs containing PPA are fairly common (Greenwood 1983) and include hypertensive crisis, cerebrovascular accidents, psychotic and other reactions similar to those induced by amphetamines, acute renal failure, myocardial damage, and cardiac arrhythmias. Although these effects would occur ordinarily only in the hypersensitive individual or heavy abuser, such unpleasant surprises may result when PPA is taken in recommended doses for relatively innocent purposes.

The central nervous system stimulating effect of PPA is also used as an anorectic agent in proprietary slimming aids (Greenwood 1983) and consequently results in those preparations being abused, particularly by younger age-groups.

Non-prescription antihistamine preparations, including those for the treatment of travel sickness and allergic conditions, constitute the fourth main group of proprietary substances of abuse. Abuse of these preparations, particularly when mixed with other substances affecting the central nervous system, produces alterations in the mental and conscious states of the user with the risk of precipitating psychotic reactions and/or causing unconsciousness and respiratory depression.

SEDATIVES AND HYPNOTICS

The most commonly encountered sedative and hypnotic drugs which create problems of use, abuse, and dependence are the barbiturates (pentobarbitone, secobarbitone, amylobarbitone), the benzodiazepines (diazepam, oxazepam, nitrazepam), and chloral hydrate.

The pattern of usage usually involves initial prescription by a medical officer for treatment of anxiety or insomnia, or obtaining the substance illegally.

Of these substances the barbiturates are potentiallay the most dangerous because of their physical effects, particularly in regard to intoxication, overdose, and withdrawal. It is for these reasons, as well as the risk of dependence, that there has been a decreased use of barbiturates as a prescribed sedative. Barbiturate abuse is more often seen as part of the illegal drug scene; barbiturates are taken either for intoxication, as a substitute for narcotics when supplies are low, or as a 'downer', following the use of stimulants. Pathological use is said to exist with the frequent use (almost daily for a month) of the equivalent of 600 mg or more of secobarbitone (DSM III), as well as the other criteria for abuse and dependence defined earlier in the chapter.

The signs of intoxication are similar to those of alcohol intoxication, and in high levels, barbiturate intoxication leads to coma, hypotension, and respiratory depression. Like alcohol, the overall effect of barbiturate use is central nervous system depression. Chronic usage results in a number of nervous system problems such as nystagmus, diplopia, strabismus, ataxia, and thick speech, as well as tolerance and dependence (Gaerlan 1980). Withdrawal mimics delerium tremens, but is more severe, with a high risk of epileptiform seizures. It has been estimated that approximately 5% of dependent barbiturate users die after abrupt cessation of usage (Ray 1978). The early signs of withdrawl are anxiety, insomnia, tremor, postural hypotension, and weakness. This stage is followed by an increased risk of convulsions, confusion, disorientation, hallucinations, and agitation; the risk peaks on the second or third day of abstinence in the case of short-acting barbiturates such as pentabarbitone, secobarbitone, and amylobarbitone.

As medical barbiturate usage became more restricted to anaesthesia and epilepsy control, a potent, although arguably less lethal, sedative and hypnotic substitute was found in the benzodiazepines, particularly diazepam (Valium). Used principally as anxiolytic agents, their value to the user and abuser lies not in any intoxicating effect, as in the barbiturates, but in the sense of being anxiety-free and feeling able to manage the pressures of daily living. Pathological use usually involves daily use, for at least a month, of the equivalent of 60 mg or more of diazepam, along with the other criteria for abuse and dependence (DSM III). Over-usage and abuse occur largely as a result of the user failing to find alternative solutions to life problems. The reasons for this might be society's attitude (including that of the health professions) that pill-taking as a panacea is acceptable, as well as the lack of adequate counselling resources.

Intoxication will result in central nervous system depression leading to the possibility of coma and even death. As with any sedative, there is an additive effect with other CNS depressants, including alcohol.

The pattern of chronic usage involves either the person taking a prescribed amount long after any therapeutic effect has been lost (psychological dependence has occurred), or dosage increasess with tolerance. Chronic use may cause weight gain, skin rashes, sexual dysfunction, dizziness, and menstrual problems (Gaerlan 1980).

Sudden cessation of a sedative may, in light users, result in anxiety and related symptoms such as insomnia and agitation. In heavy users, effects similar to alcohol withdrawal, including seizures, may occur.

OPIATES AND RELATED COMPOUNDS

The most commonly used substances in this group are the narcotic analgesics such as opium, heroin, morphine, meperidine, methadone, and codeine. Legal use of these substances relates to the relief of pain, usually over a short period and in moderate dosages. An exception to this rule is their use in high dosages over long periods for individuals with intractable pain caused by carcinoma, which is well-justified.

The reason for restricting use is that these substances quickly lead to both physiological and psychological dependence. Abuse of these substances is usually restricted to non-medical usage, where they are obtained illegally. For these people the pay-off in the early stages is the euphoric effects these substances produce — followed by dependence. Increased tolerance leads to heavier usage and a very real risk of overdose, the usual cause of death among these people. The resulting unconsciousness, hypotension, and respiratory depression may be considered a medical emergency. Overdose is usually accidental and occurs due to the 'illegal drug system'. Heroin is available in powdered or crystal form and in a variety of grades, increasing in potency. The heroin may be diluted (cut) a number of times with other white substances such as dextrose, baby powder, or baking soda. It takes only a small mistake in the system for the user to give himself twice the tolerated dose.

Intoxication with narcotics is manifested by: confusion and other signs of impaired consciousness; slow, shallow respirations; hypotension; muscular flaccidity; and pinpoint pupils. Withdrawal is not dangerous but is highly uncomfortable and resembles an infection with rhinorrhoea, lacrimation, sweating, sore throat, and pyrexia. In more severe cases, hypertension, muscular aches and pains, abdominal cramps, insomnia, restlessness, anxiety, muscular spasms, hot flushes, tachycardia, nausea, and vomiting may occur. In addition the person literally craves for the drug, or an equivalent, and feels as if every nerve ending is crying out. This latter sensation may exist long after overt physiological withdrawal has been completed and signals a particularly vulnerable period for re-establishment of the habit.

Since the use of these substances is usually very expensive, many users are in poor physical shape, with anorexia, malnourishment, chronic fatigue, vitamin deficiencies, and any number of physical problems. Socially these people are often isolated apart from a small circle of acquaintances, unemployed, have few possessions, have difficulty relating to the usual lifestyle, may be destitute, and have poor family relationships. Other aspects of social and personal disintegration include prostitution, crime, and a general disregard for other people, manifested by egocentrism and manipulation.

All of this of course applies also to the reasonably wealthy user who, although not having the same problems of supply, still succumbs to the effects of chronic usage.

HALLUCINOGENS

This group of substances includes LSD, mescaline, psilocybin, and phencyclidine (PCP or 'angel dust'). Marijuana also contains a hallucinogenic compound, tetrahydracannabinol (THC), which may cause hallucinogenic effects in high or concentrated doses.

The psychological effect of these drugs occurs due to a breakdown in ego boundaries, and personality disintegration. This results in altered states of consciousness, hallucinations, delusions, and extremes of mood of a euphoric or dysphoric nature. Physical effects are autonomic and include tachycardia, pyrexia, hypertension, dilated pupils, piloerection, and tremor. A good 'trip' may consist of bizarre hallucinations, euphoria, and grandiose delusions in which the person feels capable of achieving anything. On the other hand, a bad experience, involves dysphoria and paranoia, with frightening thoughts, stupor, and fearful hallucinations. Of the drugs listed above, mescaline and THC tend to be less potent than LSD. PCP has particularly nasty toxic effects and may result in coma and death with overdose.

One of the more interesting motives for taking these substances is as a 'mind expander' — a metaphor for searching for truth, God, or other metaphysical solutions to the 'meaning of life'. What is more likely is that people use the hallucinogens in a search for self and it is as equally likely that the self becomes increasingly disintegrated in the process. The substances produce in the individual an enhanced sensitivity and feeling of aliveness not available in non-drug-induced states.

A most disturbing aspect of these drugs is that prolonged personality disintegration may result from excessive use, and in susceptible individuals from single use. Manifestations of this disintegration are psychosis, withdrawal, personality changes, and altered social functioning. Another common occurrence is known as 'flash-back', which usually consists of a brief depersonalization and hallucinatory experience weeks or months after the use of LSD. Susceptibility to adverse reactions, particularly psychosis, could relate to the mental stability of the individual prior to usage and to pre-morbid personality.

MARIJUANA

Although having some hallucinogenic properties, marijuana and hashish in moderate doses cause alterations in the sense of time, a feeling of heightened sensitivity to stimuli, euphoria, disjointed thoughts, free-flowing ideas, and an overall change in perception of reality. Physical effects include tachycardia, dry mouth, and when the substance is smoked, reddening of the eyes. Apart from nausea, the most common adverse effect, usually experienced by the relatively naive user, is panic which may be extremely disturbing for the individual, and for others.

Tolerance and psychological dependency do occur, but physical dependence and withdrawal symptoms are not normally experienced. The subject of the harmful effects of marijuana and hashish is an interesting debate, beyond the scope of this small volume since the arguments at this stage seem equivocable. Some of the proposed long-term harmful effects include: transient psychotic episodes (flash-back experiences); an 'amotivation syndrome' characterized by loss of ambition, lethargy, and apathy; brain damage (unconfirmed in subsequent studies (Graham 1977)); reduced fertility; and bronchial cancer.

Any long-term effects of the accumulation in the body of tetrahydracannibol (THC), the active principle constituent of cannabis, have yet to be found. The alleged progression from marijuana to more serious drug use, particularly opiates, has also been proposed as a possible harmful effect, although the use of one does not seem to produce a compulsion to use the other (Graham 1977).

STIMULANTS

Substances classified as stimulants include amphetamines, caffeine, cocaine, and tobacco — largely because they cause the release of adrenaline, the major sympathomimetic. The most widely used stimulants are caffeine and tobacco, the latter in recent years having been the centre of social conflict. On the one hand tobacco is highly commercial and the source of immense economic benefits in the form of employment, government revenue, and corporate profit, as well as providing a socially acceptable means of getting an artificial 'high'. On the other hand there is increasing medical evidence that it is detrimental to health and potentially just as dangerous, perhaps more insidiously, as the so-called 'hard' drugs. It is an interesting paradox that the user of amphetamines or cocaine is often considered a social outcast and criticized for his use by the pack-a-day cigarette smoker, when the characteristics of abuse are really quite similar.

Amphetamines are powerful stimulants taken for their euphoric effect and the sense of confidence and sympathetic reaction they produce. This reaction causes hyperalertness, a sense of well-being, the ability to resist fatigue, hypersensitivity, and a general sense of being 'switched on' (which indeed the user is, even when amphetamines are taken in the low doses found in some appetite suppressants). Taken intravenously, there is an immediate 'rush' in which the person suddenly feels alert.

Adverse effects are severe anxiety and increasing tolerance and dependency. In high doses and with chronic use, hallucinations and paranoid delusions may occur in a state resembling paranoid schizophrenia (Gossop 1978).

Aggressive behaviour may also occur. Withdrawal effects are usually not dangerous, with a small risk of seizures; but short-lived depression and fatigue may occur.

Used clinically for narcolepsy and in appetite suppressants, amphetamines became popular because of their ability to assist the user in combating fatigue. Long distance truck drivers, students, medical practitioners, soldiers, sailors, and nurses on night duty are examples of those who have found the effects beneficial. Used legally and illegally, 'speed' (slang term for amphetamine) has fairly obvious pay-offs which make abuse a likely proposition.

In its physical effects on the user, cocaine in high doses is potentially more dangerous than amphetamines, leading to convulsions and (when used intravenously) possibly having a direct action on heart muscle to produce cardiac arrest. The usual method of use is by sniffing, which over a period of time causes permanent damage to the nasal mucosa. As with amphetamines, chronic cocaine use can cause hallucinations and delusions of a paranoid nature.

To talk of caffeine in the same sense as amphetamines and cocaine may seem strange, yet it too is a central nervous system stimulant. As such it is widely used as tea and coffee. Tolerance, dependence, and withdrawal are characteristics of usage, and toxic effects occur in high doses or in particularly sensitive individuals. These effects consist of insomnia, irritability, restlessness, and cardiac arrythmias, particularly tachycardia and extrasystoles. Many people will suggest that they can't get by without their daily dose of caffeine, a socially acceptable 'high'.

The problems associated with the use and abuse of nicotine are now well known, not just within the health professions but also in the community. This publicity has been due to a strong and united campaign mounted by the medical profession as evidence about the harmful effects of smoking has been gathered.

The toxic effects of nicotine have been experienced by most smokers and include dizziness, nausea, and tachycardia. Chronic use at the very least decreases exercise tolerance and is linked to a whole range of cardiovascular, pulmonary, and neoplastic diseases. Psychological and physical dependence is very common and like any other substance abuser the smoker is usually aware that he is the victim of his habit.

VOLATILE SUBSTANCES

Volatile substances are readily available in a wide range of industrial and domestic products and include aerosols, paint and lacquer strippers, polishes, petrol, degreasing agents, modelling glues, fire extinguishers, propane and butane gases, and office typing correction fluids. These substances are sniffed or inhaled in various ways in order to obtain brief euphoric effects and altered psychological states.

The abuse of these substances has become a serious problem of this decade, particularly among young children of the 12–16 year agegroup. The most worrying aspect of the practice is the profound toxic effects of the substances, which include hepatorenal damage, cerebral damage, polyneuropathy, and aplastic anaemia. A number of fatalities have been reported, death resulting from cardiac arrhythmias. Although physical dependence is rare, psychological dependence does occur and gradual tolerance develops.

The characteristics of the substances mentioned in this chapter are summarized in Table 16.2.

ASSESSMENT OF THE SUBSTANCE USER

CASE ILLUSTRATION

Mrs S. A., a 38-year-old married housewife with 3 children, is referred to hospital by her general practitioner. For a period of time the general practitioner has been attempting unsuccessfully to control Mrs S. A.'s anaemia,

Table 16.2 Characteristics of substances of abuse.

Substance	Legal status	Desired effects of abuse	Method of abuse	Dependency potential		Tolerance	Toxic effects	Long-term harmful effects
				Physical	Psychological			
Benzodiazepines	Legal on prescription	Relief from anxiety, promote sleep	Orally	Mild	Marked	High	CNS depression, ataxia, paradoxical excitement	Weight gain, skin rashes dizziness, sexual dysfunction, menstrual problems, teratogenic effects
Analgesics	Legal, non-prescription and prescription	Relief from pain as well as insomnia, anxiety	Orally	None	Yes	Mild	Nephropathy	Peptic ulceration, anaesthias, nephropathy
Caffeine	Legal	Stimulant, resistance to fatigue	Orally	None	Yes	Moderate	Agitation, tremors, rapid breathing, tachycardia, arrhythmias, grand mal seizures, hyperesthesia	Exacerbates heart disease, peptic ulcer, bladder cancer, birth defects, menstrual cramps, insomnia, anxiety, depression
Nicotine	Legal, age-restricted	Relaxation	Inhalation	Yes	Marked	Moderate	Dizziness, nausea, tachycardia, anxiety, restlessness	Decreased exercise tolerance; cardiovascular, pulmonary, neoplastic diseases
Barbiturates	Legal on restricted prescription	Relief from anxiety, 'downer' after use of stimulants, substitute for narcotics	Orally and injection	Yes	Yes	Extreme	Respiratory depression, weak rapid pulse, hypotension, coma, death	Nystagmus, diplopia, ataxia, slurred speech
Amphetamines	Legal, on restricted prescription	Stimulant, euphoria, resistance to Fatigue	Orally and injection	Yes	Yes	High	Restlessness, tremors, insomnia, delirium, nausea, tachycardia, panic, psychotic symptoms, sweating	Predisposes psychosis; weight loss, dermatitis
Opiates	Heroin illegal, others controlled medical use	Sense of warmth and intense pleasure, euphoria, a 'buzz' detachment	Orally, Inhalation, injection	Marked	Yes	High	Impaired consciousness, respiratory depression, hypotension, flaccid muscles, pin point pupils, death	Constipation, hepatitis, endocarditis, general deterioration in self-care
LSD	Illegal	'Mind expander', hallucinations, euphoria	Orally and injection	None	Yes	Extreme	Illusions, fear, panic, hallucinations, tremors, hypertension, tachycardia, hyperthermia, muscle weakness	Memory impairment, passivity, 'flashbacks'
Cocaine	Illegal	Orgasmic highs, elation, hallucinations	Inhalation, injection	Mild	Yes	Moderate	Confusion, headache, vomiting, convulsions	Psychosis with delusions paranoia, ulceration of nasal mucosa
Marijuana	Illegal	Intoxication, distortion of time, tranquility	Inhalation	None	Mild	None	Tachycardia, increased peripheral blood flow, conjunctival infection	Precipitate psychosis, reduced fertility, bronchial cancer
Solvents	Legal	Euphoria, perceptual disturbances	Inhalation	None	Yes	Mild	Excitement, aggressiveness, respiratory failure, cardiac arrhythmias, death	Profound, hepatorenal and cerebral damage, polyneuropathy, anaemias.

mild uraemia and hypertension, and has referred her in order to establish the cause of these symptoms. Investigations in hospital also reveal hyperproteinuria, fluid retention, and an electrolyte imbalance.

Nursing staff note that Mrs S. A. appears moderately anxious. On the day after admission she asks a nurse for two of her 'pills', a supply of which she keeps in the drawer of her bedside locker. The nurse discovers a quantity of a proprietary analgesic preparation and Mrs S. A., in a matter-of-fact manner, states that she takes two of these tables every two hours to keep her calm and prevent migraine; a practice she has maintained for a number of years. This analgesic abuse has resulted in renal damage.

The above case illustration depicts a possible situation which nurses may commonly encounter, involving a substance abusing individual.

GENERAL CONSIDERATIONS

The identification of the substance user's possible problems, particularly abuse and dependency, depends on obtaining important information about usage. More specific problems relate to the particular type of substance involved and these are discussed following this section. A schedule of the information required and the rationale is given below to aid the nurse in the assessment of problems.

- Name of substance(s) used. This is vital and provides a guide to the types of problems to look for.
- How often is the substance used? Frequency of use may provide a clue to the possibility of psychological abuse or dependency. A person may indicate that sedatives or hypnotics are taken only when stress threatens or when he feels anxious, rather than at prescribed times. At the very least this may indicate misuse. Heavy use (60 mg/day of a benzodiazepine) suggests abuse or dependency (DSM III).
- Is the substance prescribed? If so: by whom, when was it prescribed, and for what reason? Long-term and non-therapeutic use may be determined.
- When is the substance used? Again, this can help ascertain if it is being used palliatively or at the onset of certain symptoms, feelings, moods, or events. Taking aspirin to prevent the likelihood of a headache, or to cope, may indicated abuse. That is not to suggest that palliative treatment of pain with analgesics is always wrong usage. The nurse should be attempting to identify proper or improper use of the substance.
- Duration of usage. Long-term use of substances should alert the nurse to the possibility of abuse or dependency, as well as the likelihood of cessation of the substance's therapeutic value. A sedative, for example, might have been prescribed two years previously at the time of acute crisis, such as bereavement; and despite the event having long passed the person still takes the substance.
- Why does the person take the substance? This is an attempt to identify the pay-off, whether it be pain relief, suppression of anxiety, elevation of mood, simply coping, or getting high. Some users, particularly of cocaine, marijuana, barbiturates, amphetamines or alcohol, may indicate a social pay-off by saying they feel part of a group. Opiate users frequently state the reason and effect as being just to escape.
- What is the person's understanding of the effect (good and bad) of the substance on his mental and/or physical functioning? Here knowledge deficit may be identified as well as a clue to the reason for using the substance.
- Could the person give up using the substance and has he ever tried? These are important factors in dependency.
- Is there any evidence of tolerance, withdrawal (present or past), or intoxication?
- Have there been any detrimental physical, psychological, or sociological effects related to substance use? These may include illness (i.e. bronchitis in smokers), loss of job, marriage breakdown, disturbances in interpersonal relations, financial troubles, or impaired habits of daily living.

- What relationship is there between the use of the substance and current illness?
- What are the person's intentions in regard to use?
- Is the person motivated to reduce/cease drug usage?

As well as indicating a wide range of possible problems, these data may also identify any number of mental health problems related to drug usage. Problems may include anxiety, depression, withdrawal, anger, self-destructive behaviour, disordered thinking, hallucinations, confusion, delusions, and poor social functioning. Other mental health problems may be either the result or the cause of substance usage.

Substance abuse and dependency are important problems and indicate the need for urgent intervention. People may present in a crisis state that has occurred largely as a result of their substance use and may involve physical illness, withdrawal, intoxication, or overdose. Emotional crisis (Casselman 1980) may also occur, precipitated by an event such as being arrested, family breakdown, loss of job, financial problems, or destitution. From our experience of working with substance abusers these crisis states are more often than not the reason for admission, there being little or no motivation for substance abuse until a crisis eventuates. This is also true of alcoholics.

Occasionally a person may indicate that he has made a decision to give up or do something about his substance use in the absence of crisis. This decision-making can be facilitated by other people and, in the case of hospitalization, by the nurse. The nurse can act, however, only if the problem or potential problem has been identified by the abuser or some other person.

NURSING CARE

Lewin (1978) has suggested that the nurse should utilize the following strategies in the fulfilment of a therapeutic role with substance abusing individuals.

1. A non-judgmental attitude. This is most important, particularly in the light of the sense of frustration that nurses often feel in caring for substance users.
2. A careful collection of a wide range of information about the individual which should be recorded in the nursing notes and shared with other members of the health team.
3. Recognition of the stress points for each person and readiness to provide support.
4. The desire to discover where each individual stands in terms of physical, intellectual, and emotional development, and to proceed from there.
5. The knowledge that they can proceed only at the person's own pace and that his strengths must be found, and used productively.
6. The realization that people are irrational, and nurses must not feel personally affronted or lose confidence where there is disruption, regression, or no evidence of clinical progress.

This last point is probably one of the principal reasons for the development of frustration and a judgemental attitude among nurses towards these individuals. It is an interesting human characteristic that we tend to personalize other people's actions when they should have little real (logical) impact on us at all. This may come about because we like others to fit into our scheme of what we believe they should be like, often the belief being that they should be just like us. When things do not turn out the way we expect we feel personally affronted and respond accordingly.

As a health educator the nurse needs to be able to describe clearly to the person the physical, social, and psychological implications of his substance usage. It is possible that the user is unaware of the effects of his habit both in the long- and short-term. Although often remorseful generally regarding the trouble caused during intoxication, the person is ignorant about the actual details of the behaviour manifested at that time. In addition the nurse needs to be able to discuss factors such as stress, diet, exercise, and other aspects of healthy living.

One of the problems in treatment is that substance use is a psychosocial problem rather than simply an illness. The substance user has a whole set of values related to his substance abuse, and patterns of behaviour which are alien to the non-substance abusing individual. This is particularly true of those who have been involved in the particular subculture associated with narcotics and other 'hard core' substances. The nurse needs to resocialize the individual by reinforcing values that are more reflective of a drug-free life and covertly discouraging those values that are counter-productive. This feature of treatment also applies to cigarette smokers and other substance users. A smoker, for example, may be able to associate his habit with such factors as alcohol, other smokers, meals, stress, work, driving, or drinking tea and coffee. In identifying these factors the smoker can take appropriate action.

The management of the substance user is a difficult task for nurses, especially within a general hospital. Success, however, which in such a setting may be measured perhaps only in short-term behaviour change, is especially rewarding.

NURSING ACTION

The problems of the substance abuser may be conveniently categorized into four main groups consisting of those relating to

- intoxication
- overdose
- withdrawal
- continued cessation of use.

Intoxication

Providing care for a person who is intoxicated with any substance is perhaps one of the most difficult tasks that a nurse can encounter, particularly if the scenario is enacted in a general hospital rather than in a specialized detoxification unit. The principal problem involves the difficulty in communicating effectively with these people in an attempt to achieve some desired response or goal. The person who is severely distressed or in a state of panic will not easily be convinced that the effect is short-lived. Similarly, a person with bizarre hallucinations or flight of ideas, and who behaves quite unpredictably, is not likely to be sensitive to the need to be still and quiet down. The helper's frustration often leads to the decision to leave the person alone or to use some form of physical restraint. Unfortunately neither of these approaches is desirable.

The primary goal of care, then, is to see through this period of intoxication with the person, knowing it will end, and in so doing to achieve the following short-term goals.

1. Provide maximum safety for the individual.
2. Minimize the individual's distress.
3. Prevent any possible complications resulting from intoxication.
4. Control behaviour.
5. Preserve dignity and privacy.

The most effective means of achieving these goals is for the nurse to stay with the person until the effects of intoxication wear off. In this period the nurse should attempt constantly to reinforce to the person that his behaviour and symptoms are a result of intoxication and that they will wear off in time. This process is called 'talking down' and is designed to develop the person's awareness that his behaviour is not usual for him. Communication is facilitated by listening to what the person is experiencing, attempting to understand, and responding appropriately. In fact the skills involved are no different from those used in any helping situation — they are just more difficult to implement and it takes longer to achieve even a moderate amount of progress.

The nurse needs to remain calm, interested, and firm when the intoxicated person is resisting control. The most common mistake is to try arguing rationally with the person; this causes the situation to escalate, with the nurse subsequently becoming backed into a corner having to think up more arguments. It is important to listen and communicate rather than to act hastily in an attempt to exert control. This of course does not apply when there is immediate danger to the person or others around him, and there is no time to talk. Where the person is very aggressive either towards himself or others, the nurse should have no hesitation at all in calling for help. Most hospitals have a procedure for obtaining assistance in cases of non-medical emergencies.

Basic behaviour modification, reinforcing positive behaviour and decelerating undesirable behaviour (Carter 1980) is an important tool available to the nurse in managing the intoxicated person. The person should be informed when behaviour is unacceptable and that if he wants to discuss his problem he must behave appropriately. Statements of this kind need to be made unemotionally and firmly. This strategy is most useful when the person is abusive, aggressive, or making unreasonable demands.

Overdose

A serious overdose of most of the substances described in this chapter is a medical emergency and as such is beyond the scope of this book.

Withdrawal

To a large extent withdrawal is a medical problem after which the real treatment of the drug-free individual can commence (Gossop 1978). There are a number of reasons why withdrawal may occur. The person may have abstained from using a substance because of physical illness or an accident. In these cases the withdrawal may be anticipated when abuse is known or may occur without any prior warning. Some people may make a decision to stop taking a substance due to crises involving finance, family, or employment. Others, in the absence of any precipitating crisis, just decide it is time to refrain

from using the substance and attempt to overcome the withdrawal as a part of this decision. The most common example of this type is the smoker. In his or her educational role the nurse may facilitate the decision to stop smoking by presenting the facts relating to the detrimental effects of smoking, and then be in the position of supporting the person through the initial experiences of withdrawal. Another pertinent example relating to hospitalization is that of assisting people to cease using hypnotics and sedatives which may have been used over a long period of time.

The reason behind abstinence and ultimate withdrawal is an important consideratioin in the direction of psychological care, since it raises the question of intent to permanently refrain from using a substance. If withdrawal occurred due to circumstances other than a desire to stop a habit, then the goal needs to be helping the person to make the decision to remain abstinent. Unfortunately this is not often achieved and is one of the reasons nurses find caring for substance users so frustrating. During a period of withdrawal the symptoms are so bad that the individual will 'swear off' narcotics or barbiturates only to relapse when the painful memories have waned. Another reason for this phenomenon of temporary abstinence might be the desire to provide some reinforcement to helpers for all their hard work and the inconvenience caused to them by the substance-dependent person during withdrawal. As a result of this often repeated withdrawal/relapse scenario, it is quite common for the dependent user to be in considerable anguish over his habit.

With those who are withdrawing due to a genuine desire to stop using a substance, the principal goal of care is to support their decision. Even at this early stage the person can talk about his problem, its causes, and even make some decisions regarding changes in lifestyle. The craving for a substance can be combatted using a number of techniques such as relaxation and purposeful sublimated activity as a substitute. The person can learn to substitute unwanted thoughts about using a substance with more positive thoughts, pleasant images, reminding self about set goals, and stopping the thoughts as they arise.

Continued cessation of substance use

The single most important factor in the rehabilitation of the substance user is his motivation (Glatt 1976, Gossop 1978). Although this is an intrinsic quality, a concerted effort by all members of the health team can be made to generate and sustain this motivation. This is the principal goal of care for these people.

One of the most important roles of the nurse in a general hospital setting is acting as a means of referral for the individual. This is particularly true when the person is abusing or dependent. Specialized treatment facilities are available for managing those involved with hard drugs such as narcotics, tranquillizers, and hallucinogens. Similarly, there are programmes and agencies for the smoker and alcohol user who may not require intensive treatment. General hospitals are not usually well equipped to handle these problems, especially on the long-term basis that treatment often requires. It is vital that referral be made, giving the person the opportunity to try, at least initially, to cease his habit. The difficult task may to obtain the person's compliance and motivate him towards action.

For many substance abusers, and particularly substance dependents, continued cessation requires an enormous amount of change and personal growth. In effect the individual has to learn to live substance-free, to manage life without a destructive crutch on which to lean. Where a sufficiently close relationship exists the helper may act as a model, reflecting the type of behaviour that is necessary in order to surmount life's problems. Many drug treatment programmes are based on this notion, with the most potent models being people who, previously having been dependent, now live drug-free.

A very difficult but important aim of counselling is to assist the person to identify his motives for using a substance, and to explore the relief it gives him. With some this opens a Pandora's box of psychological problems that are often beyond the scope of nurses in a general hospital setting. However, this should not deter the nurse from engaging in a voyage of self-discovery with these people, and at the very least being a willing listener. The types of problems encountered may include depression, anxiety, hostility, inwardly turned anger, self-destructive desires, denial, withdrawal, poor communication and social skills, and indifference.

Many substance users need to re-evaluate their lives in terms of being drug-free and to set some meaningful goals towards which they can channel their energy. It is important that these goals be valued as well as socially desirable. In other words there must be an identifiable pay-off for the individual, an achievable reward. One early and fairly simple goal is a sense of well-being that is achieved by sleeping well, exercising, relaxing, eating well, and just being substance-free. Goal-setting and decision-making in general should be reinforced positively both by encouragement and by encouraging the person to reflect on how his actions have made him feel. The most satisfying reward available is a sense of achievement.

REFERENCES

American Psychiatric Association 1980 Diagnostic and statistical manual of mental disorders, 3rd edn. American Psychitric Association, Washington DC

Carter F 1980 Dealing with the disruptive patient. The Canadian Nurse, November

Casselman G 1980 Breaking the cycle of abuse. The Canadian Nurse, November

Charlesworth E A, Dempsey G 1982 Trait anxiety reduction in a substance abuse population trained in stress management. Journal of Clinical Psychology 38:4

Chein I, Gerard D L, Lees P S, Rosenfeld E 1964 The road to narcotics, delinquency, and social policy. Basic Books, New York

Drew L R M 1978 Alcohol and drug related problems: a challenge for nurse educators. The Lamp, July

Gaerlan M 1980 Living and working with drugs. The Canadian Nurse, November

Glatt M M 1976 Motivation in alcoholics and drug addicts. Nursing Mirror, January 15

Gossop M 1978 The pattern of drug use. Nursing Times, June 15

Gossop M 1978 Treatment and nursing care. Nursing Times, June 22

Graham J D P 1977 Cannabis now. H.M. & M. Publishers, London

Greenwood J 1983 The case against phenylpropanolamine. Pharmaceutical Journal 230: 585–6

Lewin D C 1978 Care of the drug dependent patient. Nursing Times, April 13

National Information on Drug Abuse 1984 Technical Information Bulletin, No. 71

National Standing Central Committee on Drugs of Dependence 1971 The use and abuse of drugs. Australian Publishing Service, Canberra

Ray O 1978 Drugs, society and human behaviour. Mosby, St Louis

Stimson G V 1973 Heroin and behaviour: diversity among addicts attending London clinics. Irish University Press, Shannon

Thorley A 1979 Drug dependence. In: Hill P, Murray R, Thorley A (eds) Essentials of postgraduate psychiatry. Academic Press, London

17

And lately, by the tavern door agape, came shining through the dusk an angel shape bearing a vessel on his shoulder; and he bid me taste of it; and 'twas — the Grape! The Grape that can with logic absolute the two-and-seventy jarring sects confute: the sovereign alchemist that in a trice life's leaden metal into gold transmute.

The Rubáiyát of Omar Khayyam

Alcohol use and abuse

ALCOHOL, HEALTH AND SOCIETY

ALCOHOL AND SOCIETY

Recent years have seen the start of a most important revolution in the concept of health and the function of the health care system. In brief, this innovation has taken the form of a growing awareness of preventive medicine and the development of the belief that health is something more than simply the absence of disease. Instead, health can be seen as involving optimum functioning. In addition we have seen more and more attention paid by health workers to what can be called the 'modern epidemics', such as cardiovascular disease. One of the features of many of the more common health problems of the second half of the 20th century is that they are, to a certain extent, avoidable. Although, for example, genetic factors may play a significant part in the individual's susceptibility to cardiovascular disease, there is little doubt that smoking, obesity, poor exercise habits, stress, and alcohol use are contributing factors. All of these are avoidable and some reflect the self-indulgence that has become a feature of our lifestyle.

This chapter and the previous one deal with the problem of substance use and abuse in the context of a health problem that

- is preventable
- is a significant feature of our lifestyle, contributing to disease

- contributes not only to disease but also to deteriorating physical, social, and psychological functioning of the individual.

It is important to note at this juncture that singling out alcohol use and abuse for special treatment is entirely artificial. It can and should be thought of in the same context as general substance usage and abuse. However we give it special treatment because of the sheer size of the problem as a health issue.

The revolution in our thinking about health has led to an increased awareness of the dangers of alcohol use and abuse both to the individual and to society. The significance in this seemingly innocuous statement lies in the attempt by health workers to create an impact on what has become an accepted part of most people's daily living — the consumption of alcohol. Its social acceptance makes any attempt to change group or individual behaviour in a more positively healthy direction very difficult.

ALCOHOL AND HEALTH

From the health perspective alcoholism is probably seen by many as being the most significant danger from the use of alcohol. In fact the risks are more far-reaching, with an estimated one-third of all general hospital admissions being alcohol-related (Bradsley 1982). Only a small percentage of these will be alcoholics or suffering acute intoxication or withdrawal. Instead, their presenting problem tends to be physiological, resulting from long-term exposure to alcohol. There are may estimates as to what constitutes an excessive alcohol intake, but Table 17.1 provides a guide from the Drug and Alcohol Service of New South Wales (1980).

It is quite possible that this is a conservative estimate, with the amount, with the amount required to actually cause problems being lower. Individual variations will also occur for age, size, health, tolerance, and drinking pattern.

The physiological and psychological prob-

Table 17.1 Alcohol intake and health risks

Intake in grams per day	Health risk
Up to 60 g for males and 40 g for females	Low physical, mental, and social risk
Between 60 g and 120 g for males and 40 g to 80 g for females	High risk of physical, mental, and social problems
Over 120 g for males and over 80 g for females	Definite physical and mental damage with inevitable social problems

10 g of alcohol is equivalent to roughly, 30 ml of spirits, 60 ml of port or sherry, 120 ml of wine or 285 ml of beer. In other words, 10 grams = 1 standard drink.

lems associated with alcohol abuse are given in Table 17.2.

For the health care worker it is quite clear that in the assessment and treatment of people suffering from any number of physical and psychiatric conditions, excessive alcohol intake should be at least considered as a contributing factor. In addition there is a very great need to increase public awareness about the problems as a preventive measure.

Table 17.2 Alcohol: mental and physical problems arising from abuse

Cardiovascular	Hypertension Arrhythmias Cardiomyopathy leading to cardiac failure
Hepatic	Cirrhosis Hepatitis Fatty liver Portal hypertension
Pancreas	Panreatitis Cancer of head of pancreas
Stomach	Gastritis Ulceration Cancer of stomach
Oesophagus	Oesophageal varices Cancer of oesophagus Oesophageal reflux Oesophagitis
Haematopoietic	Splenomegaly Haemachromotosis
Fluid and Electrolyte	Water imbalance Hypokalaemia
Pulmonary	Pneumonia Influenza Pulmonary tuberculosis

Table 17.2 (cont'd)

Intestines	Folate malabsorption
	Diarrhoea
	Ulceration
	Enteritis
Central nervous system	Hallucinations
	Memory loss
	Confusion
	Disorientation
	Sleep disorders
	Peripheral neuritis
	Tremor
Dietary	Vitamin B_1, B_6, and B_{12} deficiency
	Decrease in fat soluble vitamins
	Folic acid and amino acid deficiency
	Decrease in calcium and magnesium
	Increased fat deposits
	Wernicke's encephalopathy
Reproductive	Impotence
	Fetal alcohol syndrome
Bones and joints	Gout
	Myopathology
Trauma	Road accidents
Psychological	Anxiety
	Depression
	Dementia
	Paranoia
	Suicide
	Personality changes
	Aggressive behaviour
	Other substance abuse

ALCOHOL — THE DRUG

Alcohol is a central nervous system depressant and not, as many think, a stimulant. This confusion is probably due to the sensations it creates; generally a feeling of well-being, sociality, and relaxation. In large doses the conscious level of the individual will fall and can result in coma and death.

Alcohol is absorbed through the stomach and small intestine very rapidly. Taken up by all body organs, it is most concentrated in organs having a very rich blood supply, such as the brain. It also has the ability to pass across the blood-brain barrier easily, making the brain a principally affected structure.

Table 17.3 Blood alcohol level and behaviour

Blood alcohol level	Effect
1000 mg/l	Decreased social inhibition Loud voice
1000–2000 mg/l	Slurred speech, mood swings, decreased attention span, memory impairment, gait is affected
2000–3000 mg/l	Tremors, ataxia, stupor, irritability, unconsciousness
4000–7000 mg/l	Coma and death

Table 17.3 shows the effects that certain blood concentrations have on behaviour (Garelan, 1980).

The liver is responsible for catabolizing more than 90% of alcohol absorbed into the blood, with small amounts being excreted in urine, sweat, and the breath. Metabolism involves the break-down of enthanol into acetate which is then taken up in the Kreb's cycle to leave CO_2 and H_2O which are excreted in the normal way. Alcohol is energy-rich, its only rather dubious dietary value. It contains no vitamins and actually uses up copious amounts of niacin in the body.

The general pathophysiological effect of alcohol is to cause inflammation of a number of body tissues, including a potential for causing irreversible damage to brain cells. Other problems can be related to: the inhibiting effect it has on antidiuretic hormone; central nervous system depression; behaviour changes; and poor nutrition.

Alcoholism

The most recognized disorder relating to alcohol abuse is alcoholism. The World Health Organization (1952) has defined alcoholics as

'. . . those excessive drinkers whose dependence on alcohol has attained such a degree that it shows a noticeable mental disturbance or an interference with their bodily and mental health, their personal relationships and their smooth economic functioning or who show the prodromal signs of such development.'

DSM III (American Psychiatric Association 1980) also contains a sub-category among the description of dependencies which includes habitual drinkers as well as alcoholics. It should be clear from the previous discussion that one doesn't necessarily have to be an alcoholic to suffer the effects of alcohol use. The popular myth that an alcoholic or alcohol abuser belongs to a special social group who have no job, no motivation, take handouts, sleep on park benches, and drink methylated spirits, is far from accurate.

Jellineck (1960) has described five different varieties of alcoholism: alpha, beta, gamma, delta and epsilon.

Alpha. Continued psychological dependence on alcohol as a means of lessening physical or psychological pain. Being purely symptomatic drinking, the individual does not lose self-control and can abstain, although there may be effects on relationships, work, and health.

Beta. Heavy drinking which is characteristic of the normal social behaviour of many communities. Although no physical or psychological dependence may be evident, physical damage is the principal feature of this group. Disorders such as gastritis, neuropathy, and liver disease are the result of drinking and poor nutritional habits.

Gamma. Involves the individual losing control over drinking, the acquisition of tolerance, developing physical dependence, · and experiencing withdrawal.

Delta. Most commonly seen in societies where wine is a popular drink. The individual cannot abstain and drinks intermittently without necessarily getting drunk. Mild intoxication may be a day-long experience for these people, and they have no idea that they have a problem. These individuals will develop withdrawal symptoms when alcohol is withheld for a few days, yet such an event is poorly anticipated. The picture here usually involves admission to hospital for surgery and during the period of abstinence withdrawal develops. The individual, relatives, and the hospital staff are all surprised by the withdrawal because of the person's apparent normality.

Epsilon. This consists of periodic binges of a few days or weeks with long intervals between bouts.

In terms of dependency the most serious types are gamma and delta, in which withdrawal is a feature. An individual may also progress from being an alpha or beta type to a gamma or delta as dependency becomes more pronounced. According to Lewin (1978) 'The fundamental feature in alcoholism is a loss of freedom: the addict loses the ability to decide, of his own free will, whether or not to drink alcohol.'

SOCIAL PROBLEMS

There are two ways in which we should view the social problems related to alcohol abuse. In the first instance there are those problems that affect the individual and those close to him immediately. Relationships deteriorate as alcohol becomes more and more important in the individual's life. Sometimes drunkenness may lead to acts of violence within the home as the addict vents frustration and anger. Some of the difficulties that significant others face include: broken promises between drinking episodes; uncertainty; the addict's guilt, depression, remorse, and sense of failure; seeing a loved one deteriorate physically and mentally; poor sexual relationships; poor relationships with children; and generally deteriorating ability to communicate.

Other problems are largely economic. Maintaining a habit may stretch the family budget to the limit, if not beyond. In addition decreased work performance may result in loss of job and concomitant financial difficulties.

Secondly, on a wider social front, there is the enormous cost to the community, involving such factors as: hospital costs, lost days at work, traffic accidents, and crime.

Alcohol abuse is a problem that involves more than just the individual. Treatment must extend far beyond simply effecting symptomatic cure for the person in the hospital bed. Instead health professionals should be educating the community, making alcohol a public issue on a large scale in much the same way as the anti-smoking campaign. It is interesting that the most successful treatment programme for alcoholics and their families is a community group — Alcoholics Anonymous; that is, alcoholics themselves, not a health care agency.

ALCOHOL WITHDRAWAL

Abstinence from alcohol following prolonged heavy intake may produce a state of withdrawal. It is a condition not infrequently seen in those admitted to general hospitals, when it arises to complicate other diseases or post-surgical recovery. The severity of withdrawal ranges from a sense of vague anxiety through to a toxic psychosis known as 'delirium tremens' (DTs), which should be considered as both a medical and psychological emergency.

Symptoms of withdrawal start to occur between 24 and 72 hours following cessation of alcohol intake. Initially the person becomes irritable, anxious and experiences difficulty in sleeping. In severe withdrawal early signs also include profuse sweating, increasing tremulousness, elevated pulse, increased blood pressure, and slowed pupil reaction to light.

These symptoms increase as the person becomes confused and disoriented. A feature of DTs is extreme irritability and fearfulness. Vivid visual and tactile hallucinations are particularly terrifying, consisting of snakes, rats, spiders, ants and insects. Auditory hallucinations of a paranoid nature may also occur, adding to an already intense fear. Epileptiform seizures are common and, along with dehydration, muscular rigidity, incontinence, and the inability to take nutrition, place the individual at considerable physical risk. Hypostatic pneumonia, for example, is a common complication which, in the past, claimed many lives.

Severe withdrawal may last for around 3–5 days, after which the individual is usually exhausted and feels absolutely wretched. It is interesting that many people can remember the experience of an acute toxic state very well. For this reason many detoxification programmes allow the person to withdraw without sedation as an incentive to change while providing support from agencies such as Alcoholics Anonymous.

The reader is referred to an insightful account of a personal experience with DTs provided by McQueenie (1984). Two extracts, however, may assist in understanding how the person undergoing withdrawal feels:

'When I awoke next morning it was to see a tall, thin, woman, dressed like a nun standing over me. She only had one eye, a huge affair in the centre of her forehead. She was accompanied by three nurses I knew. They just stood and looked at me in sorrow, hanging their heads in mourning, the nun hovering over me, her single eye boring into me. She never said a word. Then, dramatically and suddenly, the whole bed became alive with rats and mice.
I complained bitterly to my wife who wearily told me it was untrue. I could not believe her. They ran helter skelter all over my pillow and I tried to get out of bed, but somehow swarms of wasps had invaded my head and I frantically tried to get them out.'

McQueenie also gives us an idea of how the person feels about self:

'Many other things happened that night and next day but I am unwilling to talk about the degradation of it all. Suffice it to say that my behaviour deteriorated to that of an animal and any pity the young nurses had for me turned to contempt. I can remember drinking my own urine — that example is all I can give. The terrible shame of it all will live with me for the rest of my life. Just you, the reader, remember this — although the patient may deny all knowledge, this is his defence against shame. He remembers a lot.'

It should be noted that the nursing care of a person in DTs is not covered here since the problems — hallucinations, disorientation, confusion, anxiety, aggressiveness — are covered in the various chapters of this book and the general principles are the same for any diagnosed condition.

Physical problems such as incontinence, dehydration and so on are medical problems common to many conditions.

NURSING CARE

CASE ILLUSTRATION

Mrs A. L., the 34-year-old wife of a prominent public figure, had been admitted to hospital for a minor operation. She was cheerful, pleasant and interacted well with the staff. The surgery was performed on the third day after admission and was uneventful apart from requiring additional anaesthesia, and an unusually prolonged recovery. Three hours after returning to the ward Mrs A. L. became agitated, her vital signs were elevated and she was becoming increasingly more confused. She was disorientated to time, place and person, her mounting agitation changing to extreme restlessness and fear. She reported bizarre, and frightening hallucinations and became aggressive towards staff who were concerned she may harm herself.

Mrs A. L. was diagnosed by the attending physician as being in delirium tremens. On recovery Mrs A. L. gave a history of her social and drinking habits suggestive of chronic alcohol abuse, although neither she, her husband, nor any of her friends had ever considered that she had a drinking problem.

ASSESSMENT

The relationship between a person's drinking habits and the reason for admission is an important aspect of initial assessment. As Cohn (1982) points out, however, this is not an easy task for nursing staff. As an area of obvious sensitivity, the subject should be brought up non-judgementally, but nonetheless raised as a standard component of assessment. It is often too late when symptoms of withdrawal have commenced. Nevertheless it has to be said that denial and rationalization are defences commonly used by alcoholics, hence a true response may not be forthcoming.

Bradsley (1982) has proposed six questions which can be put directly to the individual and are much the same type of questions usually asked about medications. They are

1. What do you like to drink?
2. How much do you take?
3. How frequently do you drink?
4. When you drink, about how much do you have in 24 hours? What is the most you can drink in 24 hours?
5. When was your last drink?
6. What was it, and how much did you have?

Relatives and friends may in some circumstances be the best source of information regarding the person's drinking habits. They are less likely to be using defence mechanisms, although this is possible, and may provide a more realistic appraisal of the situation. Involvement of the ill person's significant others in care also provides an opportunity for the nurse to evaluate the dynamics of relationships which may be contributing to abuse or interfering with health restoration. In many cases the spouse, children, or others have significant problems or knowledge deficits that require action by the nurse either directly or by referral.

If the nurse suspects that alcohol use may be a problem the ground has been laid for discussing the issue further. In some cases it may be necessary to discover whether the person has experienced DTs, intoxication for long periods, benders, mild withdrawal, admissions for abuse, contact with Alcoholics Anonymous, and involvement with other treatment programmes.

During routine physical examination of the person on admission, physical signs of the effects of alcohol may be identified. These include: alcohol on the breath, bruising, cigarette burns, hyper-reflexia, vascular facial engorgement, cardiac arrhythmias (including T wave changes on the ECG), neuropathy, and toxic amblyopia. In addition the presenting disease may be the most obvious clue (see Table 17.2).

A wide range of behavioural problems have been associated with alcohol abuse and are helpful guidelines in establishing a diagnosis of alcoholism. Some of the more important indications are listed in Table 17.4.

Establishing that an individual does have a problem with alcohol use or that it is contributing to a state of ill-health is only the first step in the assessment. The most difficult part is to establish what type of problems are precipitating abuse.

In the non-alcoholic the reasons may be many, but in general a stress reduction factor should be considered. For many people drinking alcohol has become a part of their normal daily activity; it is a learned behaviour. This is particularly true of business people and salespersons who entertain a great deal. Others simply imbibe at the end of a day's work, using a few beers at the local hotel or

Table 17.4 Indicators of alcohol abuse

A daily intake of alcohol exceeding four standard (10 g alcohol) drinks
Early morning drinking
Boasting about capacity to hold alcohol
Increased tolerance
Blackouts and/or regular drunkenness
Repeated arrests or misdemeanours involving alcohol
Major family disruptions involving alcohol
Job loss
Frequent job changes
Increasing sick leave
Interest centred around drinking activities
A pattern of day-long drinking
Drinking in response to stress
Anxiety
Depression
Paranoia
Mental deterioration
Acts of alcohol-related violence
Acts of self-harm

a bottle of wine after a couple of whiskies at home. The place of alcohol use as a pastime in our social activity cannot be overstated as a vital determinent of alcohol abuse. Try holding an alcohol-free party or barbecue and see what happens!

In alcoholism or heavy abuse psychological dependence gives way to physiological addiction.

Problem list

Our problem list deduced from the nursing assessment for someone who drinks excessively might include

1. A number of physical problems related to alcohol abuse, e.g. gastritis due to alcohol, peripheral neuropathy due to long-term alcohol intake.
2. Alcohol abuse/use due to (stress factor).
3. Excessive alcohol intake as a habit of daily living.
4. Lack of knowledge regarding the effects of excessive alcohol intake.
5. Inability to socialize without alcohol.
6. Depression/anxiety or some other severe psychological problem as a result, or as a cause, of alcohol abuse.

NURSING ACTION

The intoxicated person

Effective management of the intoxicated person who appears in casualty or is encountered in community nursing situations requires a considerable amount of skill, patience, and self-control. In the first instance a thorough individual assessment must be made to ensure that reduced consciousness and behaviour is indeed due to alcohol and is not the result of a problem such as hypoglycaemia, electrolyte imbalance, cerebral hypoxia, or some other physical cause. The presence of alcohol on the breath is not always sufficient evidence of intoxication, and following trauma it may be misleading in indicating a reason for impaired consciousness.

Intoxicated people may exhibit any number of behaviours, including anger, violence, playfulness, sarcasm, garrulousness, passive and active resistance, anxiety, and depression. Staff perceive such behaviour as resistive or unco-operative. Drunks are seen as being 'difficult' and in many respects a nuisance. Naegle (1983) suggests that this 'nurse/patient' relationship is marked by ambivalence and negativity due to social and professional attitudes. As a result nurses fail to realize their potential as care-givers to abusers. Most intoxicated people present to casualty with some other problem and hence require all the attention and skill that would be given to any other individual.

Lowence et al (1984) note that one of the principal barriers to managing these people effectively is their ability to manipulate the nurse. This manipulation either results in the intoxicated person taking control of the situation or in a negative emotional and behavioural reaction on the part of the nurse. Becoming angry, for example, and telling the person to behave creates further resistance in the guise of righteous indignation. The nurse may feel better for venting his or her feelings, but communication is not likely to be improved.

The nurse should refuse to be drawn into argument, be direct and firm, and give direct unambiguous instructions about what is required. Physical contact is sometimes useful in counter-manipulation, although care should be taken to ensure that this contact is not perceived as a threat. It is also helpful to direct the person's attention to immediate events, providing brief explanations and reminders about where he is and how he got there. When the person's behaviour becomes difficult it is useful to use some distraction or diversion intentionally.

Many people become hostile when intoxicated and may engage in verbal abuse or other personal harrassment towards the nurse. Where possible this behaviour should simply be completely ignored. People are astute in identifying another's vulnerability and when intoxicated are more likely to use this understanding due to reduced inhibitions. It is not easy to ignore personal affronts, but on the other hand there is more danger, and nothing to be gained, in responding with hurt behaviour. If the person's behaviour becomes excessively aggressive, personal safety and that of others is of primary concern.

One of the writers recalls accompanying an intoxicated woman from casualty to X-ray for investigation of possible skull fractures due to a fall. Close observation was important since it would be important to differentiate between the effects of alcohol and cerebral irritation or changes in consciousness due to cerebral trauma. During this hour-long episode this person was in turn verbally abusive, physically aggressive, tearful, tremulous, melancholic, sexually provocative, cheerful, drowsy, and finally quite co-operative. By refusing to respond to negative behaviour, not engaging in excessive verbal or physical restraint, and being firm without being aggressive there was little confrontation despite frequent threats by this woman to leave. Listening for and giving maximum attention to important cues such as family conflict provided an excellent opportunity to discuss some of her problems. Despite her previously negative behaviour she eventually talked freely, and although nothing was resolved she was confronted with the

relationship between her stressors and her maladaptive behaviour.

It must be remembered that intoxication is self-limiting and that in time the person will eventually become tired, even sleepy. At this juncture the person is thinking most of his or her own comfort. This can be used to encourage co-operation with the promise of rest, food, and drink when admission or assessment has been completed.

The hospitalized person

As indicated by assessment, the psychological management centres around identifying the principal reason for abuse and the effects abuse may have had on the individual's life.

There are two essential elements required in the resolution of the problem of alcohol abuse. Firstly, the individual must be aware that alcohol constitutes a real threat to his physical and psychological health. Secondly, and most importantly, the person must have motivation to change.

Providing the alcohol abuser with all the relevant information about alcohol and its effects is an important consideration. Many people are quite unaware that they drink too much and do not fully realize the risks involved. Although it is a sensitive issue it can be broached with care and a non-judgemental approach. If the person has a physical, psychological, or socioeconomic problem that relates directly to alcohol it is much easier to bring up the subject directly because there is a specific focus of concern. The nurse and the individual can together explore drinking behaviour and determine to what extent it is a problem. In addition the reasons for drinking can be identified, which may in itself provide valuable insight and impetus for future change.

In some cases alcohol abuse may be caused, at least in part, by some underlying psychopathology, in the shape of anxiety, depression, or schizophrenia, for example. If this is suspected then referral to more expert help may be required. Discharge from hospital or community care without some attempt at helping the person should be avoided since the next opportunity to intervene may occur only when further physical or psychological damage has taken place.

Motivation for change is entirely the alcohol abuser's responsibility. The desire to change must come from within the person. The nurse's role is to provide counselling, support, and encouragement. Counselling takes the form of exploring alternative means of living without alcohol or at least of reducing intake to two drinks a day or less. There are of course tangible rewards to be considered as reinforcers that result from controlling the habit. These include better health, improved relationships with the family, raised self-esteem, and relief from a host of socioeconomic problems.

The individual should be encouraged to set personal goals regarding control of alcohol. These goals may include a time-scale as a basis for measuring achievement. Alternative social activities that do not involve alcohol can be explored. Exercise programmes, sports activities and hobbies are useful in providing purposeful activity and a sense of well-being. Relaxation techniques have been shown to have a positive effect on self-control in the management of substance abuse in general (Klajner et al 1984).

Family support is vital for the alcohol abuser and he should be encouraged to discuss desired changes with family members. A problem arises when one partner decides to change yet the other wishes to continue heavy drinking. Sometimes family therapy may be required. The difficulty lies in helping the family generate the motivation to take such a step.

In the general hospital setting, where length of stay is usually short, the nursing intervention at a psychological level necessarily stops at about this point. Long-term therapy, counselling, and support is usually required for the alcohol abuser. For the heavy user or alcoholic, management in specialized rehabilitation centres is the treatment of choice. A relatively new innovation is that of detoxification units which are able to start psychological treatment straight from the 'drying out' stage, including the management of DTs.

Alcoholics Anonymous is an important referral agency that should not be overlooked. Most hospitals have a list of contact people who provide a visiting service whilst the alcoholic is still hospitalized and embryonic motivation makes him vulnerable to hope of conquering his drink problems.

ATTITUDES AND THE NURSE

Like those who self-harm, and substance abusers, the alcoholic is very often the victim of the judgements made by society. To health professionals working outside the specialized units that care for these people, the prevailing attitude tends to be one of derision and lack of interest. Mirroring society's attitudes, the reasons for this probably rest in the antisocial nature of these behaviours. In addition health workers see very little reward in caring for someone who is more than likely to keep on abusing alcohol until it kills them. One of the reasons for the lack of reward is that we tend to personalize the individual's failures, attributing them to a lack of appreciation for our efforts on his part. The parental role that nurses tend to assume, with the alcoholic as the child, may also contribute to this sense of frustration. Even in specialized units the burnout rate for staff caring for alcoholics tends to be high (Lowence et al 1984), indicating the 'stress' in caring for these people.

The effective management of alcohol abusers relies as much on the nurse's self-awareness as on his or her skills. Without it the nurse is a victim of his or her own emotions and resultant behaviour.

REFERENCES

American Psychiatric Association 1980 Diagnostic and statistical manual of mental disorders, 3rd Edn. American Psychiatric Association, Washington DC

Bradsley L 1982 Avoiding a crisis: the assessment. American Journal of Nursing, December

Cohn L 1982 The hidden diagnosis. American Journal of Nursing, December

Drug and Alcohol Service of New South Wales 1980
Alcohol. Government Printer, New South Wales
Gaerlan M 1980 Understanding the physiology of alcohol
abuse. The Canadian Nurse, November
Jellinek E M 1960 The disease concept of alcoholism.
Millhouse Press, Newhaven
Klajner F, Hartman L M, Jobell M B 1984 Treatment of
substance abuse by relaxation training: a review of its
rationale, efficacy and mechanisms. Addictive
Behaviours 9
Kurose K, Anderson T N, Bull W N, et al 1981 A

standard care plan for alcoholism. American Journal of
Nursing, May
Lewin D C 1978 Alcohol can be addictive: care of the
dependent patient. Nursing Times, April 6
Lowence F, Freng S, Barnes B C 1984 Admitting an
intoxicated patient. American Journal of Nursing, May
McQueenie K J 1984 The day the strangers came.
Nursing Times, June 27
Naegle M A 1983 The nurse and the alcoholic. Journal of
Psychiatric Nursing and Mental Health Services 21:6

18

Aspects of daily living

MENTAL HEALTH AND EVERYDAY LIVING

Most of the nursing care described in this book is directed towards the management of specific acute and long term problems that people experience as a result of mental ill-health. What should not be ignored in taking this approach is the role of the nurse in assisting the individual to carry out the activities of daily living; this role is central to the nursing concept described in many authoritative definitions of nursing, and is important in two respects.

Firstly, many of the indicators that suggest mental ill-health, either acute or more long-term, may be found in an assessment of the individual's ability to carry out satisfactorily normal, everyday tasks. One of the major measures that society uses to determine both physical and mental health is a person's capacity to cope with everyday living. The ability to function independently is probably the most important factor in the decision to discharge a person from institutional care. People who are confused, disorientated, depressed, anxious, withdrawn, thought disordered, or angry, are likely to have problems in carrying out what are usually automatic, almost habitual, activities involved in living from day to day.

Secondly, being able to engage successfully in healthy habits plays an important part in maintaining a sense of well-being, in turn contributing to mental and physical health.

It is not our intention to deal with the overall nursing care involved in assisting individuals to carry out these activities, since this is an integral part of nursing that is adequately described in many general nursing textbooks. Rather the accent here is on the associated psychological care. In addition the notion of healthy living will be considered as an important aspect of mental health.

HEALTHY LIFESTYLE

In recent years increasing emphasis has been placed by health care workers on promoting community awareness of healthy living. The principal aim is to prevent ill-health by providing people with the knowledge, skills, and opportunity to make sensible changes to their lifestyle (see McMurray 1980). An increased social awareness of the importance of healthy living is reflected in the contents pages of popular magazines, the enormous range of literature on the subject in book-stores, commercial health foods, anti-smoking campaigns, and marketed exercise such as aerobic exercise to music.

Importance has been placed on aspects of living which most people take for granted such as: nutrition, exercise, sleep, monitoring one's health, avoiding substance abuse, stress reduction, and recreation. The issue, for example, in western societies is now not that we eat but what we eat. The impetus for this approach has probably been the rising incidence of problems of modern living such as hypertension, obesity, atherosclerosis, cancer, substance abuse, and poorly managed stress. In preventing disease, healthy living serves to reduce many causative factors as well as supporting the body's ability to withstand stress. We suggest that healthy living may play a part in reducing susceptibility to mental ill-health in much the same way.

The nurse's role involves ensuring that the care given reflects the principles of healthy living, advocating healthy practices, and a commitment to health education. It is towards this emphasis in practice that we now turn.

SLEEP

Most nurses who have been on night duty are well aware of the physical and mental effects of lack of sleep. Similarly, working shifts with a late night finish followed by an early morning start may produce, over only a short period of time, such phenomena as lethargy, decreased performance, irritability, depression, anxiety, difficulty in concentrating, and other general signs of excessive stress. In its extreme state, sleep-deprivation psychosis may occur, with staring, tremors, hallucinations, confusion, and disorientation. Fortunately most people are overcome with the need to sleep long before this state occurs, and succumb. It would also appear that the body is affected by changes in the usual sleep rhythm or established pattern of sleep (Hilgard et al 1979).

As well as causing disturbed functioning, sleep disorder may also indicate mental and physical problems such as depression, anxiety, psychosis, drug and alcohol withdrawal, pain or discomfort, and the effects of some medications. When the cause is acute, its removal usually results in the re-establishment of normal sleep. Disturbed sleep, for example, is not uncommon following an important life event such as bereavement, change in job, or some other stress-producing change. The insomnia in these cases usually reverts when the stress subsides. Other causes include increasing age, excessive work, children, nocturnal enuresis, shift work, a restless or noisy sleeping partner, noises in general, alcohol, sleeping in a strange place such as a hospital, and excessive sleep during the day, to name just a few.

Chronic insomnia may ensue in some individuals who tend to be restless, apprehensive, and hyperactive (Milne 1982). In these people going to bed and the rituals associated with sleep become associated with a sense of unpleasantness and frustration which in turn makes sleep even harder to achieve, ending in a vicious cycle of insomnia.

Two interesting causes of sleep disorder are sleep apnoea syndrome and nocturnal myoclonus (Walsleben 1982, Milne 1982). Sleep apnoea syndrome consists of brief (up to 90 seconds) cessation of breathing caused by upper airway obstruction or absence of respiratory effort in which the diaphragm arrests. In struggling to breath the person wakes frequently throughout the night. Common symptoms include snoring and restlessness which may result in falling out of bed, sleep walking, or enuresis, as well as more general effects such as headache, personality and memory changes, anxiety, depression, and sexual dysfunction (Walsleben 1982). Nocturnal myoclonus or restless leg syndrome is of unknown cause and involves recurrent movements of the legs during sleep which tend to wake the person intermittently.

Depending on the cause, sleep patterns may be affected in a number of ways.

- sleep deprivation or insufficient sleep
- difficulty in getting off to sleep
- early waking
- restless sleep
- disturbed sleep

Approximately 7 hours of sleep seems to be the optimum amount required for healthy living, although there are individual variations. However, it is not only the amount but also the quality of sleep that is important.

There are two types of sleep, both of which appear to serve special functions. Non rapid eye movement (NREM) sleep consists of several successive stages increasing in depth to a state of virtual paralysis of the body. Depth of sleep then decreases to a state known as rapid eye movement (REM) sleep during which the individual is more easily roused and more readily experiences dreams. During the course of a normal night's sleep a person will go through four of these NREM-REM cycles. It would appear that NREM sleep is responsible for allowing the body to rest, while dreaming may be a time for sorting out the events of the day. It is also suggested that dream activity may be responsible for allowing a person to remain asleep.

IDENTIFYING THE PROBLEM

In most cases the person will complain specifically of a problem with sleeping, and care can be based on this information. At other times the individual may not be aware of poor sleeping habits and yet may complain of any of the problems described previously, in which case a more detailed assessment may be required to establish whether sleep is a problem. This assessment can be approached in a number of ways.

1. The person can be asked in depth about sleeping habits and relevant environmental factors that may interfere with sleep such as noise, children waking in the night, a restless sleeping partner, discomfort, a poorly darkened room, sleep walking, and so on.
2. The person's significant others will often be able to provide important information about sleeping problems.
3. In the hospital setting it is also possible to monitor, by observation, sleep patterns using some form of sleep chart. On this document relevant details such as waking periods, sleep periods, time going off to sleep and time on waking can be entered. Where possible, restless sleep and snoring is also monitored.

NURSING MANAGEMENT

The goal of care with individuals who have sleeping problems is to help them establish healthy sleeping habits. This goal may be desirable as a means of

- treating mental health problems
- preventing mental ill-health
- facilitating a healthy lifestyle
- reducing the effects of stress
- enhancing the recuperative powers of the body in physical illness.

The most effective way of reaching this goal is to treat the cause. Where this is not easily achieved, in chronic insomnia or where severe psychological problems exist, a healthy sleeping cycle consisting of 7 restful hours per night should become the principal goal of care. The benefit of this is the breaking of a vicious cycle in which both poor health and lack of sleep compromize each other. In chronic insomnia an effort is made to break the association the individual has between going to bed and being awake, tired, restless, and frustrated.

Useful strategies in insomnia include: waking at the same time every day, getting up when sleep does not come but remaining relatively inactive, avoiding sleep during the day unless absolutely necessary, ensuring that the bed is warm and comfortable, darkening the room adequately, and reducing environmental noise. Milk has been found to be a useful sleep inducer, containing the substance L-tryptophane. Tea and coffee should be avoided since they are both stimulants and have a diuretic effect. Alcohol, a central nervous system depressant, tends to interfere with normal sleep.

Good exercise habits also aid sleep as well as reducing stress, one of the most common causes of sleep disturbances. Care should be taken in not exercising immediately before bed-time, since the body will be energized for some time. An exception to this rule is sexual activity, which usually has a powerful relaxing effect. It is worth noting that too much exercise beyond the individual's level of training (jogging or swimming too far, for example) may cause restlessness and insomnia. This phenomenon is frequently reported by those in the early stages of an exercise programme and the treatment is simply to reduce either the duration, distance, or effort.

Relaxation training is especially indicated for sleep disorders and is probably the best treatment available, being easy to learn and free of any side-effects. The basic technique is described in Chapter 5. It is simply a matter of transposing the situation to bed-time. Relaxation can also be practised if, after waking in the middle of the night, there is difficulty in getting back to sleep. Practice and perseverance are essential to the success of relaxation; the more it is used the more easily the individual achieves a state of relaxation and the less time it takes. Although less effective, listening to soporific music and reading may be helpful.

Where anxiety is preventing sleep, some people find benefit in talking out their problem or at least in letting someone know that they are worried. Night-time for the sleepless is a particularly lonely time, accentuated by the alien environment of a hospital ward and the personal effects of physical disease and disability.

It is clear that the hospital environment hardly supplies the necessary conditions for good sleep. Quiet and darkness are rarely ever features of the average hospital ward; hospital beds are functional, yet alien and often uncomfortable compared to the bed at home. The nurse can be aware of these problems and attempt where possible to lessen their effects. Some hospital routines still include strange rituals such as waking people very early to take temperatures or give medications, instead of matching these activities to individual needs. The early morning cup of tea is an even stranger practice that defies common sense. Schedules for these and other activities should be rearranged on an individual basis to provide maximum opportunity for healthy sleep. Day-time activities should be organized to provide an optimum amount of exercise for the individual; as well as aiding sleep this practice prevents excessive day-time napping and boredom.

For the person who has slept poorly, a nap during the day can be remarkably recuperative, particularly if work performance is essential. A good strategy is to use a relaxation technique, close the office door, and take the phone off the hook. With a little practice a short refreshing doze can be easily achieved virtually in any quiet moment. Auto-suggestion, which involves telling oneself that you will feel refreshed and full of energy, able to achieve any task on waking up, may also be employed. Again, it is a matter of practice.

Many people with sleeping difficulties are

prescribed hypnotics or sedatives rather than these more effective treatments described above. Most hypnotics, although initiating sleep, actually disturb the normal sleeping cycles and it is not uncommon for people to complain of feeling hung-over, heavy-headed, and washed out after their use. Some hypnotics may cause confusion, disorientation, and even hallucinations in susceptible individuals, particularly the aged. When they are used the nurse should monitor their effectiveness carefully and report any problems to the prescriber. In addition it is important that people do not take these medications over an extended period. They are mostly ineffective after a short period, other than being psychologically rewarding, and interfere with efforts to deal with the cause.

If the usual methods of treatment fail, or if assessment fails to identify the cause, referral is essential. There are psychologists and psychiatrists who specialize in the treatment of sleep disorders; they are also able to identify disorders such as sleep apnoea where there may be considerable risk to the person.

EXERCISE

The physical benefits of exercise are well known (Hedlin 1980) and it has been popularized by several writers (Cooper 1970, Fixx 1977, Hewitt 1978) where good explanations for exercise education can be found. Although some controversy exists regarding the effects of strenuous exercise on longevity, there is little doubt that it increases the capacity of the individual to function at work and play. It also instigates a profound improvement in the sense of well-being and health in general. Those engaging in aerobic activities such as running and swimming on a regular basis are less likely to smoke, drink less alcohol, tend not to be overweight, and are more likely to have a nutritious diet. Exercise is an excellent means of dissipating the negative effects of stress such as anxiety, anger, and depression, as well as being relaxing and even meditative.

Many people who take up aerobic exercise (walking, running, cycling, or swimming) claim positive psychological benefits from regular work-outs (at least 3 or 4 times a week). The runner's 'high' would appear to have some physiological basis. Strenuous exercise seems to release endorphins which attach themselves to receptors in the brain, producing analgesia and a sense of euphoria similar to the effect of morphine. Aerobic exercise has been suggested as an effective treatment for depression (Knowles 1981). At the very least being fit facilitates carrying out other aspects of living as well as enabling the most to be made out of sporting activities or anything else which requires energy.

Most people, whatever their age, can involve themselves in an aerobic exercise programme after a physical check-up by their doctor. Many useful exercise programmes exist and the three books mentioned at the beginning of this section are excellent aids for those wishing to start out. Perhaps one of the most important points to note is that exercise needs to be relaxing rather than competitive. The latter tends to negate the positive benefits that most people are trying to obtain, such as relief from stress, anger, anxiety, depression, or simply being unfit.

For most hospitalized people jogging for miles is obviously out of the question. However, some exercise, depending on the tolerance of the individual, should be a part of every nursing care plan as a means to maintaining muscle tone and cardiopulmonary efficiency. From a psychological point of view exercise can be a goal-directed behaviour with positive rewards: it facilitates sleep, it is a substitute for boredom, and it is certainly recuperative in the right amounts. It is not so long ago that post-surgical and myocardial infarct patients would be confined to bed for long periods. Modern management sees cardiac sufferers undergoing graduated exercise programmes only days after infarction, and post-surgery the individual is motivated to get out of bed after only one or two days despite the discomfort that this entails.

One of the most difficult aspects of obtaining compliance with aerobic exercise programmes is that it often involves a dramatic alteration to lifestyle and in the early stages requires some perseverence. It is certainly a lot more demanding than taking medication or alcohol as a means of obtaining pleasurable feelings. The most the nurse can do is to provide information and encouragement; the motivation to commit both time and effort despite difficulties has to come from the individual.

HYGIENE

The maintenance of good personal hygiene for most people is a habit accomplished with relative ease and success. It is interesting, however, to reflect on the amount of time and energy that is invested in caring for the body. In some cases, such as preparing for a special date or occasion, the rituals can be quite complex to get things absolutely right. We have, in fact, strict formal and informal rules about hygiene and dress for virtually every occasion — from balls and banquets to beach and bedroom. More importantly, rules exist for hygiene and dress for quite ordinary activities such as work. Social acceptance may hinge on the ability to conform to the rules of the group.

Mental ill-health often interferes with a person's ability to care for self even in the simplest of ways such as bathing, shaving, combing hair, and even dressing. This may be the result of a psychotic phenomenon in which reality is disturbed in some way. Depressed and withdrawn individuals lack the drive to bother with normal habits; severe anxiety may produce a similar result. Poor hygiene and dress may be one of the first signs available to the nurse of a psychological problem in an individual. Flamboyant or bizarre choice of clothes, make-up, or hairstyle may indicate that changes have occurred in thinking, symptomatic of deteriorating mental health.

The nursing responsibility in regard to normal hygiene is much the same as for a person who is physically ill, the difference being in the approach. The goal of care should be to enable the person to regain the motivation to carry out these basic activities. It is important to understand the psychological reasons behind the individual's apparent lack of interest in hygiene and to use this understanding to encourage compliance with a positive approach. Careful instructions regarding hygiene and its benefits should be given and all the requirements made available when motivation is very low. The routine of bathing, shaving, and washing hair, should not be hurried; the person should be encouraged and prompted to do as much as possible, with as much privacy as possible. Positive reinforcement may be given when a measure of independence is observed, to facilitate autonomy and a sense of positive self-regard. In general hospitals the emphasis is often on completing bathing and toileting quickly, and during set, routinized times. Unfortunately this does little for those who are confused, disoriented, depressed, or similarly incapacitated.

Toileting for these people must include providing motivations towards activities such as shaving, hair-styling and, in women, the application of appropriate make-up, talc, and perfumes. Clean, attractive and comfortable attire, including footwear and where necessary dressing gowns, is also necessary. Special attention may be required in regard to menstruation, which the individual may ignore or fail to manage herself. Irregularity of menstruation should be noted, since this may not be reported.

During bathing and its associated activities the nurse can discuss the individual's problems and carry out physical and psychological assessment. This, in fact, may be the optimum time for observing changes in behaviour, emotion, thought content, and other signs that indicate improvement or deterioration.

The benefits of paying such close attention to these activities go beyond generating a sense of well-being, although this in itself is significant. In psychotic individuals reality is reinforced by reinstating habits and directing attention towards self. Depressed people obtain some measure of accomplishment and are able to identify with previous sensations of wellness. Caring for one's body is also goal-directed behaviour providing the opportunity for decision-making and immediate rewards.

ELIMINATION

Problems of elimination, such as incontinence, retention, or constipation, may sometimes have a psychological basis. It is important, however, to ensure that no clear physical cause exists before assuming a psychogenic origin.

Constipation is a frequent symptom of depression, particularly in severe cases, and may result from: reduced gastric motility, psychomotor retardation, poor nutrition and hydration, and lack of concern about normal habits. Constipation is exremely uncomfortable and, when severe, may cause bowel obstruction with all the concomitant effects. A careful assessment of normal routine, how it has been disturbed, and for how long, should be obtained as a basis for the determination of treatment.

In the initial stages aperients and even enemas may be required to remove impacted faeces. A great deal of tact and understanding is required when giving a depressed person an enema because the procedure is likely to accentuate negative feelings. It is an intimate procedure associated with dependence and childhood rather than adulthood and self-esteem. Other nursing measures include providing adequate hydration and a diet with roughage, fresh fruit, and fibre such as bran. The principal aim is to restore normal habituation. The individual should be reminded to go to the toilet and a record kept of the regularity and result. Compliance is facilitated by careful explanation of the effect of depression on bowel routines and the importance of their return to normal.

Bowel problems often reinforce the person's ideation about being dirty (or full of dirt) and contribute to an overall sense of regression. The nurse should treat bowel activities as routine, yet respond empathically to the individual's reaction to the problem.

Probably the most common problem of elimination found in those who have a mental illness in general hospitals is incontinence. A common feature of delirium and dementia, incontinence can create an enormous workload for the nurse in changing beds and washing those who have lost bowel or bladder control. Although this is a routine activity for the nurse, frustration is often generated that may result in less than positive care. The effect on the person is also significant, incontinence doing very little to aid a sense of reality and self.

One of the most effective methods of management, particularly with those who suffer from dementia, is regular toiletting, using a commode chair or the toilet if possible. The effect of this is to forestall incontinence and to reinstate normal bladder habits. This process is in effect a retraining programme. Other strategies involve an effort to keep individuals in touch with themselves and their environment. Ambulant people may also experience incontinence and should be toiletted regularly. It can be surprising how mental state may improve when incontinence is prevented, and in turn the improved mental state reduces the risk of incontinence. People feel better when they are not incontinent, and nurses are less likely to feel negative towards them.

Other causes of incontinence include boredom, frustration, anger (Alchin & Weatherhead 1976), and anxiety. It is one way, however negative, of getting others to take notice. The provision of stimulation and attention may be all that is required to solve the problem. The nurse should also be aware of cues that the person has a need to express feelings and respond to them.

Retention, diarrhoea, and frequency of urine, may result as a side-effect of some psychotropic medications.

NUTRITION

One of the most difficult nursing activities is

to ensure that withdrawn people receive an adequate diet. Time, effort, and considerable patience are required to obtain compliance with eating, since it is one of the few activities that cannot be done for a person. Demented and delirious people may be too confused to concentrate on meals. Similarly hyperactive individuals may have little time for eating, and consequently lose weight very quickly. Stress and anxiety interfere with normal gastric functioning, producing dyspepsia, nausea, and anorexia.

Meals should be small and nutritious, consisting of the individual's preferrred foods. Unless it is absolutely necessary, food should not be mashed or puréed, but presented attractively to stimulate appetite. Preparation of the person in a comfortable, upright position, and preferably out of bed, is important. Overall, meal-time should be a pleasant experience rather than a rushed, uncomfortable period of frustration on the part of both the individual and the nurse.

Where possible, eating should be accomplished with no assistance from the nurse other than prompting and empathic encouragement. In some cases it may be necessary to feed some individuals; this should be unhurried and carried out at the person's own pace with a minimum of distractions. It is vital not to talk to the person as if to a child, although a degree of firmness may be required. There is no benefit in threatening someone with insertion of a nasogastric tube or intravenous therapy; this will only result in increased anxiety and most likely, decreased compliance. Food may sometimes be the object of delusions, with a person perhaps believing food is poisoned or that it will have some effect on his or her thinking and behaviour.

The nurse can attempt to solve these problems with eating by identifying motivations for individual reluctance to eat. By undertanding the reason for non-compliance the nurse is more likely to develop problem-solving strategies.

Problems are not just confined to non-compliance but may extend to other areas

such as vitamin deficiencies in alcoholics, overeating, and generally poor nutrition. It is up to the nurse to educate and advise the individual regarding a diet that will contribute to well-being. Referral to a dietitian or nutritionist may be necessary to institute weight reduction programmes, and to obtain information regarding the right foods to eat. It is probably true from a mental as well as physical point of view that 'you are what you eat'.

Although detailed discussion is beyond the scope of this book, at this stage it is worth mentioning eating disorders (DSM III, 1980). The most frequently encountered eating disorder is anorexia nervosa, which consists of a fear of becoming obese, disturbance of body image, and refusal to maintain body weight. The person becomes emaciated, malnourished, and develops system dysfunction resulting eventually in death if treatment is not instituted. People with this severe disorder are not uncommonly encountered in general hospitals where they may be receiving treatment for their physical disability. Special care needs to be given to these individuals and referral to both a psychologist and psychiatrist is essential. Staff will need to obtain advice on how to treat the person, who may be placed on a behaviour modification programme even in the early stages of management. Treatment usually requires referral to special agencies with highly specialist and skilled staff.

CONCLUSION

The ability of the person to carry out normal habits is often excellent evidence that mental health is improving. Conversely, healthy habits promote mental (and physical) well-being. In the busy environment of the general hospital it is important that nurses do not abnegate their responsibilities in ensuring that the activities of day-to-day living are carried out with the attention, time, and application they deserve. Last but not least, the hospital routine should be geared towards individual requirements, thus making hospitalization the least disruptive experience possible — a forlorn hope, perhaps, but a very good argument for the development of community health systems that can enable early discharge

from hospital. There is no doubt that living in one's own environment on one's own terms is more likely to result in normal habits and normal behaviour.

REFERENCES

Alchin S C, Weatherhead R G 1976 Psychiatric nursing: a practical approach. McGraw Hill, Sydney

American Psychiatric Association 1980 Diagnosis and statistical manual of mental disorders, 3rd edn. American Psychiatric Association, Washington DC

Altschul A, Simpson R 1971 Psychiatric nursing. Bailliere Tindall, London

Berry P D 1984 Psychosocial nursing: assessment and intervention. Lippincott, Philadephia

Burr J, Budge U V 1976 Nursing the psychiatric patient. Bailliere Tindall, London

Cooper K H 1970 The new aerobics. Bantam Books, New York

Fixx J F 1977 The complete book of running. Outback Press, South Australia.

Hedlin A 1980 Exercise: how the body responds. The Canadian Nurse, April

Henderson V, Nike G 1978 Principles and practice of nursing. Macmillan, New York

Knowles R D 1981 Handling depression through activity. American Journal of Nursing, June

Milne B 1982 Sleep-wake disorders and what we can do about them. The Canadian Nurse, April

Stuart G W, Sundeen T S 1979 Principles and practice of psychiatric nursing. Mosby, St Louis

Walsleben J 1982 Sleep disorders. American Journal of Nursing, June

Index